CW01066909

Abortion in the Ancient World

Abortion
in the
Ancient World

KONSTANTINOS KAPPARIS

Duckworth

Second impression November 2002
First published in June 2002 by
Gerald Duckworth & Co. Ltd.
61 Frith Street, London W1D 3JL
Tel: 020 7434 4242
Fax: 020 7434 4420
inquiries@duckworth-publishers.co.uk
www.ducknet.co.uk

A catalogue record for this book is available
from the British Library

ISBN 0 7156 3080 6

Typeset by Ray Davies
Printed and bound in Great Britain by
Bookcraft (Bath) Ltd, Midsomer Norton, Avon

Contents

Preface

Abortion is one of the few social issues in our times with the potential to agitate public opinion to the point of violent street protests and acrimonious discussions in television studios, law-courts and lecture theatres. For a historian the study of an issue as complex and diachronic as the debate on abortion is intriguing in itself, but it also illustrates the profile, values and beliefs of the particular society under discussion. My objective, when I decided to study abortion in the ancient world, was twofold. First, I set out to investigate the link between the ancient and modern debates on abortion, and second, I expected that the study of this multifaceted phenomenon would shed further light upon important legal, religious, political and cultural aspects of the ancient world.

From the outset it was clear that the main arguments in the modern debate are not really new, but rather the latest manifestations of an old, inconclusive debate that started thousands of years ago and still continues today. Some of the arguments and issues explored in this book, such as the close link between attitudes to abortion and demographic trends, or the controversy over the human status of the foetus, are as relevant today as they were 2,500 years ago. Accordingly, each chapter of this book starts with a brief outline of the issue under discussion now and then goes back into the past to follow the argument in Greek and Roman medical, philosophical and literary works, from the fifth century BC to the end of pagan Graeco-Roman antiquity in the fifth century AD. I am primarily a historian of classical Athens, so I was particularly interested in the evidence from that place and period. However, I realised that it would be unwise to ignore the wealth of information from medical and literary sources concerning other periods of Greek and Roman history, not least because their study would help us place the facts concerning Athens in context. This book would be much poorer if I had not referred to the achievements of hellenistic[1] medicine and philosophy, the highly significant references to abortion in the literature of the republican and early imperial era, the accounts of Soranus, Galen and other medical sources from later antiquity, and finally the works of early Christian authors. However, an in-depth approach to such diverse historical settings, and a full discussion of the large, complex topics involved would be unrealistic objectives. This is why my presentation is sometimes limited to points directly relevant to attitudes to induced abortion and its ethics. The focus is on the Greek world (in particular the classical period), with frequent parallels and references to comparable practices and attitudes in Rome, and occasionally Byzantium and the Near East. I hope that the book will prove useful to those interested in the literature and history of Ancient Greece, and also to students of the Roman world, to those with an interest in the history of medicine and medical ethics, and to a wider audience interested in the debate on abortion throughout history. Christian views on abortion, which play a major role in the modern debate, were forming during the period studied here, and this book thus provides a basis for a more profound understanding of these views.

In the course of this challenging task I received generous help. My colleagues at Queen's University Belfast, Dr J.B. Campbell and Dr J.C. Curran, assisted me with a variety of issues related to Roman history and law. Professor M. Mullett, Dr Janet Rutherford and Mr James George were always there to assist me with early Christian literature and Byzantine history. Dr Ruth Macrides, from the University of St Andrews, offered substantial help with Byzantine canon law. Professor D.M. MacDowell, Professor D. Whitehead, Professor F.B. Williams and Dr M. Alden helped me to refine a number of points. Dr C. Panayotakis sent me a number of papers from the University Library in Glasgow, and gave unconditional friendship and support. Professor Susanna Morton Braund, Ms Deborah Blake, and Duckworth's anonymous referee offered valuable assistance with the publication of this book. I am indebted to all these colleagues and friends for their assistance.

I am aware that this still is a very controversial subject, and that one person's strongest convictions may be absolute anathema to someone else. My main objective has been to investigate the historical data with an open mind, beyond entrenched positions or confrontational politics. Objectivity, even if unattainable, is perhaps the most desirable quality in a historian. However, in the process I discovered that with an issue such as abortion, emotional participation, empathy and a personal perspective can only add to one's understanding and interpretation of history.

Gainesville, Florida   K.K.
April 2002

Introduction

An English doctor who in the 1930s performed an abortion on a fourteen-year-old raped by four men, risking his career and freedom in the trial that followed the operation, said of abortion that it is 'an insoluble problem, because it has bothered mankind for at least 2,500 years'.[1] The liberalisation of the abortion laws in many western countries in the second half of the twentieth century did not put an end to this controversy. This very old debate is still running, as intense and acrimonious as ever. Medical advances in our understanding of the cycle of gestation, the development of the foetus, and the process of reproduction have not altered substantially the core of this debate. We may understand the process of foetal development much better than Aristotle or Galen, but we are still far from agreeing on the point at which we are prepared to treat a foetus as a human being in its own right. We may pride ourselves on the steps we have taken to create a more humane society, and we may even claim that we recognise the right to life for every person, but in practice we are still far from recognising the sanctity of human life without qualifications. Our society may allow women far greater control of their own destiny than the ancient world did, but women are still subject to political, social and personal restrictions, norms and rules that make motherhood not always desirable. So, despite the fact that a modern woman may be in control of her own destiny to a greater degree than a woman in classical Athens, she may still have to face the conflict between her own interests as an individual and those of the unborn. Progress over the past 2,500 years may have changed some variables in the debate, but these new variables have not produced a solution; the core issues and dilemmas remain unresolved.

Many of the points now made in public debates are not new. The essence of the argument has been discussed for thousands of years, since the first practitioners of rational medicine and natural philosophy started debating such matters in the fifth century BC. The process of procreation and gestation, the nature of the unborn and the point at which it becomes a living human being with a set of rights and duties, the rights of the mother as an individual versus those of the unborn, the rights of the mother versus those of the father, the right of a pregnant woman to choose her lifestyle – all these questions attracted the attention of the pioneers of rational medicine. Even before Hippocrates philosophers were discussing matters such as the soul and the essence of life, speculating on the way the phenomenon of life works and trying to understand how it is created. They were intrigued by these great mysteries, and were trying to unveil and control them.

The first handbooks of medicine as an independent discipline, based on clinical observation and seeking to provide rational explanations for health and disease, were contained in the huge and diverse collection of medical literature conveniently named 'the Hippocratic Corpus'. Scholars in later centuries believed that all these works had been written by Hippocrates of Cos, the father of rational medicine, whose life and activity can be placed in the second half of the fifth century BC. However, content, style and even chronological clues unambiguously suggest that this is a collection of works written by several different hands and brought together over a fairly long period. The Corpus is a very important source of medical theory, practice and ethics in the classical period. In it we find a substantial number of references to drugs, substances and techniques allegedly capable of procuring an abortion. The reliability of this information has been the subject of several studies in recent years, but lack of clinical evidence means that we are still far from conclusive answers.

We also have evidence that explores issues related to the ethics of induced abortion. The best known among these texts is certainly the Hippocratic Oath. For many years after the monumental study of L. Edelstein on the Oath this document was believed to be a text of Pythagorean origin, that is, an incorporation of the beliefs of a marginal sect, unrepresentative of mainstream views on abortion and its ethics. However, in 1984 C. Lichtenthaeler produced a very substantial critique of Edelstein's views. His objections and arguments have certainly influenced my views to a considerable degree, and even though I do not agree with some of his conclusions, I am prepared to follow him in his belief that the Oath could be a mainstream document from the late fifth century BC.[2]

From the hellenistic and imperial eras we have a considerable amount of medical literature concerning abortion, most notably the detailed account of an abortion procedure in the *Gynaecology* of Soranus, and several references in Galen. Both authors are concerned not solely with medical facts, but also with the ethics of abortion. Their views, which are presented in Chapter 3, were probably in line with growing anti-abortion attitudes in the early empire, as these are illustrated in Chapter 5. The Galenic Corpus, in particular, is an important source for ancient embryology, the stages of foetal development and the beliefs of ancient medicine on the human status of the unborn. In the words of R. Flemming, Galen's 'medical woman is not just rich in description but also in explanation'.[3] Flemming, in her lucid account of Galenic scholarship, presents the great man not only as a physician, but also as 'a moral and rational being, as a social and medical practitioner, as an epideictic advocate of his art'. Accordingly her presentation of Galen's medical woman goes beyond anatomical theory into social and cultural concepts. Galen's attitude to upper-class Roman women was frequently critical, on account of their vanity, insatiable appetites and undisciplined way of living that needed to be corrected with a regime intended to restore the health of the body and soul. All this is valuable background knowledge, but it is in some of those treatises that have been mistakenly attributed to Galen that we find most of our information on attitudes to induced abortion in the Roman empire. These works have little to do with medical writings; they are primarily philosophical and rhetorical in character, and, precisely for these reasons, constitute rich sources of information. Two Pseudo-Galenic studies deal specifically with this issue, and one of them, *Whether what is carried in the womb is a living being*, is translated and briefly discussed in Appendix 1. Among medical studies in Latin perhaps the most important sources are Celsus and Priscianus. The former gives us a very detailed account of an operation for the removal of a dead foetus, discussed in Chapter 1, while the latter presents yet more literature on abortion drugs.

The work of Priscianus comes near the end of an era, a long tradition that probably started as empirical wisdom, and preceded rational medicine. I have no doubt that the roots of ancient pharmacology go deep into popular wisdom on illness and healing substances available long before the first works of the Hippocratic Corpus. The pioneers of rational medicine probably incorporated much of this wisdom, and the subsequent pharmacological studies by Theophrastus, Dioscorides and Pliny continued this line. Pliny is an interesting and valuable source, for alongside more conventional pharmacological science he incorporates much oral supernatural belief and superstition on allegedly abortifacient substances – topics absent from the more rational studies of the Greek medical authors and natural philosophers.

To this specialised literature we must add a number of Graeco-Roman literary sources. Some of the accounts are quite substantial, such as two poems by Ovid (discussed in Chapters 4 and 5) and a lengthy scene from Chariton's novel *Chaireas and Callirhoe*, the oldest European novel. One of the most important sources dealing with legal and ethical issues, a law-court speech attributed to Lysias from an abortion trial in the early fourth century BC, is unfortunately lost. However, the speech was still available in late antiquity and the rhetoricians studying Attic oratory were obviously intrigued by it. They were impressed by the skill of the orator when he turned a medical issue into a rhetorical topic. Statements from a number of scholars and rhetoricians concerning the narrative and argument of the speech have been preserved, and from these a limited reconstruction of the main points of the case is possible. I have attempted to interpret these statements and reconstruct the details of this intriguing trial in Chapter 6.

The references to abortion in Plato and Aristotle are fairly brief, but extremely important for our understanding of ancient demographic trends and the general attitude of the classical Greek world towards abortion. Moreover, Aristotle's biological works shed light on aspects of ancient embryology and contemporary opinions on the human status of the foetus.

References to abortion in other literary sources, for example Euripides' play *Andromache*, are usually brief, but still offer valuable information. In addition to this evidence we have a substantial number of texts that illuminate other important aspects of law, society and daily life in ancient Greece and Rome. The speeches written for trials before Athenian courts, the great works of the Greek tragic stage, the comedies of Aristophanes, Menander and Plautus, the speeches of Cicero and the satires of Juvenal be singled out as particularly important for our understanding of ancient culture. The study of these sources is crucial for our understanding of abortion in the ancient world, for they provide the background against which we can place attitudes on this and related topics.

The available evidence allows us to form a picture of ancient societies which, despite the inevitable gaps, is reasonably clear in its general lines. However, the picture is less satisfactory when it comes to our understanding of women's personal situations. Except for a few truly great and highly emotional verses by Sappho[4], and a few scraps of poetry by female poets such as Corinna and Telesilla, we do not possess anything written by women. We must rely on men's accounts of women's situations, and however honest an effort they may make to put themselves into women's shoes, one must acknowledge that the evidence we have comes from male hands and male minds, and often reflects male perspectives.

The difference between a male and a female point of view has less to do with biology and more to do with upbringing, culture and perceived roles of the sexes.[5] Male authors sometimes attempt to present female concerns, but on an issue such as abortion a man's feelings and perceptions could be very different from those of a woman. When, for example, Euripides places in Andromache's mouth a concern about the continuation of the family line, he is probably reflecting something we can identify as a stereotypically male concern (see Chapter 5).[6] So, in this case, even though the speaker is female, her point of view is chiefly male. However, more genuine attempts have been made to identify with a woman's point of view. When Chariton makes his heroine Callirhoe[7] express an intense dilemma, whether she should give birth to her child in slavery or attempt an abortion, even though her maternal instinct goes against it, he is presenting a dilemma which a woman in the situation of his heroine might genuinely face, and in this respect one could say the male author has identified quite successfully with a female point of view. I am aware that some scholars might disagree with this style of analysis of a literary text; some might even argue that male authors cannot present female points of view, and others might say that what is male and what is female is very much arguable. It is outside the purposes of this book to engage in such controversy. Aware of the possible objections, I will still employ some literary texts, as well as other sources, as a basis for my attempt to understand the woman's point of view, her personal situation and motives behind the desire for an abortion. These texts may not be the best resources for these purposes, but they are all we have.

Moreover, there is an inherent danger when one tries to explore fields so broad and diverse. We could forget that we are dealing with a millennium of history, two civilisations, two very different religious systems, a number of different nations, and hundreds of different small worlds and local cultures. If we did so, we could carelessly crush all this diversity together as if the ancient world were one coherent political, economic, religious, ethical and cultural system. As far as I know, every single study of abortion in the ancient world produced so far, has, to a larger or smaller degree, done exactly this, namely treated the ancient world as one unit with a single system of values. This is a serious methodological fault. On certain issues, the political, economic and cultural parameters of the Greek city states may be very different from those of the hellenistic kingdoms, or the Roman empire. A set of cultural values that applies to democratic fourth-century Athens may not necessarily apply to Julio-Claudian Rome. But I do not need to labour the obvious: if we want to understand what would be the reaction to an induced abortion in classical Athens, we need to place the act against the legal, political, historical and cultural setting of classical Athens. And if we want to understand what the Romans thought about abortion, then we need to investigate abortion in the historical setting of the Roman empire.

Among previous scholarship on the subject the monumental work of Enzo Nardi, *Procurato aborto nel mondo Greco-Romano*, needs to be singled out, since it provides a thorough and methodical study of the topic. Nardi meticulously classifies a wealth of evidence by period and place. However, in doing so he becomes subject to a fault that has been pointed out by S.K. Dickison in her perceptive review of his book: he fails to synthesise the rich material that he provides.[8] Dickison correctly writes: '*Procurato aborto* should hence be considered as a manual for future work, which should result in a more readable and synthesized treatment of the material.'

I have tried to respond to these challenges and produce a 'readable and synthesized' treatment of the available evidence, without losing sight of time and place. When discussing a certain piece of evidence I have tried to keep in mind when it was produced, where, by whom, and for what purpose. As such it should be evaluated against its own background, and in the context of its own literary genre. This has not always been easy. Abortion is an issue that enters many different disciplines. It is certainly a medical issue, and one of the most difficult areas of medical ethics from antiquity to the present day. It is also a matter that raises serious legal problems, and as such it is studied by lawyers and legal scholars. It is a social issue, related to gender relations, perceptions and stereotypes. It is an economic issue, since the decision to continue or terminate a pregnancy is quite often related to economic factors. It is a political and philosophical issue, for it raises some very important questions about the value of human life. It is a theological issue, at least for a number of people who believe that the destruction of a foetus is against divine will. It is a demographic issue, since it may have repercussions on population control policies. And finally, it is a moral issue, because the prohibition or acceptance of induced abortion mirrors the ethical beliefs of a particular society. Abortion is a complex subject, and a historical analysis of the evidence must take all these factors into account.

I have tried to explore abortion in the ancient world in all its complexity – thematic, temporal and local. Moreover, I have studied the subject not as an issue of historical interest that has little relevance for the present, but as part of the modern debate. To the extent that my limited knowledge of modern medical, ethical, legal and sociological data has allowed, I have presented the facts and debate over induced abortion in the ancient world as an extension of the modern debate. I am convinced that the study of ten centuries of history, from 500 BC to 500 AD, can indeed bring wisdom to the modern world. It can allow us to understand better some of the contentious issues of the present, and if it cannot provide us with definite answers, at least it can make us think and perhaps re-evaluate some of our convictions. What makes Graeco-Roman antiquity an intriguing period to study is the fact that, paradoxically, it contains the closest system of cultural values to our own, and yet is so different in certain ways. The pagan Graeco-Roman world had concepts of ethical, legal, moral, and cultural issues that were advanced enough to match our own, but based on a different view of life, one that removed ultimate moral authority from Heaven and brought it to Earth. Each human being had to evaluate his or her actions on the basis of rational thinking, upbringing and personal understanding of moral standards, and consider what was good and expedient for the individual and society as a whole. Surely they have much to tell us.

1

Methods of Abortion:
Science and Superstition

The wide variety of methods used to procure abortions attested by ancient authors suggests that abortions were neither a novelty in the classical period nor an invention of Hippocratic medicine. If we are to believe Euripides,[1] abortions took place in the time of the Trojan wars, and a fragment of Sophocles[2] also places abortion in the mythical past. In reality, it was probably a very old practice indeed. By the end of the fifth century BC, when the first works of the Hippocratic Corpus were published, a substantial amount of knowledge regarding techniques and issues related to abortion was already in circulation. L. Dean-Jones says that gynaecology in particular probably incorporates a large amount of folk-practice, perhaps more than other branches of ancient medicine, and similar conclusions were reached by A. Rouselle, N. Demand and J. Riddle.[3] On the other hand H. King is less keen to accept that women knew so much about pregnancy and childbirth.[4] The dispute is not over the fact that women knew about such matters, but over how much they knew, and this question is not easy to answer. No matter how hard we may speculate, the absence of relevant literature written by women makes it impossible to quantify. But one thing is certain: the medical knowledge incorporated in the Hippocratic Corpus was not exclusively the enterprise of a few pioneers, but also, to some degree, based upon wisdom collected through the centuries. A. Preus[5] correctly relates the origin of knowledge concerning abortion to the experience and observation of women during pregnancy. Midwives, doctors and elder women might know about substances or situations that could be harmful to pregnancy and lead to a spontaneous abortion (miscarriage). This knowledge could be used in two ways: it could be employed to safeguard a pregnancy or to terminate an unwanted one. The number of references to abortion in the ancient world clearly suggests that women and their helpers would attempt to induce an abortion when one was desired, and that they could and did perform them, in one way or another, despite medical risks or negative ethical perceptions.

Greek and Latin frequently do not differentiate between a spontaneous and an induced abortion. Greek has a specific word for miscarriage (*apobolê*), but it is rarely used. The terms most frequently employed for a spontaneous or an induced abortion are *amblôsis*, or *ektrôsis* (or *trôsis*, *trôma, trôsmos*), or *phthora* (or *apophora*) for the noun, and *ambloun* (or *ambliskein* and *amblottein*), or *ektitrôskein*, or *phtheirein* (or *apophtheirein*) for the verb. *Phtheirein* is an ordinary Greek verb meaning 'to corrupt' or 'to destroy', which was sometimes employed in this particular sense. The other terms are more technical and primarily used to indicate an abortion (but *trôma*, the same stem as trauma, is often used to indicate any kind of wound, as does the simple verb *titrôskein* 'to wound'). Grammarians and lexicographers were intrigued by the simultaneous use of the terms *amblôsis* (stem *ambo-* 'blunt, dull') and *ektrôsis* (stem *trô-* 'wound, injure'), and attempted to understand the difference between them without success. Eustathius believed that *amblôsis* is wider and can be used for any kind of abortion, while *ektrôsis* could only be used if the aborted foetus was unformed. But we cannot put much faith in this explanation, because it is flatly contradicted by Galen, when he says that *amblôsis* is the *ektrôsis* of an immature foetus (as opposed to birth, which is the delivery of a mature foetus). Phrynichus thought that one (*amblôsis*) is Attic, because it is used by Lysias (see Chapter 6.iii), while the other (*ektrôsis*) is non-Attic, and therefore bad Greek (*adokimon*). But this probably is not true either, because one finds *ektrôsis* often in the Hippocratic Corpus, and, even if not in its entirety, at least for the major part the Hippocratic Corpus is Athenian literature. But actually, we may be able to find the answer in modern Greek usage. Nowadays one would usually write *amblose*, and use it in a rather formal context, while most people would say *ektrose* in everyday discourse. This stylistic difference was probably the same in antiquity and has not changed through the centuries. Thus Lysias, Antiphon, Plato and other sophisticated authors had the sensitivity to see this difference and use the more formal word *amblôsis*. But some of the less sophisticated authors of the Hippocratic Corpus were unaware of such niceties of style, and employed the everyday, colloquial word *ektrôsis* and its compounds. If this is so, we can understand why Phrynichus reached the conclusion that *amblôsis* is good Attic Greek, while *ektrôsis* is not.[6] In Latin things are much more straightforward: D.R. Langslow writes: '*abortus* (Cels.), *aborsus* (Theod.), *abortio* (Cass.) "a termination of pregnancy", accidental or deliberate from the verb *aboriri* specialized from its basic meaning "to pass away, disappear, be lost".'[7]

The lack of terminological distinctions between spontaneous and induced abortions is probably related to the fact that from very ancient times, well before the advent of rational medicine, for women experience with miscarriages went hand in hand with knowledge about induced abortion. Women had obviously experimented with terminating unwanted pregnancies from time immemorial. Soranus, a second-century AD physician and perhaps the most authoritative figure in ancient gynaecology, provides us with a valuable summary of most available knowledge concerning the termination of pregnancies in the ancient world:

After the conception one must refrain from any exaggeration and agitation, physical and mental, for the sperm is expelled as a result of sudden fear and sorrow and joy, and on the whole as a result of a powerful shock of the mind, and strenuous exercise and violent intermissions of breath, coughs, sneezes, beatings, falls – and in particular on one's back –lifting weights, jumps, hard seats, use of drugs, administration of pungent drugs and sternutatories, malnutrition, indigestion, drunkenness, vomiting, looseness of the bowels, loss of blood through the nose, the haemorrhoids or another outlet, relaxation through an agent which can increase the temperature, and because of high fever, and shiver and spasm, and in general anything which can cause a violent motion, that is, the means to cause an abortion.[8]

However, as the true causes of many miscarriages were not well understood and irrelevant factors were often linked with a spontaneous abortion, this traditional wisdom contained inaccurate information. The issue was further complicated by factors such as religion and superstition. The pioneering study[9] *Sacred disease* demonstrates clearly that in the years before Hippocratic medicine tried to provide rational explanations for the causes and cures of illness, supernatural elements were prevalent in medical issues.

In the words of Celsus, a Roman author of the first century BC, Hippocrates was the first to separate medicine from philosophy and establish it as a discipline in its own right.[10] Nevertheless, despite the steady progress from the sphere of the supernatural to the world of reason in the classical period and afterwards, superstitious beliefs in dark forces capable of causing harm to the unborn foetus are preserved even in serious medical texts, and surely much more than what it is preserved for us in writing must have circulated orally in the ancient world.

As a result of the often confused understanding of the true causes of a spontaneous abortion, we find that information concerning abortion techniques and related health issues is often of dubious quality. It is frequently the case with ancient medical texts that a piece of sound advice is immediately followed by irrelevant or even harmful information. Hippocratic medicine inherited an accumulation of traditional wisdom and much of it was employed by Hippocratic doctors, while part of the popular wisdom concerning pregnancy and abortion was rejected by serious medical practice as irrelevant or harmful. Hippocratic doctors and their heirs made an honest effort to learn about the human body, how it works, what is good and what is bad for it. But this effort alone often proved insufficient to lead them to the truth. Clinical observation and experience with patients was the ultimate source of wisdom, but these alone could not tell decisively which drug or substance was useful or harmful, and why. The Greeks and the Romans did not have a good understanding of chemistry, and their knowledge of biology was quite often nothing more than wild syllogistic deduction. When ancient medical authors talk about the qualities of a certain substance, it is possible that they have the backing of some clinical experience, but probably no scientific data of any significance. So what they say could be based on accurate observation, and therefore be correct, but there is an equal chance that it was just rough extrapolation based upon flawed data and arguments, or totally superficial reasoning.[11]

There are numerous theories on female biology and anatomy to be found in the works of ancient medical authors, and these have been discussed in a number of studies in recent years. In particular, women classical scholars such as L. Dean-Jones, H. King and R. Flemming, with a strong interest in women's history, but also with thorough grounding in traditional classical scholarship, have produced remarkable accounts of ancient theories and perceptions of the female body.[12] Considering the extent and nature of these theories, ranging from accurate observation to wild imagination, it is curious to see that in most cases where a reference to induced abortion is made in ancient medical literature, theory on female biology seems hardly to affect the course of the operation. One may ask why the beliefs in the wandering womb, or the discussion of the effects of virginity on the body, had almost no impact upon actual practices and procedures of induced abortion. The answer I believe is simple: abortion was a hands-on experience and skill. One could either do it or not, and the effects would be seen immediately. Theoretical arguments concerning female biology and anatomy would not help; practical wisdom and skill would. Probably this is why so little of those ancient medical theories that fascinate modern scholars, and were held as the corollary of medical knowledge for millennia, has transferred itself into advice related to abortions.

Moreover, even if a few prominent physicians, whose work has been transmitted to us, understood a certain aspect of human biology fairly well, there is no guarantee that their wisdom was transmitted to the majority of physicians in the ancient world. One would have good reason to question the credentials of many people who practised medicine throughout antiquity (see also Chapter 3).[13] Much as we may admire the often precise knowledge of Soranus, it would be a fallacy to believe that all those who were offering gynaecological advice and performing abortions in his time (early second century AD) and afterwards, were aware of or able to profit from the achievements of the great physician. The approach of Soranus is to some degree tied to the teachings of the Methodist sect, but he scrutinises his information with solid rational arguments. Thus his *Gynaecology* is the most famous surviving work of Greek medicine on this subject, and undoubtedly does credit to the clinical knowledge and sober judgement of a man who on the basis of this work was named *medicorum princeps*. However, Soranus did not mean to write just another manual for a small circle of well-educated Greek physicians; he intended the *Gynaecology* to serve as a manual for the large number of midwives providing basic healthcare for women in the Roman empire. Yet, even though the intention was good, whether this valuable manual ever reached the majority of midwives is highly questionable. There are good reasons to believe that many of them, particularly midwives serving small rural communities, could not read at all.[14]

The lack of uniform standards and controls regarding the professional qualifications of medical practitioners, socio-economic factors which prevented members of small, remote communities from going to study in Athens, Alexandria or Rome with experienced and learned doctors, the limitations in the circulation of books and acquired wisdom, suspicion of the effectiveness of new methods and treatments, and, in general, the slow and inconsistent implementation of scientific advances, hampered the progress of medical science over the centuries.[15] Although one cannot doubt that Hippocratic medicine and its heirs moved the knowledge of the human body and its functions from the world of the supernatural to the world of reason and science, the practical benefits of this transition were limited for a large number of medical practitioners. For example, one finds that when Aetius[16] compiled his handbook of prescriptions in the sixth century AD, after ten intense centuries of medical science and despite all the considerable progress made thus far, similar inaccuracies and superstitions to those that we encounter in the fifth century BC, when Hippocratic medicine was still in the cradle, were widespread and part of the approved practice of the time. The overall picture is not a uniform one, and medical science was not moving forward with a steady pace, building up precise information and making the treatment of gynaecological conditions ever easier and safer.

In addition, it is important to stress that the medicine of the time did not have a monopoly on abortions. The author of the work *Diseases of women* complained that women often induced abortions themselves and points out the impending dangers:

> If the woman in the process of inducing an abortion receives a large wound, or causes ulcers to the uterus as a result of the application of pungent drugs – and women experiment all the time with such things – and the foetus is killed ....[17]

The furtive nature of the operation, especially when the woman wished to hide the existence of the pregnancy in the first place, often meant that even if she decided to ask for help, she might not visit a well known and experienced practitioner, but rather persons with obscure credentials, who were not in the habit of asking too many questions. These could be other women, midwives, abortionists who practised for profit, religious figures, magicians, or, in fact, anyone who professed to possess some form of knowledge and would be willing, for any reason, to assist a desperate woman. Certainly the advances in medical science from the fifth century BC onwards had not reached some of these practitioners.

Abortions were performed throughout the ancient world by a variety of methods, some relatively safe, others life-threatening, some efficient, others perilously ineffective, and by a wide range of practitioners, from the

women themselves to skilful practitioners such as Soranus, with largely
different degrees of knowledge and understanding of gynaecological issues, expertise and skills. A mass of information, mainly from medical
texts but also from other sources, has reached us suggesting that a wide
range of techniques was used in antiquity. Dating these techniques and
placing them into a pattern of development is a difficult task. Some
prescriptions and potions can be dated since they are ascribed to a certain
person,[18] and the same can be said about techniques which can be ascribed
to a certain medical author. The main difficulty, however, is that we do not
really know how much of this information was new at the time and how
much derived from long established practice. For example, when Galen
speaks about the antidote of Orbanus the Indian, it cannot be said with
certainty whether Orbanus invented the potion, modified a traditional
recipe, or simply recorded a potion used by practitioners before him over
a long period of time. Equally, when Celsus describes in detail an operation for the removal of a dead foetus (see Chapter 1.v), it is impossible to
tell which parts of this procedure were devised by whom and whether a
certain technique described there was a new breakthrough or a centuries-
old skill. The knowledge of an author like Celsus was broad and could have
originated from a number of sources. He was writing not only on medicine
but also on other liberal arts suitable for the education of a Roman
gentleman, and had collected a substantial amount of material from Greek
medical authors, which he arranged to suit his educational and intellectual purposes.[19] Thus an attempt to trace and describe the development of
the methods and techniques of induced abortions in the ancient world
would be a difficult and complex task. Here I have tried to place this
information into rough chronological order, when at all possible, and only
to such an extent as can enable us to see what Hippocratic[20] medicine
knew, as opposed to what later doctors achieved.

i. Orally administered drugs

Modern science has been unable so far to produce an agreeably efficient
and safe abortion pill.[21] Although research continues, such a pill is still in
the experimental stages.[22] Ancient medicine employed a wide range of
substances allegedly capable of harming the foetus and causing an abortion from common herbs, found in plenty in the Greek countryside, to
exotic substances imported from the fringes of the ancient world. Herbs or
their extracts would be processed and blended into potions, believed to
have abortifacient qualities. The prescriptions were sometimes simple,
but on other occasions very complex recipes were suggested. The range
varied from substances as common and simple as the cyclamen to a
number of complex potions, called antidotes (*antidota*), made of ingredients sometimes only available in the metropolitan centres of the ancient
world. Even making allowances for the fact that one author often borrows
information from another (for example, Pliny and Dioscorides often seem

to be borrowing from the same source, perhaps Theophrastus), a number of herbs and substances to which abortifacient qualities are attributed consistently appear in ancient medical and pharmacological studies. Some of these, although possibly unsafe for the mother, might have worked if administered properly, in appropriate dosages and combinations.

Careful authors, like Soranus, precisely describe the qualities of a certain drug or cocktail as contraceptive, emmenagogue or abortifacient, and give instructions concerning the way it should be administered – that is, whether it should be used as an oral drug, a pessary or an ointment. Soranus draws some distinctions:

> A contraceptive is different from an abortifacient, because the first prevents conception, while the second destroys the product of conception. Thus, let us say that the abortifacient is one thing and the contraceptive is another; on the other hand, some say that the expulsive is the same as the abortifacient, while others say that it is different.[23]

Soranus was not the first to make these distinctions. Hippocratic medicine was well aware of these differences, and the author of *Diseases of women* describes various drugs as abortifacient, that is, drugs meant to kill a live foetus (*phthoria*), expulsives (*ekbolia* or *elatêria*)[24] and contraceptives (*atokia*).[25] There are also a number of references to emmenagogues and awareness that these could be used as abortifacient drugs.[26] The distinction between oral drugs, pessaries and ointments is made clear in the following list:

> For it is not possible to destroy the foetus without violence, by means of a potion, some edible substance, or pessaries, or any other means.[27]

The author of *Diseases of women* gives an endless list of prescriptions of various potions and pessaries, meticulously providing instructions regarding the method of administration. Most of the substances mentioned in later medical and pharmacological studies are already listed in this work. Here I provide a few examples of substances with allegedly abortifacient qualities recommended by Hippocratic doctors and subsequent medical and pharmacological studies. Clover (*trifylon*[28]) mixed with white wine is recommended as an emmenagogue and abortifacient.[29] Edderwort (*drakontia* or *drakontion*) mixed with vinegar and water was believed to be such a strong potion that even the smell could be poisonous.[30] The abortifacient qualities of the mountain rue (*agrion peganon*) were highly praised throughout antiquity.[31] Birthwort (*aristolochia*: literally, 'excellent birth') mixed with pepper and mint was believed to hasten the birth and to be an efficient abortifacient.[32] White hellebore (*elleboros leukos*), bryony (*ampelos leukê*), bracken (*thelypteris*), shepherd's purse (*thlaspis* or *thlaspi*), calamint (*kalaminthê*), Cretan poplar (*diktamon*), gilliflower (*leukoion*), base horehound (*stachys*), and many other herbs, were well known as abortifacients from the time of Hippocrates.[33] Even a poisonous fish the colour of a hare (*lepus marinum*: literally, 'sea-hare'), which can cause nausea and violent sickness, was used as an abortifacient, according to Pliny.[34]

A large number of cocktails and prescriptions are recorded in ancient medical texts. Their ingredients could be toxic substances such as copper, known abortifacients like those mentioned above, or harmless substances like leek or honey. I give a few examples of such potions recommended by Hippocratic medicine.

Mul. 174: 3 inches of soap-wort (*stroutheion*) root boiled in honey.

Mul. 180: 1 obol of poplar from Crete powdered in water. It was supposed to expel a dead foetus.

Mul. 180: Leaves of chaste-tree (*agnos*) in wine.[35]

Mul. 182: Mashed leek (*prassou chylos*) with myrrh (*smyrna*) and sweet wine.

Mul. 182: Fennel (*marathon*) root in oil, wine and honey.

Mul. 184: A small bunch of mint (*minthê*), rue (*peganon*), coriander (*koriannon*) and sawdust of cedar or cypress tree in aromatic wine.[36]

This is only a small sample of an endless list of herbs and potions, used in numerous combinations and cocktails. As the centuries went by, these recipes became more complex and the antidotes described in Galen's *Peri antidoton* are truly difficult recipes, which would be blended in the laboratory of the professional pharmacist, rather than on the kitchen table of an ordinary housewife (see §ii below). The blending of these drugs required knowledge, skill and a supply of materials, some of which would be hard to find. The following example is an antidote attributed to Orbanos the Indian:

Myrrh 15 drachms;[37] saffron 16 drachms; Indian spikenard 16 drachms; cinnamon, cassia, panacea 13 drachms of each; amomon 8 drachms, garlic germander 25 drachms, in another one 5 drachms; flower of camel-hay 8 drachms; meum athamanticum 3 drachms; rose essence 12 drachms, 3 obols; wild nard 5 drachms, 3 obols; St. John's wort 5 drachms, Arabian ginger 6 drachms; black pepper 6 drachms; white pepper 8 drachms; storax 5 drachms, 3 obols; wild fennel seed 3 drachms, 4 obols; long pepper 5 drachms, according to others 6 drachms; costos root 7 drachms, 3 obols; clover seed 5 drachms; gentian 4 drachms, round birthwort 4 drachms, hulwort 5 drachms, clover root 5 drachms, 3 obols; cardamon 5 drachms; echion root 4 drachms; incense 6 drachms; parsley 6 drachms; mullein 6 drachms; hartwort 5 drachms; Aethiopian cumin 3 drachms; balsam fruit 4 drachms; Celtic nard 4 drachms; opium 4 drachms, 3 obols; porched barley seed 3 drachms; Egyptian incense 4 drachms; Illyrian iris in equal quantity; mandrake juice 6 drachms, obols; sagapenon 4 drachms; opopanax 3 drachms; anise 4 drachms; hypocystis juice 6 drachms; turpentine 5 drachms, 3 obols; castor oil 5 drachms; balsam tree juice 16 drachms; wild rue seed 3 drachms; juice of all-heal 4 drachms; equal amount of turnip; marrow from deer 6 drachms, 3 obols; nard essence 20 drachms; dried goat's blood 5 drachms, 3 obols; equal

amount of goose blood; duck's blood 3 drachms, 3 obols; Egyptian bouphthal-
mon juice 8 drachms; Chian athamantic wine as much as it takes.[38]

The availability of materials for these potions must have been an important factor and it may often have been the case that individual doctors or
pharmacists replaced one substance which they could not find with another, or omitted it altogether, thus altering the chemical composition of
these potions with unpredictable consequences. Sometimes the alteration
of a traditional antidote was deliberate, intended to enhance the powers of
the drug. Galen, for example, modifies the antidote of Mithridates Eupator
by adding traditional abortifacients such as Cretan poplar, mountain rue
seed, or clover seed, in order to boost the abortifacient action of this
antidote. He describes the action of the modified drug as following:

By adding these the use of the drug serves many purposes, for it destroys
four-month-old foetuses and expels three-month-old ones.[39]

The fact that so many different substances and cocktails were suggested
has to do with two factors. First, as none of these drugs could be totally
reliable, doctors and pharmacists continued experimenting through the
centuries with increasingly complex recipes and combinations in their
effort to produce the most efficient abortifacient, that is, a drug which
could be trusted to induce an abortion with as little agony and danger to
the woman as possible. Second, the inconsistent availability of materials
forced doctors and pharmacists to be inventive and resourceful. A herb
very common in one part of Greece, might be absent elsewhere and have
to be replaced by one which allegedly had similar qualities.

It is hard to tell how efficient these drugs were in reality, but as Nardi
points out,[40] some could indeed harm the foetus and prove efficient, even
though they could be detrimental for the mother too. Based on a study by
G. Negri,[41] Nardi mentions that the cyclamen, the birthwort, the bryony
and the squirting cucumber[42] (*elaterion*) actually possess the qualities
attributed to them by ancient doctors and pharmacologists. Several other
scholars in recent years have pursued this line of research. The studies of
J. Riddle, a specialist in ancient pharmacology, may represent the culmination of research into the contraceptive and abortifacient qualities of
several plants and substances mentioned by ancient authors. Riddle has
argued that many of these herbs and plants actually possessed contraceptive or abortifacient qualities.[43] Pushing the argument to the limit, he
concluded that women in antiquity had a much more accurate knowledge
of the qualities of these herbs than one might imagine at first glance, and
that this knowledge was forgotten in later centuries. The conviction that
'women in antiquity knew what only a few women know today' is crucial
for Riddle's argument.

The reaction to his views has been mixed.[44] Riddle certainly succeeded
in making a credible case for the capabilities of ancient pharmacology.

However, how far these capabilities could go remains questionable, and will remain so until proper clinical testing proves or disproves the contraceptive or abortifacient effects on humans of the large number of substances and herbs mentioned in the sources. I am not prepared to engage in proper speculation without data, or embrace theories about the supposedly 'forgotten knowledge' of ancient women. However, it is sensible to conclude that unless some of these substances had some degree of effectiveness, faith in the potential of abortifacient drugs would have eventually faded away, rather than being included in the most advanced medical handbooks available to the world for two millennia. It is clear at a glance that many of the suggested substances would have been truly harmless on their own. Items such as honey, goat's blood or deer marrow apart from influencing the taste of the drug, they would have no serious effects. However, a cocktail of basically harmless substances with drugs such as opium, mandrake or mullein could produce a powerful mixture with serious side-effects and prove detrimental to both the pregnancy and the health of the woman. Galen assures his readers that the antidote of Aelius Gallus, which in his opinion was a safe abortifacient drug, had been effectively used by Caesar and Carmes as a lethal poison.[45] This assurance is characteristic of the perception of those potions. It was well understood that those of the substances which could prove efficient were toxic drugs with potentially lethal qualities. A passage of Galen illustrates very clearly the reality surrounding the employment of abortifacient drugs.

> Most of the drugs ... are too weak to be efficient for such an undertaking, but some, even though potent, are dangerous for human life.[46]

Doctors since the time of Hippocrates were aware that many of the drugs cause serious side-effects. Perhaps the most striking reference is a medical record from the *Epidemics*. The author explains with chilling precision what happened to a woman known as the wife of Simos, after she had an abortion:

> The wife of Simos had an abortion after 30 days. This happened either spontaneously, or after she drank something. Pain. Plenty of bilious, pale, green vomit every time she had something to drink. She had seizures, and she was biting her tongue. I visited on the fourth day, and her tongue was swollen and black. The white on her eyes was red. She was sleepless. On the fourth night she died.[47]

The attending physician cannot pinpoint the precise reason for the abortion, but he suspects that it was deliberately induced by means of drugs, to which the serious complications could be attributed. Throughout antiquity it was well understood that abortions could usually be induced by means harmful for the mother too, and that they were more dangerous than normal childbirth:

Abortions are more dangerous than normal births, because it is not possible to kill the foetus without violence ..., and violence is a dangerous thing.[48]

In a similar mood Soranus states that contraception is safer than abortion.[49] The possible damage to the uterus, the dangers of septic abortion and, on the whole, the potential danger for the mother's health were clearly understood from the time of Hippocrates. Moreover, Soranus points out that the symptoms before an abortion are far more violent if this is induced by means of drugs.[50]

References to abortions in non-medical literature confirm that the ordinary person had a clear awareness of the dangers from the use of abortifacient drugs. Plutarch relates how Lycurgus, the mythical lawgiver of Sparta, persuaded his sister-in-law to avoid an abortion:

He said that she should not have an abortion and poison her body with drugs and put her life at risk[51]

Ovid wrote some intriguing verses concerning a woman fighting for her life after an abortion:

Aiming to end her pregnancy – so rashly –
Corrina lies exhausted, life in doubt.
To run such fearful risks without my knowledge
Should make me rage, but fear's put rage to rout ...
O Isis ...
Turn your eyes here; on her – and me – have mercy;
You will give life to her and she to me ...
You too, kind Ilithyia, who take pity
When girls are locked in labour, and relieve
Their hidden load, be present, hear my prayer ....[52]

In the next poem Ovid compares the dangers and wounds of war for men, with the dangers from abortions for women.

What good for girls to be exempt from warfare,
No shields, no line of march to meet the foe,
If they get wounds, in peace, from their own weapons
And blindly arm themselves to their own woe?
She who first from the womb wrenched life's beginnings
Deserved to die by her own warring hand ...
Why pick – so cruel – fruit that's green and bitter,
and steal the growing grapes the vine would fill?
Let ripe fruit fall by nature; let beginnings
Grow on; life's no slight prize for small delay.
Why poison unborn children, why take weapons
To probe the womb and delve the life away?
We blame Medea by her son's blood spattered,
For mother-murdered Itys we lament;
Both mothers cruel, but both had cause for tragic
Vengeance on husbands in that shared blood spent.

Tell me what Tereus or what Jason drives you
To violate yourself in such distress ...
But gentle girls do that, though not unpunished;
Killing their wombs' young life, they often die.
Die, and they are on the pyre with hair dishevelled,
And 'Serve them right' say all those standing by.
But may these words of mine bear no bad omen,
But vanish in the wind, and I'm content.
Ye gracious gods, let her sin once in safety;
Enough – next time impose your punishment.[53]

Saint Basil in his first letter to Amphilochios says that a woman who had induced an abortion should be treated like a murderess not only on account of the life of the unborn, but on account of the grave risk upon her own life too:

> The woman who had an abortion should be held responsible for premedita-
> tion of murder ... because in this case punishment is due not only because of
> the unborn, but also of the one who took destructive action against her own
> self, for women usually die through such an undertaking.[54]

Even if we conceded the possibility that sometimes women and medical persons were deceived over the qualities of a substance or unable to foresee the ill-effects of a certain drug, we would still be confronted by the fact that women and their medical attendants were prepared to experiment with a wide variety of drugs which they often recognised as highly toxic, and went to great lengths in their desire to have an unwanted pregnancy termi-nated. Why women put their lives at such a risk and the pressures that induced them to seek an abortion are explored in Chapter 4.

One question which inevitably arises from the preceding account is why the use of oral drugs was so widespread when doctors and patients seemed aware of the fact that safe drugs were weak and potent ones dangerous. The main attraction of oral drugs was that they did not require extensive involvement of third parties. Recipes and drugs could be handed over from one woman to another, or from the midwife, the doctor, or the abortionist to a patient. A woman wishing to have an abortion would ask someone she trusted and believed that they knew about such matters, and hopefully she would be offered some advice about the abortifacient potential of this or that herb or substance. Then in the peace of her home, away from intrusive eyes, she could mix by herself the recommended drugs, using herbs from her garden or drugs obtained from a store in the market-place. In the event that the woman had asked the assistance of a sympathetic medic, she could still take away the prescribed drug and use it at home, without many people knowing about it. The desired secrecy was guaranteed and the hope of success often outweighed prudent considerations concerning one's health.

Orally administered drugs might also be more attractive compared with other methods of abortion, because they appeared to be less dangerous, less drastic and less cruel to the woman's body. The harm they might cause to her system would be less evident than the horrors of surgical means, or the ulcers caused by potent pessaries (see below). As such oral drugs would be perceived as more humane and safer to use, regardless of their actual qualities. Besides, even if one vaguely knew that drugs could be harmful, one might not know whether a particular substance was harmful, or to what extent, or how it could affect different persons (for example, sometimes substances which might be safe for a strong young woman, could be detrimental for a woman with a certain health condition). In the popular wisdom surrounding abortions, as well as in the armoury of ancient medicine, oral drugs were the most accessible method of induced abortion and the one which appeared at first to be the least troublesome. If this method failed and the women survived the attempt, she could always resort to more drastic methods.

If the works of ancient doctors had not been transmitted to us, we might think that drugs were the only method of induced abortion known to the ancient world. In non-medical works drugs appear to be the standard method used by women to induce an abortion.[55] This surely has to do with the fact that the former works were written by men, who had an idea that drugs were used by women for this purpose, but often did not know exactly how the entire process was carried through. Considering that abortions were performed away from the eyes of the ordinary man, there was a certain degree of secrecy surrounding the entire issue, giving rise to a mythology reflecting male attitudes, fears and prejudices about various potions known and used by women along with poisons, love philtres, aphrodisiacs – all kinds of drugs with all sorts of mysterious powers. While, as I mentioned above, medical and pharmacological studies would use a more precise vocabulary (e.g. *phthorion, ekbolion, atokion, katharterion*) describing the activity and qualities of a certain drug, the word most frequently used in non-medical literature is *pharmakon* (or *pharmakion*), which was the word also used for a lethal potion, or in fact any kind of chemical blend.[56] In the eyes of male authors all the substances used by women for birth-control purposes were one and the same, that is, potent poisons with strange powers. In this context it is not surprising that Pliny places abortifacient drugs on a par with magic and love philtres and Galen places them next to aphrodisiacs, or philtres that explain dreams, excite hatred, curb the opponent's ability to speak in court, or kill (see also §vii below).[57]

ii. Pessaries

The word 'pessary' indicates a vaginal suppository and is derived from the Greek word *pessos*.[58] The use of pessaries by Hippocratic medicine is certain, as the word is mentioned in the Hippocratic oath (cf. Chapter 3) and a large number of pessaries is recommended supposedly for various therapeutic reasons in the Hippocratic Corpus, and in particular in the study *Diseases of women*. The ingredients and blending of abortifacient pessaries was analogous to that of oral drugs, with one significant difference: on average, pessaries were more potent and sometimes we find among the ingredients irritant substances which would not be orally administered, like the juice of the wild fig, a milky liquid which causes acute irritation.[59] The use of substances such as the soap-wort, birth-wort, mountain rue, myrrh, white hellebore, squirting cucumber, cyclamen, calamint, lupine (*brathy*), cedar-oil, centaury (*kentaurion to megalon*), mixed with substances such as water, wine or hot oil and made into pessaries, was recommended from the time of Hippocrates.[60] Some of the substances used in pessaries, such as white hellebore or soap-wort, produce alkaline substances, and as such they were similar in composition to Utus Paste, a method of abortion used until the 1960s, but condemned by modern medicine as unsafe.[61] Pessaries took the form of liquid to be poured into the uterus (*ekchuton*), or solid suppositories (*balanos*), depending on their composition. Here I give a few examples of pessaries from *Diseases of women*:

8,186: Saffron blended with goose fat, passed through a sieve, to be poured into the uterus and left there for as long as possible.

8,184: 1 drachm allum (*stypterie*), 1 drachm myrrh, 3 obols black hellebore mixed with red wine, kneaded and made into suppositories, which were to be left inside until bleeding started. This was a rather potent pessary, which was recommended by Hippocratic medicine in order to kill and expel a foetus which did not move.

8,186: Mashed leek and celery, 1 ladle of rose-oil, 1 quarter of goose-fat, 3 obols of pine-resin. The mixture should be melted in oil and poured into the uterus.

More recipes are provided in other Hippocratic works, intended to clear the uterus. I mention a few more recipes for powerful pessaries from the work *Superfetation*:

8,502 (*CMG* 33,6-7): Copper scum and one third of sodium carbonate, mixed with boiled honey and made into suppositories of average size and width, to be applied into the mouth of the womb. In order to make this pessary even stronger one could mix the copper scum alone with squirting cucumber. Alternatively, when the mouth of the womb appeared to be dry, one could add scraps of fig-branch processed, so that it would become smooth.

More recipes for pessaries are offered in later medical studies:

Ps.-Gal. 14,481: One obol of opopanax made into ointment and applied inside. Pseudo-Galen assures his readers that this one is safe and that it has been tried on many women.

Ps.-Gal. 14,481: Smooth soap-wort with honey, made into small pessaries. It was meant to be an emmenagogue and could also terminate a pregnancy in the second month.

Ps.-Gal. 14,481: Two and a half figs, blended with one obol of sodium carbonate.

The inventiveness and versatility of ancient medics and pharmacologists is astonishing. One of the prescriptions for pessaries even uses mouse-dung as one of the basic substances:

Egyptian salt, and mouse-dung, and wild colocynth, and a quarter of honey to be poured over half-boiled. Then take one drachm of pine-resin, add to the honey and the colocynth and the mouse-dung, mix everything thoroughly, make suppositories and insert them into the uterus, until it seems that it is time.[62]

Like orally administered drugs, pessaries could be blended by women themselves at home. Even when they were given to them by a doctor or someone else, they could be taken at home and applied by the woman alone. Thus pessaries also guaranteed a degree of secrecy and privacy and this is why they seem to have been, alongside oral drugs, a method preferred by many women.[63] The dangers from pessaries, like those from oral drugs, were clearly understood by ancient doctors from the time of Hippocrates, and pessaries are explicitly banned by the Hippocratic Oath. Ancient doctors knew that highly irritant pessaries, effective as they might be, could cause ulcers, inflammation and septic abortions, leading to sterility or even death,[64] but, as with oral drugs, often the desire to terminate an unwanted pregnancy was too strong to be subjected to reason.

iii. Externally applied drugs

A number of known abortifacient substances used in oral drugs and pessaries were also used in creams and ointments for external application on the abdomen. Galen says of the cyclamen:

Its abortifacient quality is so potent that even if one applies it on the abdomen it penetrates through and aborts the embryos.[65]

Galen also recommends various other ointments and creams. Pseudo-Galen gives an example of a poultice supposed to be able to cause the death of the foetus:

Two ladles of bruised corn to be boiled with vinegar and made into porridge. When it is half-boiled (add) one part of aloe, make it like an emollient plaster and apply towards the navel and down to the line of the ephebaeum and bind it.[66]

The following poultice was supposed to cause a safe and painless abortion while the woman was sleeping:

> Boil one part of cypress leaves with water and crush thoroughly until it becomes an emollient plaster and apply on the navel and the abdomen and bind with a strip; tell (the woman) to lie on her back ... and she has a painless abortion while sleeping.[67]

Several creams and ointments are also recommended by Soranus, but only in combination with other methods.[68]

None of these treatments can have been very effective. The main attraction of externally applied drugs was that they could not cause any serious damage to the woman's health. Women would use them hoping that they could have a relatively safe and not very agonising abortion. Naturally, when these means failed women could resort to other more potent, but also more dangerous and painful, methods. In cases of combined treatment, when external applications were used along with pessaries, oral drugs, hot baths, bleeding, etc., the effect of the external creams might be overestimated. In reality, even though it might not enhance the action of more potent treatments, it served as a reassurance to the woman and her medical advisor that more than one available method had been used.

iv. Mechanical means

Well before Hippocrates women must have been aware of the fact that violence or strenuous physical exertion could harm a pregnancy and cause an abortion. Women working in the fields in agricultural communities and hard-worked female slaves would have provided study cases in plenty. This knowledge could be employed when the termination of a pregnancy was desired and mechanical means of various types were certainly used for this purpose throughout antiquity. Hippocratic medicine was aware of the possibility of inducing an abortion by means of physical violence or over-exertion. In the study *On the seed* we read:

> I say that the child crippled in the womb was crushed either because the mother was hit where the foetus was, or because she fell or some other violent incident happened to her; if the child is crushed, it is crippled that way and if the foetus is further crushed, the membrane which encloses it bursts and the foetus is aborted.[69]

Hippocratic medicine recommended strenuous physical exercise as a means of causing an abortion. The author of *On the nature of the child* describes how he advised a woman who was practising prostitution to induce an abortion successfully by means of leaps:

> And hearing that, I advised her to kick up her heels so as to strike the

buttock, and she had already jumped seven times, until the seed fell to the ground.[70]

Soranus, discussing this passage, says that it was interpreted by some doctors as implying that Hippocrates was not against abortion and that he simply objected to the use of abortifacient drugs on account of the danger they posed for the mother, and this is why he recommended abortions by means of physical exertion (for further discussion see Chapter 3).[71] Soranus himself recommends various such means, to be used in the course of inducing an abortion:

> In order to cut off the conceptus she must <move more vigorously> walking energetically, she must be shaken about on carriages, jump vigorously and carry weights beyond her strength.[72]

Galen also refers repeatedly to physical exertion as a means of inducing an abortion:

> And if it ever happens to the woman to jump or slip and fall down or somehow to be pushed violently either physically or mentally, she can easily have an abortion.[73]

Violence against the woman as the cause of an abortion is mentioned in the passage of Theon which refers to the speech of Lysias *To Antigenes: on the abortion* (see the discussion in Chapter 6):

> Someone hit a pregnant woman on the abdomen and is tried for murder (sc. because she had an abortion).[74]

The passage in Exodus that outlaws abortion also mentions violence against the woman as the cause of an abortion (see Chapter 2 for further discussion):

> If two men are fighting and they kick a pregnant woman and she loses the child ....[75]

The last three passages speak about a spontaneous abortion, inflicted upon the woman against her intention or consent, but nevertheless confirm that violence against a pregnant woman, as well as physical exertion, were situations clearly understood to be potentially damaging to the pregnancy and possibly leading to termination (see Chapter 6 for the legal implications).

T.N. Cingomklao describes in detail the application of a massage technique in rural Thailand, which accounts for the 80% of the total number of induced abortions in this area.[76] Massage techniques were sometimes employed in the course of an induced abortion in the ancient world too. Soranus recommends massage of the entire body with hot oil, and in particular of the area around the ephebaeum:

Hot oil must be applied all over the body and rubbed in vigorously, and especially around the ephebaeum and the abdomen and the lower back.[77]

The author of *Diseases of women*[78] goes further and recommends powerful shaking of the woman by two strong men as part of the operation to remove a dead foetus from the womb.

Perhaps with the exception of the last two techniques, mechanical means guaranteed complete privacy and secrecy. Nobody needed to know about the woman's efforts to induce an abortion, or, indeed, the existence of the pregnancy. The woman did not need to implicate other people, search for any substance or send a trustworthy slave to the market to ask for suspicious drugs. An additional advantage was that an abortion induced by mechanical means could always be presented as an accident, as a spontaneous abortion, provided, of course, that the woman had no strong reasons to hide the pregnancy, but nevertheless wished to terminate it. The main drawback was that the efficacy of this method was limited and the chances of success depended very much upon the woman's courage and determination. In order to force a miscarriage she might need to exert a considerable degree of violence upon her own body, and, unlike drugs or pessaries, which once administered would take their own irreversible course, mechanical means could normally be controlled and the entire undertaking interrupted before reaching the critical point. No matter how much the woman wished to have an abortion the agony of the experience might prove too much to take, and her nerve might fail her.[79]

v. Surgical abortions

Surgical removal of the foetus and clearance of the contents of the uterus by dilatation and curettage (the so-called D&C method) was the standard abortion technique until recently, when it was gradually replaced by the vacuum suction method or chemically induced abortions.[80] This technique was known to the ancient world, although, naturally, due to the lack of anaesthetics and antibiotics, it was a dangerous and painful undertaking, employed only in extreme circumstances. The most complete account of a D&C operation is provided by Celsus, a writer of the first century AD, in the following passage, where he describes the removal of a foetus nearly at term but already dead:

> Again when a woman has conceived, if the foetus, nearly at term, dies inside and cannot get out of itself, an operation must be done, which may be counted among the most difficult; for it requires both extreme caution and neatness, and entails very great risk .... The woman should be placed on her back across the bed, so that the iliac regions are compressed by her own thighs; by this means both her hypogastrium is in full view of the surgeon and the foetus is forced towards the mouth of the womb. This, after the death of the foetus, contracts, but later on usually dilates a little. The surgeon making use of this opportunity should first insert the index finger of his greased hand, and keep it there until the mouth is opened again, and then

he should insert a second finger, and the other fingers on the like opportunity, until the whole hand can be put in. To allow of this, much depends both on the size of the vagina, and the resistance of its sinewy tissues, and the patient's constitution, and also her strength of mind, especially since on occasion even both hands have to be passed in. It is also important that the hypogastrium and extremities should be kept very warm, that inflammation should not have begun, but that the treatment should be adopted without delay. For if the abdomen is already distended, the hand cannot be inserted nor can the foetus be extracted without the greatest suffering, and fatal spasm of the sinews often follows, accompanied by vomiting and tremor. But when the hand has reached the dead foetus its position is immediately felt. For it lies head on or feet foremost, or crosswise; generally, however, so that there is either a hand or foot within reach. It is the object now of the surgeon to direct it with his hand either into a head or even into a foot presentation, if it happens to be presenting otherwise: and if there is no other course, when a hand or foot is grasped, the trunk is straightened: for grasping a hand converts the presentation into a head one, grasping a foot into a foot presentation. Then if the head is nearest, a hook must be inserted which is completely smooth, with a short point, and this it is right to fix into an eye or ear or the mouth, even at times into the forehead, then this is pulled upon and extracts the foetus. But not every moment is proper for the extraction; for should this be attempted when the mouth of the womb is contracted, as there is no way out, the foetus is torn away from the hook, and its point then slips into the mouth of the womb itself; and there follows spasm of the sinews and great risk of death. Therefore whilst the mouth is contracted we should wait, and draw gently on the hook when it dilates, and so at these opportunities gradually extract the foetus. Now the right hand should pull the hook whilst the left is inserted within and pulls the foetus, and at the same time guides it. It also often happens that such a foetus is distended by fluid, and from it a foul sanies discharges. If so, the abdomen of the foetus is bored into by the index finger, when by escape of the fluid the foetus is made smaller; then it is gently to be delivered by the hands alone. For if a hook is inserted it readily slips out of the soft little body, when the danger noted above is incurred. If the foetus has been turned to present by the feet it is also not difficult to extract; for the feet are grasped by the doctor's hands, and it is readily drawn out. But if the foetus is lying crosswise and cannot be turned straight, the hook is to be inserted into an armpit and traction slowly made; during this the neck is usually bent back, and the head turned backwards to the rest of the foetus. The remedy then is to cut through the neck, in order that the two parts may be extracted separately. This is done with a hook, which resembles the one mentioned above, but has all its inner edge sharp. Then we must proceed to extract the head first, then the rest, for if the larger portion be extracted first, the head slips back into the cavity of the womb and cannot be extracted without the greatest risk. Should this, however, happen, a folded pad is placed upon the woman's hypogastrium, and then a man strong but not untrained, must stand on her left side, and place his two hands over the hypogastrium and press one over the other so that the head is forced to the mouth of the womb, when it must be extracted by the hook as described above. But if one foot presents whilst the other remains behind with the trunk, anything which has been drawn out must be cut away piecemeal; and if the buttocks begin to engage in the mouth of the womb they are to be pushed back and the foot of the foetus found and then drawn forwards. There are also other difficulties, which make it necessary to cut up and extract a foetus which does not come out whole. Now as soon as the foetus has been extracted it should be handed to the assistant to hold on his upturned hands, and the surgeon with his left hand must draw gently upon the navel cord, so as not to rupture it, whilst he passes his right hand along it up to what they called the secundines, which was the envelope of the foetus within the womb. When his hand has grasped the secundines including the whole of the blood vessels and membranes he brings them down from the womb in the same manner, and extracts the whole together with any retained blood clot. Then when the thighs have been tied together the woman is put to bed in a moderately warm room, which is free from draughts. Over the hypogastrium is placed greasy wool, dipped in vinegar and rose oil. The rest of the treatment followed is the same as for inflammation and for wounds which are in the sinews.[81]

The technique described by Celsus was not new in its entirety. Hippocratic medicine was aware of dilatation techniques and direct intervention into the uterus.[82] A surgery for the removal of a dead foetus is described in considerable detail in the work *Diseases of women*, but the technique is more crude and primitive than the one described by Celsus: it is mainly based on powerful shaking of the woman in the hands of two strong men, so that the gravity would drive the dead foetus out.[83] Another technique with the physician trying to extract the foetus with his hands is described in the work *Superfetation*:

> If the embryo remains inside dead and it is not possible to drive it out, either automatically or by means of drugs, grease the hand with wax, so that it becomes very slippery, then insert it into the womb and separate the shoulders from the neck, pressing heavily with the thumb: a nail fastened on the thumb is also necessary for this operation; after the hands have been separated, remove them; then cutting through the abdomen pull out gently the little guts, and after they have been removed crush the little ribs, so that the tiny body becomes compressed, more manageable and easier to drive out, since it will have less volume.[84]

Both direct intervention into the uterus and shaking are also described in the study *On the excision of the foetus*, written specifically to explain such procedures. In this study too the recommended procedures lack the precision and expertise of the techniques described by Celsus. Surgery as the means of emptying the uterus from its contents was practised throughout antiquity, and there is even a reference to a surgical instrument specifically employed for such purposes called *embruosphaktês* (literally: 'embryo-slayer'), probably something like the sharp hook described by Celsus. However, the name of the instrument implies that it was used rather to kill a live foetus than remove a dead one.[85]

One of the main dangers of a D&C operation is the perforation of the uterus. The danger of perforation was well understood from the time of Hippocrates, and Soranus advises that an abortion induced by means of sharp objects be avoided:

One must avoid ... destroying the embryo by means of a sharp object, for there is a risk to inflict injury upon the nearby area.[86]

To these risks add poor sterilisation techniques and the lack of anaesthesia and antibiotics, and we can see that such an operation would always be an excruciating and life-threatening ordeal, and certainly not a course of treatment to which ancient doctors and their patients can have resorted on a regular basis. In fact, as far as I know, in all attested cases the purpose of the operation is the removal of a dead foetus, not the elimination of a living embryo. This does not necessarily mean that surgical methods were not used to induce abortions, but I think we can safely conclude that surgery, when it was used to eliminate a living foetus, would only be employed as a last resort, perhaps almost invariably for therapeutic reasons, when the woman and her doctor had no choice. In situations where the continuation of a pregnancy posed an immediate threat to the woman's life and all other means had been exhausted, a surgically induced abortion might seem to be the only course of action. Equally, when the existence of a dead foetus, which could not be expelled by other less drastic methods, would inevitably result to the mother's death, a D&C operation might be the woman's only hope.

vi. Ancillary techniques

Several treatments were recommended by ancient doctors in the course of an induced abortion, none of which would have the desired effect on its own, but all of which were thought to assist to this end. Bleeding is recommended by Galen and Soranus. The latter acknowledges that this technique originates from Hippocrates.[87] Soranus recommends that plenty of blood should be let out. This in fact could weaken the mother and prove harmful for the pregnancy. Hot baths, which popular opinion held as an effective method of DIY abortions until recently, are recommended by Soranus.[88] A restricted diet, again with the intention of weakening the mother, is recommended by Soranus,[89] along with various other treatments such as massages, leaps, etc., all of which were perceived to be part of one course aiming at the termination of the pregnancy. Pain, severe indigestion, flux, or even a vain endeavour to evacuate (*teinesmos*), were thought to be potentially pernicious for the pregnancy.[90] Galen upholds the popular belief that a strong emotional shock could cause a miscarriage, lucidly reflected in the anecdote about pregnant women who had miscarriages during the performance of Aeschylus' *Eumenides* when frightened by the horrific appearance of the chorus of the Erinyes.[91]

vii. Magic and superstition

Abortions in the ancient world were undoubtedly surrounded by tales of miraculous treatments. The most important source for this popular mythology is Pliny the Elder, a Roman gentleman of the first century AD, who dedicated his *Natural history* to the future Emperor Titus (while Vespasian was still alive[92]). Pliny mistrusted Greek doctors, and wanted medical care to return to its traditional Roman roots, when nature provided for everything that one needed in order to stay in good health.[93] Thus Pliny provides an abundance of information on traditional cures, herbs and recipes, some of it clearly borrowed from Greek sources. Amid lists of truly potent drugs, Pliny mentions the supernatural abortifacient qualities of an old serpent skin crushed and drunk in wine, or the hoof of a donkey.[94] Some plants were believed to be such potent abortifacients that simply crossing over them could cause a miscarriage. Pliny shares with Dioscorides, the slightly senior Greek herbalist (but more systematic in his organisation of the material on plants and their powers[95]), the information that if a pregnant woman crosses over the root of a cyclamen, or the stone bugloss (*onosma*), she will have an abortion.[96] Various animals, such as a viper, or an animal called *amphisbaina*, were believed to have the same effect if crossed over.[97] Pliny attests the belief that if a pregnant woman crosses over the egg of a crow, she will have an abortion through the mouth.[98] Pseudo-Galen believed that if a pregnant woman crossed over a stone bitten by a dog (*lithos kunodektos*) she would have an abortion, while Aelian speaks about a stone called *aetetis* (eagle-stone) that could safeguard the pregnancy against an abortion.[99] The menstrual blood of another woman was also thought to have abortifacient qualities if crossed over, and the fiery thorn (*oxuakanthê*) could cause an abortion if the abdomen was hit with it gently three times (Dioscorides, however, seems doubtful about this, using the verb *historeitai*, i.e. 'the story goes').[100] Yet, perhaps the most famous among such substances was the wine of Keryneia. Theophrastus records the popular belief in its abortifacient qualities:

> In Achaïa, and in particular around Keryneia, there is a type of vine-tree, from which the wine makes pregnant women have an abortion; and if a dog eats the grapes, she miscarries, too. Yet, neither the grape nor the wine has any particular taste, compared with others.[101]

The same story is repeated by several other authors, with Dioscorides trying to provide a rational explanation for the mythical abortifacient qualities of this wine:

> There is also some wine with abortifacient qualities, since next to the vine-trees grows the hellebore, or the wild fig, or the scammony, from which the grape takes this particular strength; and from these the wine acquires its abortifacient qualities.[102]

Astrology was also involved in the popular mythology surrounding abortions. The astrologer Maximus (first century BC) expounds the influence of the moon on abortion following the zodiac cycle.[103] According to him, Aries will bring danger during the first day, but the woman will be fine afterwards. Taurus holds a dangerous fate for a woman who had an abortion during the first day, but things improve after the second. She will certainly die with the embryo in Gemini, unless the benign influence of another star saves her. Cancer does not hold any danger for a woman who has an abortion. The woman does not have much hope in Leo. Virgo brings bad death, and Libra brings certain death to the woman. She will not suffer much in the first day, but the second day will give her much more pain in Capricorn. In Aquarius the woman will suffer the first day, but she will be fine after the second.

These stories reflect the certainty of popular belief concerning the influence of magic and the supernatural upon human fertility. If men such as Dioscorides, Pliny and Galen, who had good knowledge of the qualities of various plants and substances, were prepared to incorporate such stories in their work, even if with scepticism or disbelief, surely women would be telling each other all about the allegedly miraculous efficiency of this or that plant. It would be reasonable to suggest that much of the popular mythology on the abortifacient qualities of various plants was left out of the more prestigious medical and pharmacological studies transmitted to us. Surely much more was said, if not written, which has been left out of these studies. Pliny dismisses the belief, attributed to two famous midwives Lais and Elephantis, that the charcoal of cabbage-root, myrtle or tamarisk had abortifacient qualities.[104] Such dismissal of traditional wisdom was not always as explicitly stated but surely a decree of critical selection preceded the inclusion of various substances into the works of Theophrastus, Dioscorides, Pliny and Galen, while there is no doubt that Soranus had scrutinised carefully and with consistent scientific criteria the information he provided. Galen complains that sometimes people are too uncritical of the drugs they recommend:

> For some of these (sc. philtres and drugs) are even ridiculous, like those supposed to tie up the opposing litigant, so that he will not be able to speak in court, or induce an abortion on a pregnant woman, or prevent conception for ever, or do this and that ... so I wonder, what went through their mind when they decided to record such drugs. For how these drugs are going to bring fame to those men after their death, when the mere knowledge of them brings indignity upon them while they are still alive?[105]

Serious medical literature was generally critical and selective. However, even in authors who were not prepared to put much faith in popular belief, one finds a fair number of treatments that amount to nothing more than superstition or mere credulity, and surely a lot more was in circulation. Women, in their desire to control their own fertility without pain or danger, would be susceptible and prepared to believe and circulate all kinds of tales about the qualities and potential of many items. Evidently there was a market out there and certain people might move in and capitalise on this demand. If serious scientists such as Galen, critical as they might be, were ready to accept the validity of some of these tales, the local doctor, chemist, or midwife would certainly be more gullible and the local abortionist perhaps even more prepared to advertise miraculous treatments, out of faith or the pursuit of profit. The desire and demand for such treatments, inaccurate knowledge, and a vivid imagination in a world which, despite enormous progress, was never entirely convinced by the potential of medical science, blurred the border between science and superstition. And if doctors and women, who had first-hand experience of abortions, were prepared to accept popular mythology to such an extent, the ordinary male, who did not have any first-hand knowledge, would be much more susceptible and ready to accept that powerful drugs with miraculous, if not supernatural qualities were used by women to induce abortions on demand, and behind men's backs. It is no wonder that such drugs, along with love philtres, poisons and potions with various other strange effects were viewed by men with suspicion, perceived as a threat to male control, and unequivocally condemned in non-medical literature.

Conclusions

The wide variety of methods and the sheer number, versatility and inventiveness of abortifacient techniques and substances employed by the ancient world are a testimony to the fact that abortions were sought and procured by women and their medical aides on a regular basis. The lack of uniform medical standards and practices, inconsistent availability of materials, incomplete understanding of related factors and health conditions, inconsistent exchange of information, and imperfect scientific knowledge were factors that encouraged experimentation, as no technique available to the ancient world was totally reliable, and certainly none totally safe. Women, doctors, midwives and other persons involved in inducing abortions were always seeking treatments and methods which could guarantee success with the least possible suffering and danger. Since the knowledge of gynaecology, pharmacology, surgery and related disciplines possessed by the ancient Greek world was lacking in many areas, a safe, painless and efficient course of treatment remained beyond the reach of Hippocratic medicine and its successors. Even though, judging by the standards of the time, one may admire the achievements of Hippocratic medicine and its heirs, or the gynaecological knowledge and shrewd observations of Soranus (in many cases comparable to nineteenth- or early twentieth-century medicine), induced abortion remained a difficult, painful and often life-threatening ordeal. Superstition and popular mythology surrounding abortions responded to the desire for safe and painless abortions with a number of allegedly miraculous suggestions. Even though miracle treatments were widespread, any woman determined or desperate enough would know that this could not happen without considerable degree of pain and danger. Women knew it, doctors, midwives and abortionists knew it, and even the ordinary male would know that abortion was a dangerous operation. Perhaps not many foetuses would be able to survive the rigorous abortion course recommended by Soranus, which is a combination of most abortion techniques known to the ancient world, but it is sufficient to read through the pages of the famous gynaecologist in order to understand that only a very determined or desperate woman would put herself through such an ordeal. Women would often attempt to terminate unwanted pregnancies with safer and less painful means, maybe at the beginning following some superstitious advice and then increasingly attempting more powerful, and painful, techniques. How far they would go depended not only upon their determination and state of mind, but also upon the reasons which dictated that the pregnancy should be terminated (see Chapter 4).

W. Krenkel, after a thorough study of the methods employed in the ancient world has concluded that nearly all techniques available to medicine until the 1950s were already known in antiquity.[106] The drugs used might not be as efficient as those employed by twentieth-century medicine for chemically induced abortions, and a D&C operation in the ancient world might resemble the suffering of Prometheus, bound to a pillar while his liver was eaten by an eagle, but the principles of each technique were adequately understood. If we notice that the suction method was only developed in the 1960s, when the liberalisation of the abortion laws in many countries allowed for research and permitted the perfection of a simpler and safer technique, we are bound to accept that induced abortion did not move forward with the same speed and vigour as most other fields of medicine. Abortion remained a conservative medical practice which changed very little throughout the centuries, and the reasons for that are probably partly social and partly political. For many centuries this was a women's issue viewed with suspicion if not active disapproval by men – a matter with which serious (male) medical researchers might be reluctant to be associated.

When Does Human Life Begin?

Is the embryo a human being in its own right, or, so long as it cannot live independently, ought it to be treated as an extension of the mother's body? Should a potential person receive the same treatment as an actual person? When does someone become a person? These are important questions with profound legal and ethical implications which are still at the centre of the debate on induced abortion today.[1] Those who are prepared to accept the legitimacy of abortion, for whatever reason, are inclined to treat the foetus as only a potential person while it remains attached to the mother. Those who reject abortion consider the unborn to be a person in its own right, with an independent right to life, even though it has not yet realised its full potential (which, at any rate, does not happen before one reaches adulthood). Modern medicine has not been able to provide a conclusive answer to these very old questions. Science nowadays, with the assistance of sophisticated equipment, can describe the stages of foetal development more accurately, but it cannot define when a person acquires his/her identity in the eyes of society and the law.[2] What complicates matters further is that different people approach these issues from different perspectives and diametrically opposite points of view. These different approaches are connected with religious, ethical, philosophical, political and economic considerations, and intensified by parameters such as possible differences in the understanding of matters related to pregnancy and foetal development between men and women. A recent study concluded that 'women tend to define new life as being human earlier than men and by a different set of characteristics than men. They tend to regard it as human when they know it is growing. On the other hand, men do not identify the new life as human until they can see it or communicate with it.'[3] These findings, as well as the rest of the findings of this survey, which reveal a striking diversity of perspectives among various social groups, clearly suggest that this plurality of opinions is rooted in the fundamental difficulty of defining a universally agreed point in the life and development of the embryo that marks the beginning of its existence as an individual.

The birth of a child is a convenient point for most societies to acknowledge and formally recognise the arrival of a new human being. The new person is registered under a certain name and thereafter acquires the same rights and protection accorded to all other members of his/her community. However, convenient as this point may be, it reflects no universal certainty about the beginnings of human life. Many mothers (and fathers) would not think that the lives of their children, carried and carefully looked after for months before birth, started at this point, but that birth is only a step in a process that had started much earlier. The majority of legal and political systems are prepared to recognise to a certain extent that life starts before birth with a number of provisions aimed at the protection of the unborn and support for the mother. Similarly most religious and ethical codes recognise the unborn. It is evident that, even though birth is considered to be the convenient starting point of an individual's life for legal and economic purposes, the firm belief that birth is not the real beginning of a human life is common.

Some people, legal codes and religious/ethical systems (particularly those that try to define the beginnings of human life with definite certainty) consider fertilisation to be the obvious starting point. However, a considerable number of scientists argue that it would be premature to speak about 'human life' from a time as early as fertilisation or even implantation of the fertilised egg, considering the large extent of spontaneous embryonic loss in a normal couple.[4] Moreover, if 'human', with all the legal, theological, political and philosophical implications of this term, is understood in a sense that exceeds narrow biological definitions and describes certain qualities of a human being, it might be premature to characterise the zygote as human, as it has not yet acquired any of these qualities (even though it has an in-built potential). Thus, in the perception of many the embryo is not a self-defined human being from the moment of fertilisation or implantation, but acquires its human identity at a later stage.

The theory of gradual development of the foetus into an independently defined human being has found many followers from antiquity to the present day. The gradualists may come from very different backgrounds and have very diverse beliefs, but they agree on this one point, that the embryo acquires human identity while growing in the womb, that is, some time after conception but before birth. Beyond this point opinions diverge and factors such as the viability of the foetus, its formation, the acquisition of sense, the beginning of movement in the womb, or, in more abstract terms, the animation of the embryo, have often been used as arguments in a long and inconclusive debate. Modern medical science has been in a position to influence the debate by re-defining some of these factors in recent years. Observations through advanced equipment have described more accurately the stages of formation of the foetus and shown that an embryo has the capacity of feeling and moving at an earlier stage than was commonly believed in the past.[5] The contribution of modern medicine especially to the problem of the viability of the foetus, an issue which has occupied a central place in the debate, is having far-reaching consequences.[6] The chances of survival of a foetus separated from the mother's body even as early as the second trimester of the pregnancy have increased and this has affected the entire debate on abortion. An aborted foetus which comes out still alive and perhaps viable may pose difficult legal and ethical problems for those concerned,[7] but medical science cannot be expected to respond to these problems unaided. These questions are not simply medical issues, but more complex ones. Apart from the doctor, they concern the lawyer, who has to decide upon the moment from which a being should be treated as human and its destruction as homicide. They also concern the theologian and the moral philosopher who wish to advance an opinion on the ethics of the destruction of a human foetus. Finally, society in general might have a legitimate concern over matters which affect its present and future composition, and may wish to know the moment that it should admit new members. The complexity and importance of these questions have placed them in the heart of a debate which continues with the same vigour today as in the ancient world.

The difficulty with these issues was certainly more intense in the ancient world, with its rather limited, and often mistaken, understanding of the development process of the human embryo. The scientific uncertainty not only caused legal, ethical and philosophical uncertainty, but also encouraged speculation and intense discussion, resulting in a wide diversity of opinions and theories. Doctors, philosophers, scholars, religious leaders and intellectuals had their own certainties and their own ideas about the beginnings of human life. Ancient perceptions of the beginnings of human life and human identity can be classified into three groups divided along the lines stated above: there were those who believed that human life begins at conception, those who believed that it begins at birth, and those who believed that it starts at some point between conception and birth, while the embryo is growing in the womb. Thus, it would be fair to say that the origins of the current debate go back to the beginnings of medical science and to the first enquiries about the human being as a self-defined biological, political, legal, moral and spiritual unit, in classical Athens.

Ancient perceptions of the beginning and definition of human life certainly influenced the attitudes of individuals and groups towards induced abortion. Often (but not always) those who believed that human life begins at conception considered abortion to be a crime. Gradualists were against abortion only if it took place beyond some point in the pregnancy and under certain circumstances. Those who believed that life begins at birth might find abortion a deplorable practice, but they had no good reason to perceive it as a crime equal to homicide. The origins of the debate along these lines can be clearly traced in works from the classical period, when medicine took its first steps as an independent discipline and was in a position to observe foetal development and make scientifically based observations about it. When the desire to interpret the world on the basis of reason encouraged philosophical quest for the origins of human life, medical certainties and uncertainties were taken over by scholars, philosophers, writers and religious leaders. In their hands the medical data were transformed into arguments and certainties or uncertainties of a different, more complex nature, giving rise to an inconclusive debate destined to continue in the forthcoming millennia and influence law codes, theological discussions, ethical inquests and social attitudes.

i. What is 'human'?

The answer to this question may seem self-evident, in the sense that we know a human being when we see one, but a brief yet comprehensive theoretical definition of a human being seems to be out of reach. The reason is that a human being is a complex entity with many aspects. It is possible to distinguish between a human and a non-human in relation to one of these aspects, but it is not possible to render this complexity in a few words. A modern doctor or biologist would be able to speak about human genes, as opposed to genes with different DNA. A lawyer would be able to speak about a person as an entity with certain rights and duties. A moral philosopher would be able to speak about a being, who can and has to make choices and take decisions. Thus, it is often the case that different people speak about a different thing when they refer to human identity, because one places emphasis upon one aspect and builds his/her argument around this, while another has in mind a different aspect. However, a human being is each one of these things and all of them at once, and there lies the root of a very old controversy.

The ancient Greeks, like ourselves, knew a human being when they saw one, but ancient Greek doctors, philosophers and authors could not agree upon a clear and comprehensive definition of human identity. The difficulty of providing such a definition is reflected in the diversity of vocabulary used in their discussions about human identity, as well as the investigation of the meaning and content of the terms employed. It is outside the purposes of this study to try to cover this large field in its entirety. Here I limit myself to the presentation of the views on human identity held by ancient authors in the context of the debate on abortion.

Greek authors would often use words such as *embruon*, *kuêma*, *to kuoumenon*, or *to kata gastros* (literally 'what is carried in the womb'; Latin: *quod in utero geritur*), and Roman authors would use terms like *foetus* or *embryo* to describe the human foetus.[8] These are rather neutral, scientific terms with no particular moral or philosophical quality. Yet one could argue that in a certain context even neutral terms like these could be charged, because they might imply an unwillingness on the part of the speaker to define the foetus as human. Terminology in this instance can be significant; even 'pregnant'. For example, the use of the word *anthrôpos* (or *homo* in Latin), implicitly if not explicitly, amounts to attribution of human identity to the unborn, usually accompanied by critical attitudes towards abortion. Let's say, when Juvenal speaks about 'humans in the womb' he implicitly acknowledges the human identity of the unborn, and criticises wealthy Roman women for having abortions.[9] The Hippocratic study *Fleshes* illustrates even more lucidly an understanding of *anthrôpos* as a continuity, from conception to death.[10] However, as I mentioned above, the term 'human' is vague and too encompassing to make it a suitable basis for discussion when the nature and acquisition of human identity are debated. Caution is necessary: the use of terms like 'child' (*paidion* or *teknon*: Latin *infans* or *puer*) or 'human' (*anthrôpos*; Latin *homo*) may often be connected with negative attitudes towards abortion, but this is not always the case. The term 'child' to describe the unborn is often employed by authors with a critical attitude towards abortion, with the implicit understanding that a foetus, like a born child, is a person in his/her own right.[11] However, in the Hippocratic study *On the nature of the child*[12] the term is employed to describe the second and final stage in the development of a foetus, and in a similar manner in Galen's study *Semen* the term describes the last stage of a four-fold process (semen, *kuêma, embruon,* child).[13] There also times when the term 'child' is used conveniently without any particular significance: for example, the Greek translation of the Torah[14] differentiates between an unformed and a formed foetus, treating the abortion of the latter as homicide, yet it uses the word 'child' (*paidion*) in both instances.

The vague, indecisive nature of these terms is probably the reason why another term, the word *zôon* (literally 'living being', Latin *animal*), appeared in a number of medical, philosophical and rhetorical studies discussing the human status of the unborn. The content and understanding of this term are far from self-evident, and this is why we often find that authors who use it feel the need to explain what they mean by it. Sometimes it is simply used as a synonym of *anthrôpos* with all the characteristic complexity of this term,[15] but in most cases it encompasses a narrower, more specified field. The author of *Whether what is carried in the womb is a living being* defines it as following:

> A living being is an essence with soul and sense, as far as the general characteristics of all its categories are concerned.[16]

Clement gives the following definition of the term in relation to the question whether plants are 'living beings':

> What is called a living being? ... If one calls 'living being' something that eats and grows, we should ask again whether he thinks that plants are 'living beings' ... for Plato calls 'living beings' the plants too, which share only the third part of the soul, the one which is the seat of the desires, while Aristotle[17] thinks that the plants share the vegetative and nutrient soul, but he does not go as far as calling them 'living beings', for he only calls a 'living being' the one which shares the other, the sensate soul .... Thus, according to Plato, the plant has a soul and is a living being, but according to Aristotle, it is not a living being yet, because it does not have sensation, but it has a soul .... But according to the Stoics the plant is neither animated, nor a living being, because a living being is something with a soul.[18]

The search for an interpretation of the term *zôon* in the context of defining human identity is summarised by the author of the Pseudo-Galenic study *Medical terminology*:

> Some called it a living being, others did not. Those who said that it was a living being based this assumption on movement, because the embryo, too, moves, and (they said) that it feels pleasure and rejoices when the mother feels pleasure, while it shrinks and contracts, sensing like a living being, when she is distressed. For sense is not a natural characteristic of anything else, except a living being. However, those who believe that it is not a living being (say) that it feeds and grows like a tree, but it does not start or stop moving by itself, like living beings do. Not only it does not move spontaneously, but also it does not move deliberately, but (it moves) like the trees and the plants, for the wind is the cause of their movement, while the moist and slippery environment, as well as the shape of the uterus – since it becomes like a sphere as it fills out, and the shape of a sphere facilitates all movement, because it lacks any base – are the causes of the movement of the embryo. On the other hand, Asclepiades said that the embryo is neither a living nor a non-living being, and maintains that it resembles those who are asleep, because as they have senses but are not making use of them, the embryo in the womb does not either.[19]

These passages illustrate the diversity of opinions as to what a living being is, and highlight the lines along which the definition of this term was sought. These lines are nutrition and development, movement, sensation, animation. As different people understood the term in connection with a different line of argumentation, there was no agreement among ancient medics and philosophers as to what a living being was, but, all the same, the term was used in relation to the status of a foetus.

Already in the Hippocratic study *On the nature of the child* the development of the foetus is compared with that of a plant, and similar comparisons can be found elsewhere in medical literature.[20] Later authors tended to attribute this comparison to Plato.[21] Ancient doctors and natural philosophers had observed that a foetus attaches itself to the wall of the uterus, and from there feeds and grows like a plant, but beyond this point opinions diverged. Some understood the movement of the foetus in the womb to be like the movements of a plant, that is, mechanical, not conscious;[22] others, however, take movement to be a proof that the foetus is a living being.[23] Some Greek philosophers understand the term in connection with animation rather than movement: According to Plutarch, the Stoic philosopher Chrysippus understood that the soul was what distinguished a living being from a plant. Thus the embryo was living like a plant in the womb, but at birth, chilled and tempered by the air, it became a living being.[24] Similar views were put forward by Philo, who considered the embryo to be part of the mother, but after birth it became a living being in its own right.[25] Philo connected the concept 'living being' with formation.[26]

The evident conclusion is that, on the whole, the term *zôon* as a technical term is no clearer than any other, nor does it succeed in defining the status of the foetus in more specific terms. The debate has remained active from the time of Hippocrates to the end of the ancient world and down to the present day. When various authors speak about the foetus as a living being or 'non-living being', as a 'child' or a 'human', each of them understands these terms in his/her own individual way. Bearing this in mind, we can now explore in more detail ancient theories about the status of the embryo and the beginnings of human life.

ii. Human life begins at conception

The theory that the embryo acquires human identity (namely, a soul) from the start, that is, from the moment of conception,[27] was certainly popular among early Christian authors[28] (but not universally accepted[29]). However, this theory did not make its first appearance in the Christian era. As Edelstein and Carrick have pointed out, the Pythagoreans believed that the embryo acquires a soul from the moment of conception, and that the seed contains the full code of a human being, body and soul, simultaneously activated at the moment of conception.[30] This is clearly attested by a number of sources. There is a reference to Pythagorean views in *To Gauros, on how embryos are animated* (2,2), wrongly attributed to Galen:

> It would be difficult to tell whether the embryo was potentially a living being, since it had exhibited the possession (of the power to become one), or actually a living being, because it would be difficult to specify the moment of the infusion (of the soul). And whatever moment one might set, it would be nothing more than a conjecture, as one who argues that it happens when the seed is implanted ... and on this much is said by Noumenios and the interpreters of Pythagorean doctrine.

Diogenes Laertius also refers to the Pythagorean views on the subject:

> The soul is a fragment of aether, cold and hot, and the soul is different from life because it contains cold aether. It is immortal, because the essence from which it has been cut off is immortal. Living beings are born from each other from seed, and birth from earth is impossible. The seed is a drop of brain containing hot steam inside. When it is deposited in the uterus, ichor and liquid and blood are produced from the brain particles, from which flesh and nerves and bones and hair and the entire body is composed. Soul and sense are produced from the steam. This first creation is formed in forty days, and then, in accordance with the law of harmony, the baby is perfected and born after seven, or nine, or maximum ten months. The seed contains all the codes of life ....[31]

The Pythagoreans believed that the soul is actually contained in the seed in the form of condensed steam. At the moment of conception it is released, and this is how animation occurs and sense is installed, right from the start. This point is very important, because for many medics, philosophers and authors, abortion was legitimate for as long as the unborn had not yet acquired a soul and sense, but it stopped being acceptable after the point of animation of the foetus. Beyond that point the unborn was believed to be a person, a human being in its own right.

The theory that the foetus was fully human from the moment of conception, because the soul entered the body at that point, is associated by the author of *To Gauros, on how embryos are animated* not so much with the Pythagoreans – even though, as I mentioned earlier, their contribution is acknowledged – but with Plato. This author argues against the Platonic school of thought that allegedly held such beliefs, and concentrates much of his fire against statements of Plato on the soul. His intention is to prove that animation occurs only after birth, and he seems to perceive the Platonists as typical representatives of the opposing theory that life begins at the moment of conception. Galen is aware of this theory of animation at conception and he too attributes it to the Platonic school of thought, but then he firmly rejects it, because he cannot accept that the immortal, universal soul could be the creator of worms, spiders, scorpions and mosquitoes.[32] A treatise from later antiquity that defends this theory, *Whether what is carried in the womb is a living being*, also supports the association with Platonic thought, as Plato is the only Greek philosopher prominently mentioned by name side by side with the great Hippocrates.

Plato's own views on the subject are not so easy to classify. First, as I will explain later in Chapter 5, he does not hesitate to recommend abortion for the purposes of birth control with no regard for the human identity of the foetus; moreover I am not aware of any passage where he unequivocally states that animation occurs at the moment of conception. However, many passages in his work could be interpreted as pointing in this direction. His theories on the immortality of the soul and reincarnation could conceivably give rise to a theory suggesting animation from the moment of conception, and I think this is what has happened in this case. Those striving to prove in later antiquity that the foetus acquires a soul at conception needed a figure-head, an influential mind from the classical period to whom they could refer as the founder of their beliefs, and thus turned to Plato, interpreting his works to this end. Thus it seems very likely that in later antiquity, and certainly before the Christian era, a number of scholars and philosophers were arguing the case of animation at the moment of conception by invoking the Platonic works and scavenging through the Hippocratic Corpus for passages that could support their views.

The human status of the unborn, regardless of the stage of its development, may also be implicitly recognised by some authors such as Virgil, who refers to the souls of unborn *children*,[33] or Juvenal, who refers to 'humans in the womb'.[34] Some legal provisions, like the Athenian law allowing a pregnant woman to remain in her dead husband's *oikos* in the hope that she will produce an heir, or the Egyptian law that prohibited the execution of a pregnant woman, have also been interpreted as implicit recognition of the human status of the unborn.[35] However, these cases amount to implicit rather than explicit recognition; moreover in none of these sources is it clearly stated that human status was acquired exactly at the moment of conception (as the Pythagoreans believed) and not at a later stage of pregnancy. (For a more thorough discussion of these provisions see Chapter 6.)

On the existing evidence we are bound to conclude that before the Christian era only a minority was prepared to accept that the foetus was animated and therefore human from the moment of conception. To put it simply, the Greeks and the Romans would generally speak about a human being when they could see one, or at least be in the position to feel manifestly its presence and imminent arrival. Thus it seems that authors with a generally hostile attitude towards abortion often did not adopt this point of view because they positively believed that the fertilised egg (or, speaking in contemporary terminology, the withheld semen) was a human being, but for a variety of other reasons, expounded elsewhere in this book.

iii. Human life begins at birth

Whatever views individuals or social and legal systems may take on abortion and prenatal existence, one thing is certain: birth is a very significant point in the life of a person. In our times a human being acquires a name, is registered, and becomes a member of society with prescribed rights and duties when he/she is born, and not before or long after that. Likewise, in the ancient world a child would be given a name and recognised as an independent person only after it was born, even though matters were more complicated with regard to status (slave/alien/citizen), right to life, and admission of this child to the community (see Chapters 5 and 6). The majority of doctors, philosophers and intellectuals perceived birth as a determining point, but not necessarily the beginning of human life. However, for a significant minority birth was the actual beginning of life in a human form, while antenatal existence was a different state of affairs. The theory that human life starts at the precise moment of birth precedes the days of Hippocratic medicine: in the extant literature it appears first in Empedocles, who, according to Galen, denied that the embryo was a living being:

> Empedocles (said) that the embryo is not a living being but (accepted) that it breathes in the womb; however, it breathes like a living being only after birth.[36]

Similar views were put forward by another Presocratic natural philosopher, Diogenes of Apollonia, who considered air to be the basis of life and the soul to be cold air, entering the body with the first breath after birth. Simplicius, the sixth-century AD Neoplatonist philosopher quoting a passage of Diogenes says:

He concludes that humans and other animals live and obtain a soul and mental faculties from this principle which is the air, saying the following:

'... Humans and the other breathing animals live in the air, and this is their soul and mental faculties, as it will be clearly demonstrated in this study. And if this is removed, they die and their mental faculties abandon them.'[37]

In another passage Diogenes clearly defines the soul as cold air:

The soul of all animals is this thing, air warmer than the external by which we are surrounded, but much colder than the one near the sun.[38]

As a consequence, Diogenes and those who shared similar views in later centuries were not prepared to accept that human life can start before birth. That Diogenes perceived birth to be the beginning of life is explicitly confirmed by the author of the study *On the preferences of philosophers*, attributed to Plutarch:

Diogenes (says) that the infants are born without a soul, but in a warm condition. Thus the naturally hot attracts the cold into the lungs immediately after the exit of the infant.[39]

Diogenes, as far as I know, was the first advocate of a theory which was going to become dominant in later centuries and occupy a central place in the debate, as the main opposition to the theories of the gradualists. The views of Diogenes were later taken over by the Stoics and formed the core of the belief that the unborn cannot be considered to be a human being in its own right.

The theories of Empedocles, Diogenes, Anaximenes[40] and others, were partially sidelined for most of the classical period. According to the existing evidence, most classical authors seem to be gradualists, namely supporters of the theory that life begins at some point between conception and birth as the embryo is maturing in the womb. This change of approach is probably due to the fact that Hippocratic medicine, by observing that the foetus had already acquired a sufficient degree of formation in the later stages of the pregnancy to qualify for human identity, changed perceptions regarding the beginnings of human life (see §iv below). Thus, it seems, the theory that human life begins at birth subsided in the classical period in favour of the theory that human existence starts at some point before birth as the pregnancy advances.

The theory that life begins at birth was reinstated by hellenistic doctors and promoted by the Stoics in later centuries with such vigour that it became a respectable rival of gradualist theories. H. von Staden, in his learned edition of the fragments of Herophilus, states that the great anatomist and physician departed from the Aristotelian emphasis on the sentient soul.[41] Aetius and Plutarch attest that, according to Herophilus, the movement of the embryo is mechanical, not pneumatic, and since pneuma does not enter the body before birth, the embryo could only be considered as a living being after birth:

> Herophilus grants foetuses natural motion, but not pneumatic motion. And the nerves are responsible for the motion. They [sc. the foetuses] become living beings whenever they are poured forth and take in some air.[42]

I am not so sure that Herophilus departs from Aristotelian theory on sensation and animation of the foetus as sharply as von Staden believes (see §iv below for a more elaborate presentation of the views of Aristotle). Both Herophilus and Aristotle would agree that the motion of the foetus and basic life functions are not evidence of a sentient soul, and do not prove that the foetus is a living being. Where they depart from each other is that while Aristotle, in accordance with gradual development theories that were dominant in the medical circles during the classical period, concludes that the sentient soul develops before birth, Herophilus returns to Presocratic perceptions of air as the vital essence of life and thus is bound to conclude that animation can only take place after birth.[43]

The view that animation occurs at birth, with the first breath of air, was championed by the Stoics and found wider acceptance in later antiquity. Similar views were held by a significant minority and as we have seen there is an entire treatise, erroneously attributed to Galen, entitled *To Gauros, on how embryos are animated*, champions the view that animation occurs at birth, and even refers by name to the Stoic philosopher Chrysippus, one of the early advocates of this theory.[44] The Stoics, whatever their individual beliefs about the condition of the unborn, claimed that the baby is born hot, but without a soul. Then the soul, which is cold air, is attracted to the body by the heat, enters through the mouth (*aer conceptus ore*),[45] and thus animation takes place immediately after birth.[46] Therefore, one can be considered a human being only after birth. A perception of the unborn as part of the mother's body was quite common[47] and, according to Philo, enjoyed considerable support among learned men:

> That those carried in the womb of are part of the pregnant women is supported by natural philosophers and by the most authoritative among doctors.[48]

Philo compares pregnancy with the work of a sculptor: nature keeps the unborn in her workshop, as a sculptor keeps a statue, until the creative process is complete and the time comes to bring it into the light.[49] The concept that the unborn was kept in a state of suspension until birth, and as such could not be considered fully human in its own right, was also advocated by Asclepiades.[50]

This brief summary suggests that the concept of birth as the starting point of life was a respectable alternative, which many authoritative professionals and intellectuals were prepared to accept in later antiquity. The scanty evidence concerning the classical period suggests that some people might be prepared to embrace this theory, but these would only represent a small minority compared with the gradualists, who apparently represented the majority view on the subject. Yet to say that all those who believed that life begins at birth had a favourable attitude to abortion would be an erroneous oversimplification. The case of Philo, who clearly saw the unborn as an extension of the mother's body, but, on the other hand, vehemently disapproved of abortion, is a clear example of this. Those who believed that human life begins at birth might not see the destruction of a foetus as an act equal to homicide, but they did not necessarily see it as an acceptable practice either.

iv. Human life begins while the foetus is growing

Hippocratic medicine made the first systematic observations of the human body and its development, and meticulously noted the results of these observations. The achievements of Hippocratic medicine were limited by the reluctance of its practitioners to study anatomy by dissecting human bodies; in the area of embryology this limitation was undoubtedly debilitating. The human foetus and the stages of its development were a matter of great interest to doctors and natural philosophers of the classical period, but the methods available to study them were inadequate, which is why one observes a great diversity of opinions regarding the stages in the development of a human foetus. Doctors drew parallels between the stages of development of animal foetuses and those of human ones, and tried to outline the development of the latter based on observations of the former.[51] Naturally another important source of observation was aborted foetuses.[52] The methods employed by ancient doctors for the observation of foetuses are summarised by Galen as follows:

> This is apparent in abortions and in the dissections of pregnant animals.[53]

Limited as this information was, at least it allowed the conclusion that the formation and development of the human foetus to maturity was a gradual process. Hence doctors and philosophers were prepared to acknowledge that human life did not start at birth but beforehand, at some point when the pregnancy was sufficiently advanced. Hippocratic doctors seem to retain the Presocratic theory that air is the force that brings the foetus to life. However, they refine it by arguing that life can begin before birth, since the embryo breathes in the womb (as Empedocles had argued, see also Hip. *Genit.* 17).[54] In the understanding of many, the acquisition of human identity was not something that happened at birth but well before that, when the foetus was sufficiently formed to be considered a human being. Formation was a crucial concept in connection with the human identity of the unborn in Hippocratic medicine. This concept was sometimes linked with movement; later it was taken over by philosophers and often joined with other concepts, such as animation, in the debate over the beginnings of human life.

The precise moment of formation was a much debated issue from the time of Empedocles, who maintained that formation started on the 36th day and was completed on the 49th. These numbers are multiples of 9 and 4 in different combinations (9 x 4 = 36; 9 x 5 + 4 = 49).[55] The Pythagoreans believed that formation is completed in 40 days, and made no secret of the fact that they reached this figure by means of mathematical calculations, not anatomical or clinical observations.[56] In *Nutriment* the time given for formation is 35 days.[57] Galen reports that, according to some doctors, formation is completed by the 40th day, but according to others by the 50th. That Empedocles was the first to state that a boy matures faster than a girl was accepted by doctors and natural philosophers in the classical period, with very few exceptions, most notably Diogenes of Apollonia and the author of the Pseudo-Galenic study *Philosophical history*, who writes:

> Empedocles said that in humans formation begins from the 36th day and the limbs are perfected from the 51st. Asclepiades said that in boys, because their constitution is hotter, the formation begins on the 26th day and is completed from the 50th, while in females formation takes two months because of the lack of heat.[58]

This passage seems to suggest that Empedocles did not differentiate along lines of gender but that this distinction was made much later, being put forward by Asclepiades of Bithynia, the 'innovative rationalist physician and thinker of the second century BC'.[59] However, there is no doubt that the theory that boys mature faster than girls had been around since before Hippocrates and certainly in circulation for centuries by Asclepiades' time.

Even when writers do not differentiate between a male and a female foetus, it does not necessarily imply disagreement with the conventional view.[60] Opinions diverge to a considerable degree when it comes to the exact timing of formation. For example, according to the author of the study *On the nature of the child* a male is formed by the 30th day of the pregnancy, and a female by the 42nd,[61] while in the study *On the seven months' child* we read that a male is formed by the 40th day, but a female is still unformed. In the former study we read:

> Many women aborted a boy shortly before the 30th day and it looked unformed, but those aborted on the 30th, or afterwards, looked formed. On a girl, after the abortion, the formation of the members is accordingly visible after the 42nd day.[62]

The author continues to explain why the female foetus is formed after the male foetus:

> The reason why the female is solidified and formed later is that the female semen is weaker and wetter than the male; for this reason the female is bound to solidify later than the male.[63]

Further speculation on the reasons why the female is formed later than the male (such as a delayed flow of blood to the uterus when the foetus is female) can be found earlier in this study,[64] but these are rejected by the author. Galen also supports the explanation quoted above:

> For it is apparent ... that the male is not only hotter but also drier than the female right from the start.[65]

Soranus, with sober judgement, abandons all this traditional wisdom about differences in the formation between male and female foetuses. However, he retains the distinction between a formed and an unformed foetus:

> At the beginning, while the semen is still unformed, the conception[66] is one of semen, but after the beginning, when what is in the womb is formed and no longer is semen, the term 'conception' is still applicable, but it is not conception of semen but of an embryo, because the semen has already changed, and it is a substance, and to a certain degree a soul, and no longer semen; this is why some people introduce a different terminology calling the first phase of the conception imperfect and the second perfect.[67]

It is evident that formation was considered to be a very important point in the life of a human being by a significant number of ancient doctors and philosophers, because they saw it as the beginning of someone's life as an individual, whatever each person's views may have been as to the precise moment when this happened. According to the author of *On the nature of the child* someone 'becomes a child' (*gegonen paidion*) after formation, and the same idea is suggested in Galen's *On the use of the members*:

> That what is in the womb is already a living being when it is formed in all its members is stated in the *Commentaries on the demonstration* and the study *On the opinions of Hippocrates and Plato.*[68]

In accordance with such views it is not surprising that the abortion of an unformed foetus in the early days of the pregnancy was seen in a different light from an abortion in later stages, when the foetus was already formed. In *On the seven months' child* we read:

> Whatever survives the 40th day, generally, escapes the danger of an abortion taking place .... After this time the embryo is stronger, and individual members of the body are visible, and all the members of a boy are very clearly discernible, but only flesh with extensions is visible in the case of a girl.[69]

The information that most abortions take place within the first 40 days is also provided by Aristotle, who would not even use the term 'abortion' for the termination of a pregnancy before the 7th day:

The termination of the pregnancy is called efflux until the 7th day, and abortion until the 40th, and most foetuses are destroyed in that time.[70]

The terminology, namely calling a termination which took place in the first seven days 'efflux', rather than 'abortion', is not Aristotelian, since we encounter this word in the Hippocratic study *On the seven months' child*. It seems that the term was well established in medical vocabulary by the time of Aristotle. Soranus uses the term 'dissolution of the conceptus' (*eis to dialuthênai to sullêphthen*), when he states that an abortion should take place in the very early stages of the pregnancy (within 30 days),[71] obviously while he still considered the foetus to be unformed. The inevitable conclusion is that the most authoritative medical practitioners and learned scholars in the Greek world might not even call it an 'abortion' if a termination had taken place in the very early stages of the pregnancy, while the foetus was still unformed. They would not recognise as human something which did not yet look human.

Outside medical and philosophical literature we find a very significant passage where a distinction is drawn between a formed and an unformed foetus, in connection with abortion: Exodus 21:22-4, following the Greek translation of the Septuagint, reads as follows:

> If two men are fighting and hit a pregnant woman, and her child comes out unformed, he must pay compensation, according to the demands of the woman's husband, after an estimate, but if it was formed, he must give a soul for a soul, an eye for an eye, a tooth for a tooth ....[72]

The Latin translation, the Vulgate, is truer to the Hebrew original, from which it has been directly produced. The Hebrew original reads as follows:

> If two men strive and hurt a woman with child, so that her fruit depart from her, and yet no mischief follow: he shall be surely punished, according as the woman's husband will lay upon him; and he shall pay as the judges determine. And if any mischief follow, then thou shalt give life for life, an eye for an eye, a tooth for a tooth ....

In the Hebrew original and the Vulgate abortion is not treated as homicide; only the death of the mother is treated as such. In the translation of the Septuagint abortion is not treated as homicide if the foetus was not formed, but amounts to homicide if it was formed. Here the death of the mother is not mentioned as a possibility, but one can easily infer that if it occurred, it would be treated as homicide. The Greek version is not an accidental mistranslation, but certainly a deliberate distortion of the original under the influence of Greek thought, so as to accord with contemporary theories about formation and the beginning of human life.

Considering that this is the only passage in the Bible that explicitly refers to abortion it should have a considerable impact upon the views of Christian scholars. One would expect that Christian theologians, in accordance with this passage, would not seek to equate abortion with murder, since the Bible does not equate abortion with homicide in this, the one and only explicit reference to it. This passage, in whatever version we take it, clearly suggests that abortion does not always amount to homicide. The Greek version suggests that it amounts to homicide only in the later stages of the pregnancy, after the formation of the foetus, while in the Hebrew original and the Vulgate abortion and homicide are two different things: abortion is to be punished by a fine, while homicide is to be punished by death.

Yet such distinctions seem to be too fine for the majority of Christian theologians. When the early Fathers of the Church started writing about abortion in the third or fourth century AD, the general climate was very hostile towards a practice that was perceived as a threat to the Roman family, if not to Rome herself (see Chapter 5 §iv below). It is no wonder that they were influenced in their views by contemporary attitudes. Many of them readily classed abortion as homicide, in accordance with the moral standards of the later Roman empire, while this passage was conveniently ignored.[73] St Basil, perhaps the most vocal critic of abortion, is certainly aware of the passage. Yet he actively defies the authority of the Bible, which he obviously reads from the Septuagint version, when he says in one of his letters to Amphilochios:[74] 'We do not fuss about such terms as "formed" or "unformed".' A line above he says 'a woman who had an induced abortion should face murder charges'.[75] But not all Christian scholars held such views: a number of them were prepared to follow the Septuagint version of Exodus and adopt a gradualist approach, according to which abortion should be treated as homicide only after formation. These scholars link formation with animation, maintaining that the reason why abortion should be treated as homicide only after formation is that this is the moment when the soul enters the body, and not before: their views are presented in considerable detail by Nardi and Noonan.[76] For the purposes of this book a few examples will be sufficient: Theodoret, bishop of Cyrrhus, accepts the distinction made in the Septuagint version of Exodus, links it with gradualist theories about animation (see below) and explains it as follows:

> They say that when the body is fully formed in the womb, then the embryo acquires a soul. For the Creator first made the body of Adam and then breathed the soul into it.[77]

In another study he supports the same idea:

> Speaking about a pregnant woman, who had an abortion as a result of blows, he says that the embryo is first formed, then animated.[78]

Augustine in a much discussed passage says:

> For in reality he did not wish to acknowledge as homicide the destruction of

an unformed foetus, actually because he did not consider what is carried in
the womb in this condition to be a human being (*hominem*). From this point
often arises the question on the soul (*anima*), that is, if something which is
not formed cannot be perceived to be animated either, and thus that it (sc.
the abortion of the unformed foetus) should not amount to homicide, because
one cannot say that the soul has left something which did not have a soul in
the first place.[79]

Some Christian authors even accept Greek gradualist theories down to the
point of numbers, and consider that formation and animation take place
on the 40th day and that an abortion would not be homicide before that
day but it would be after that.[80] In such theories I find a fascinating case
of continuity between secular pagan spirit and Christianity, an uninter-
rupted line of thought running from the pioneers of Hippocratic medicine
to Patristic Christian literature, which I would hardly have suspected
before reading these theories.

A similar degree of continuity can be observed in theories concerning
the movement of the foetus in the womb. According to Galen, it was
commonly believed that a boy starts moving earlier than a girl,[81] and this
view certainly goes back to the time of Hippocrates. In the study *On the
nature of the child* we read that a male starts moving in the third month
and a female in the fourth month.[82] According to the study *Nutriment* a
child starts moving on the 90th day.[83] Galen says that a boy starts moving
from the 70th day and a girl from the 90th,[84] and elsewhere records
another opinion according to which a child started moving from the 100th
day. Soranus dryly rejects speculation and predictions about the gender of
the child based on the timing, place and form of movement, which clearly
indicates that he did not share the views of his predecessors about different starting points of movement for boys and girls.[85]

Movement was perceived to be the beginning of life by a fair number of
ancient doctors and philosophers, with Plato perhaps being one of them.[86]
Galen, in *On semen*, distinguishes four stages in the development of the
foetus (semen, *kuêma*, embryo, child), which he attributes to Hippocrates,[87] and considers the unborn to be human from the moment it can
move, that is, at the fourth stage:

> But the admirable Hippocrates calls what is in the womb 'child' when it jerks
> and moves, as he says, like a completed living being.[88]

As I explained in Chapter 2 §i, not everyone would agree with the statement that motion is a sign of human life, because for many the movement
of the embryo was mechanical, like that of a plant, not conscious, like that
of an animal (*zôon*). But whatever the opinions of the (mostly male)
medical practitioners and philosophers of the time may have been, there
is another important dimension which we must take into account, and this
is the experience of the mother. Motion is a very important factor in the
entire debate, because from the point that the kicks and turns of the

unborn can be felt by the mother, they function as a manifestation of life
inside her. She can be aware of something that the outside world has yet
to see. Not surprisingly, the concept of 'quickening' as a legal term,
according to which human identity should be attributed to the unborn
from the moment its movements are felt by the mother, subjective as it is,
has been an important one for a number of legal systems in the past.[89] In
this respect, if we had studies written from Greek women on the issue,
they might change the entire perspective, and place a stress upon this
concept which male authors were unable to achieve.

Formation and movement were biological facts, which could be meas-
ured and empirically observed, but for many neither of these factors *per se*
was a sufficient indication that a new human life, in all its complexity, had
begun. We have already seen that a number of Christian authors sought
to link formation, mentioned in the Septuagint version of the Exodus
passage, with animation, and they were not the first to do so. Diogenes of
Apollonia, several centuries before the establishment of Christian theo-
logy, had attempted to interpret the biological fact of life as an animation
by means of cold air entering the lungs at birth. Hippocratic medicine was
prepared to accept that breathing air was essential for life, but still
believed that the foetus could breathe in the womb. On this assumption
Hippocratic doctors could speak about the unborn as a living being, or a
'child' in a biological sense. However, Hippocratic doctors did not seriously
seek to link the biological aspect with the mental and spiritual faculties of
a human being. The man to do this for the first time was Aristotle. In a
sense he was the right man for the task: he had a thorough understanding
of biological facts and as a philosopher was certainly the most active and
far-reaching mind of his time.[90] Aristotle sought to establish a clear link
between medical observations of foetal development and more abstract
concepts such as sense, animation and life.[91] He took over the gradualist
theories of Hippocratic medicine and expanded on them, placing them in
an entirely new dimension. He went beyond the fact that the embryo is
formed or starts moving at a certain point and tried to link the biological
aspects of movement and formation with psychic functions. He concluded
that an embryo becomes a living being from the moment that sense is
developed. This link between sense and the beginning of human life had a
lasting effect upon the debate on abortion, and still, in one form or another,
plays a central role in the current controversy.[92]

Aristotle believed that the embryo cannot possibly be born without
some form of psychic function, but he was not prepared to accept that
complete animation occurs at the moment of conception. Perhaps the fact
that he did not have a very clear idea of the soul as a separate entity, but
rather understood it as a pattern or entelechy, a set of functions, as P.J.
van der Eijk has suggested,[93] had something to do with it. Aristotle
observed that the embryo can perform some of the functions of a living
being, but not all of them, and this is why he came to the conclusion that
only the nutritive soul was infused at the moment of conception, in order

to allow the foetus to grow in the womb. The sentient soul, which would turn it into a living being (*zôon*), developed later, as the embryo was growing in the womb. The following passage from *Generation of animals* (736a27-b1) is a clear expression of his views on this matter:

> It is necessary to clarify matters concerning ... the soul – because a living being is defined by it (a living being possesses the sentient part of the soul) – whether it exists in the semen and the foetus or not, and where does it come from. No one should consider the foetus as soulless and deprived of life in every respect. The seeds and the foetuses of living beings are no less alive than those of the plants, and up to a certain point fertile. It is obvious that they possess the nutritive soul, ... but as they grow they acquire the sentient soul too, and thus become living beings.

Since Aristotle did not perceive the foetus in its early stages as a human being, he did not hesitate to suggest abortion as a method of population control (see Chapter 5 §iv below). However, he proposed some safeguards in order to make sure that this took place only in the early stages of pregnancy and so long as the foetus had not yet been animated. In a well-known passage from the *Politics* he recommends that, if an abortion had to take place, it ought to happen before animation and the beginning of human life:

> The abortion must be induced before sense and life are instilled, because what is permissible and what is not, will be defined on the basis of feeling and living.[94]

The precise moment when sense and life were instilled into the embryo are not clearly defined anywhere in the surviving works of Aristotle, but we obtain an idea of his views from various passages where he speaks about the time when an abortion should take place (see above, pp. 46-7).[95] Aristotle's idea that the embryo starts life as a plant with a vegetative soul and becomes animated only later in the pregnancy, is also discussed by Clement of Alexandria, while Aristotelian views about gradual acquisition of sense, soul, life and human identity had a profound influence upon scholastic writers, Christian theologians and Western European legal systems in subsequent centuries. One could say that they are still with us, and still play a part in the modern debate.[96]

We can safely conclude that in the classical period learned persons, namely doctors, philosophers and those with an interest in the matters expounded here, were predominantly gradualists. The achievement of Hippocratic medicine in describing more accurately than ever before the stages of development of the human embryo altered perceptions and made people think that birth, important as it was, need not be the starting point of someone's life as an individual, and that human life begins before birth, while the embryo is growing in the womb. This view encouraged speculation concerning the precise moment when the unborn is mature enough to be considered as an individual human being in his/her own right. In this process empirical concepts, such as formation and movement, were linked with more abstract moral and philosophical ones, such as sense and animation, and strenuous efforts to understand the beginnings of human life were made. Although in the hellenistic and imperial eras rival theories were promoted, the views of the gradualists continued to have a large following, even among Christian authors, and had a tremendous influence upon the perceptions of future generations. Considering that nowadays the majority of modern legal systems adopt a gradualist approach over the issue of abortion, these views evidently retain their appeal.

Conclusions

The legitimacy of abortion was very much a matter of concern for ancient doctors, natural and moral philosophers, and other scholars with relevant interests. The attribution, or not, of human identity to the unborn was identified as one of the key problems related to the issue and a lively debate had already been started by Presocratic natural philosophers, such as Empedocles and Diogenes of Apollonia, which would continue vigorously in the coming centuries. The observations concerning foetal development by Hippocratic doctors were a significant breakthrough and profoundly changed attitudes: ever since the results of these observations were published, doctors, philosophers and other learned persons have been prepared to accept that human life does not necessarily begin at birth, but at some point before, while the embryo is growing in the womb. Concepts such as the formation and movement of the unborn played an important role in the debate and were taken over and transformed by Aristotle, who added dimensions such as sense and animation to the debate. In later centuries rival theories were promoted, mainly by the Stoics, which revived the Presocratic wisdom that life begins at birth, because this is the moment of animation. Throughout this debate, clearer definitions of what is human and how human identity should be defined were sought, a number of theories were put forward and several terms were employed in connection with this search. However, in the end, the debate remained inconclusive, as no side was in the position to define clearly and comprehensively what makes something a human being and when a person acquires human identity. Christianity inherited this inconclusive debate and a number of early Christian scholars moved along the same lines as their pagan predecessors. However, many Christians, in an effort to provide conclusive answers, adopted an absolute position, considering as human what was conceived and its destruction as homicide, even though this attitude was not in accordance with the only passage in the Bible in which abortion is explicitly mentioned.

The Doctor's Dilemma

Current laws on abortion often put the medical profession at the centre of an intense controversy. In several countries where abortions are legal, the desire of the woman to have the pregnancy terminated is not sufficient. One or more doctors have to agree that termination is warranted by serious concerns over the woman's physical and mental health and well-being. How this provision is interpreted in practice may vary considerably from place to place and from one doctor to another. Let us take as an example the case of the Abortion Act 1967 in England, and consider how this law could be implemented:

> A person shall not be guilty of an offence under the law relating to abortion when a registered medical practitioner terminates a pregnancy if two registered medical practitioners are of the opinion formed in good faith –
> a) That the continuance of the pregnancy would involve risk to the life of the pregnant woman, or of injury to the physical or mental health of the pregnant woman or any existing children of her family, greater than if the pregnancy were terminated ....

The law requires that before a doctor consents to the termination of the pregnancy he/she must take into account the risks that its continuation would pose to the following: (i) the life of the woman, (ii) her physical health, (iii) her mental health, (iv) her existing family. A routine medical assessment should be able to define the risks to a woman's life or physical health, and in this sense the first two of the allowances made by the law are quite straightforward. However, the assessment of the risks to the woman's mental health, or the dangers to her existing family, is a much more complex procedure. A person's mental health depends upon many factors. Upbringing, background, social status, financial conditions, career, ambitions, relations with other people, and other such factors can have an effect upon a person's mental health and well-being. Thus, the doctor is required by law to investigate matters which exceed by far the limits of his/her scientific training and expertise, enter into fields such as economics, politics and the law, and become a judge of personal circumstances, contemporary social structures and spiritual matters.[1]

The doctor is not a detached being from another planet. As a person who lives in the world he has his own ideas, beliefs and convictions. These sometimes may have a strong impact upon his professional opinion, at a conscious or subconscious level. One can envisage a situation in which a doctor with religious beliefs hostile to abortion has to pronounce judgement over the termination of a pregnancy.[2] Is he expected to set aside these beliefs? Even if he is expected to do so, is he willing or able to detach himself to such an extent and try to assess the case objectively? And once a decision to terminate a pregnancy has been taken (perhaps by other practitioners), should the aforementioned doctor be compelled to carry out the operation, or expected to do so without inner conflict? There is no easy answer to such dilemmas.

Moreover, a doctor also has an identity as a professional. He may wish to pursue a career and realise ambitions in circles where reputations matter. Therefore his professional conduct and readiness to perform tasks related to his post are watched and his reputation can be built on the basis of such considerations. To perform an abortion in the days before legal reform in many countries in the 1960s and 1970s was not only an illegal but also a disreputable act. It was a practice to which a stigma was attached, and practitioners associated with it might put their professional reputation at risk.[3] A doctor who in good faith tried to help a very distressed patient might fare no better in public opinion than a back-street abortionist. Attitudes gradually changed after legal reform, but to say that abortion is no longer an issue that can ruin someone's professional reputation would simply be untrue. In particular in the United States the vocal anti-abortion lobby has targeted doctors and clinics that perform abortions in an intense effort to discourage medical practitioners by threatening to taint their professional reputation irrevocably. Strong moral and religious views on abortion have carried the issue outside the realms of pure medical practice, making it a matter which can affect a doctor's professional standing.

Before the partial legalisation of abortion doctors might be prepared to put their reputation at stake for two reasons: a deep sense of duty to the patient, or profit. I have already mentioned the case of an English doctor taken to court in the 1930s after an abortion on a fourteen-year-old victim of rape, and acquitted on the ground that the pregnancy posed a grave risk to the mental health and consequently the life of the mother.[4] In this case the doctor was prepared to put his career and reputation at risk, because he felt a strong moral obligation towards the well-being of his patient. Undoubtedly there were many cases of that kind, where doctors had to bypass or completely ignore the law because they felt that the general condition of their patient's mental health and well-being required it. The other side of the coin was the black market created by the heavy demand for an illegal practice.[5] In England alone the estimated number of illegal abortions before 1967 was 100,000 a year.[6] Not all of these were performed by qualified doctors; in fact, many were induced by unskilled people, attracted by the large profit which could be made. The enormous dangers of illegal abortions have been well described in modern medical literature and were one of the strongest arguments in favour of a regulated decriminalisation of abortion.[7] The liberalisation of the law resulted in a very substantial reduction in back-street abortions in many countries. However, the market is still flourishing in places where access to properly supervised abortions is limited due to legal, geographical or economic factors.

The legal conditions attached to abortion can still be restrictive, and some feel that the law as it stands does not go far enough. Recently, a number of ambitious career women in London working on tight timetables seemingly felt that the existing procedures in the British National Health Service were far too slow, time-consuming and cumbersome. The market responded swiftly to their needs by establishing clinics where, for a handsome fee, the entire process of approving an abortion and actually inducing it was reduced to a few hours. A London clinic was recently criticised for 'lunch-time' abortions. Whatever the implications, the reality is that where there is demand for something, someone will be quick to make a profit out of it, and human health and life are not exempt.

Doctors in the ancient world were faced with similar dilemmas to their modern counterparts. They too might find themselves having to pronounce an opinion on matters that extended beyond their professional expertise and entered the spheres of law, religion, politics and ethics. Like modern doctors, they might face a series of conflicting interests: personal belief versus professional conscience, financial interest versus moral integrity, instant cash versus reputation. And like their modern counterparts they were compelled to make up their minds and take sides on an issue that was arguably as divisive and controversial then as it is now. Many of the problems which modern doctors have to deal with, when it comes to an issue like abortion, are in fact very old and have troubled doctors from the beginnings of their discipline.

The main difference between ancient and modern doctors is not in the nature of the problems that they face, but in the intensity of these problems. Unlike their modern counterparts, ancient doctors could not protect themselves and their professional reputation behind standard policies and procedures, or precise legal provisions, and thus absolve themselves of personal responsibility by simply conforming to approved standards. Perhaps with the exception of a minority of doctors practising within the frame of strict guilds or cults, such as the Pythagoreans, each doctor was generally free to decide his course of action. Each individual had to balance his interests and reputation against the demand for abortions from patients from very different backgrounds and with a wide variety of personal circumstances. Should the doctor bluntly refuse, make allowances, or attempt to induce an abortion on demand, regardless of the circumstances? Should he take into account the high toxicity of most drugs and recommend mechanical or surgical means instead? If there was a conflict between the well-being of the patient and contemporary moral standards which of the two should prevail? These were problems that every doctor might have to face in the ancient world. The existing evidence suggests that the response to these problems was very diverse and depended very much upon the social and cultural context, external circumstances and the personal temperament and beliefs of individual doctors. In order to be able to understand more precisely how ancient doctors responded to problems, some of which still trouble the medical profession, we need to take into account the conditions in which they practised their art. This is why a schematic presentation of the conditions and the ethical standards to which ancient doctors were subject is necessary before we attempt to explore their responses to abortion and its ethics.

i. The medical practitioner in the ancient world

Medical education was not a standard process.[8] It could last only months, or take a number of years, it could be a hands-on experience or a long-term acquaintance with philosophy and cosmology, a very practical skill or a highly theoretical enterprise, a manual craft or an exercise in wisdom. The absence of established medical schools where one could go and learn the basics is one of the reasons for this diversity, but on its own insufficient to explain the large differences in theory and practice, not only from one period and place to another but also from one physician to another. Anyone remotely familiar with the surviving medical literature from the ancient world can trace the reasons behind this diversity largely back to historical factors. Greek rational medicine was born and developed from natural philosophy and retained links with philosophy up to the end of its creative period (second century AD). Medical theory remained attached to a number of philosophical movements with which it retained a reciprocal relationship. As J. Longrigg,[9] who has thoroughly investigated this relationship, puts it, 'philosophers and medical men shared a common intellectual background. They subscribed largely to the same general assumptions and, to a considerable extent, adopted the same concepts, categories and modes of reasoning. Thus there developed a close and complex correlation between medicine and philosophy.'

It is undeniable that the most prominent names of Greek medicine subscribed to a certain intellectual tradition with strong philosophical influence: Empedocles and Diogenes of Apollonia, the founders of doctrines which had a tremendous impact upon the development of medical theory in subsequent centuries, never attempted to draw a line between philosophy and science. In their works the two are inseparable aspects of one and the same wisdom. Similarly Alcmaeon of Croton, arguably the pioneer of Greek rational medicine, was associated with the Pythagoreans by Diogenes Laertius (8,83), as were most of the physicians of the Sicilian school.[10] The contribution of the Pythagoreans to medical theory and practice has been studied by Edelstein in his famous work on the Hippocratic Oath (see §3 below). In most of the works of the Hippocratic Corpus we see the strong influence of philosophical theories. Even in studies such as *Ancient medicine* and the *Nature of man*, where the strong link between medicine and philosophy is criticised as an inhibiting factor on the former, one can see the influence of contemporary philosophical theories. It is an irony that the classic theory of the four humours, very much a product of Presocratic philosophy but with such eminence and influence that it hampered the understanding of internal disease for thousands of years, is best explained in the study *Nature of man*, whose author writes at the same time:

> For I do not say at all that a man is air, or fire, or water, or earth, or anything else that is not an obvious constituent of man; such accounts I leave to those that care to give them. Those, however, who give them have not in my opinion correct knowledge.[11]

The contributions to medicine and biology by Plato and Aristotle are so strongly influenced by their philosophical systems that practical science is often indistinguishable from logic and theory.[12] The case of Aristotle is even more remarkable: he was the first, in the words of W. Detel,[13] to 'strongly emphasise that every scientific explanation has a syllogistically valid form', and at the same time the first person known to us to carry out systematic dissections of animals in his effort better to understand anatomy and physiology.[14] He had considerable practical knowledge, yet this knowledge is often so subservient to philosophical principles that it can lead to the most absurd conclusions. Diocles of Carystus, the most famous physician of the fourth century BC, probably had a strong connection with the Lycaeum and certainly moves along the same lines as Aristotle with his dissections of animals and anatomical studies.[15] One can trace a strong philosophical influence even in the works of the two great doctors and anatomists of the Alexandrian era, Herophilus and Erasistratus. For all their practical wisdom, Herophilus was a supporter of the humoral theory, while the relationship of Erasistratus with peripatetic teleology has been recently studied by H. von Stadten.[16] Soranus, a doctor famous for his sober, unbiased judgement, was a Methodist, and the cosmopolitan mind of Galen could easily accommodate detailed empirical knowledge with philosophical teleology, interests in rhetoric, and a theological system that touched the edge of superstition.[17]

Each one of the great doctors of the ancient world was a carrier of the intellectual legacy of a certain philosophical system, and this legacy influenced the exercise of his art, not only as far as general explanations of matters related to health and disease were concerned, but often in very practical ways too. The course of treatment that they suggested, their preferences over matters such as diet, drugs, healing methods and the interpretation of specific symptoms, and in general their style and perceptions as medical practitioners were certainly influenced, if not sometimes dictated by the intellectual/philosophical traditions to which they subscribed at a purely theoretical level, with little or no reference to clinical experience. The adverse effect of this powerful bond between medicine and philosophy upon the development of the former had already been noticed by the authors of some studies in the Hippocratic Corpus, and in the hellenistic period the Empiric school, with Heracleides of Tarentum (first century BC) as its leading figure, promoted a brand of medicine which was a reaction to the excessive use of philosophical theory in medicine, seeking the return to the crude beginnings of medical science.[18]

The Empiricists were not the first to subscribe to a type of medical practice that did not rely much on theory. In fact this form of medicine was very old. The art of healing was a very traditional craft. In Homer washing and bandaging wounds is mentioned, while in Pindar we find a reference to oral drugs and surgery.[19] However, in early Greek poetry (as in Egyptian and Babylonian medical texts[20]) disease comes from the gods and has supernatural causes, and this is why incantation is an indispensable part of the cure. The gods are the senders of disease and its healers.[21] The picture we obtain from early Greek literature is that, until the time the first pioneers of rational medicine tried to separate it from superstition, people primarily placed their trust in the hands of the gods, trying to help their work whenever possible. This picture is probably true to a certain extent but we must also keep in mind that, as it suited the purposes of poets to present the gods as the main agents of disease and healing, the extent to which healing was in reality treated as a rational and practical skill before the middle of the fifth century is probably understated. The number of therapies available in the early works of the Hippocratic Corpus unambiguously suggests that the wisdom concerning herbs, drugs and therapies inherited by the pioneers of rational medicine was quite substantial. Probably, observation, trial and error had led to the knowledge of many drugs and healing procedures, that had nothing to do with supernatural belief. The author of *Ancient medicine*, who wrote in the second half of the fifth century BC, is fully prepared to acknowledge this legacy and indicates in no uncertain terms that contemporary medicine should built on it rather than try to cast it aside; he writes:

> Medicine has long had everything, a principle and a way, through which many correct discoveries have been made during a long period, and many more will be made, if one is capable and continues searching with full knowledge of what has been discovered. But anyone who discards all this and disapproves of everything, searching for a new way and a new form, and claims that he has found one, he has been deceived and in turn he deceives others.[22]

The masters of the Sicilian and Coan schools had inherited a whole range of treatments and cures of various conditions from popular medicine, which they accepted and sought to recast in theoretical models in their search for wholesome and consistent interpretations of disease. Their expectation was that once the true nature of disease was understood, adequate treatment could be administered on a systematic and consistent basis. However, another contemporary school of medicine, the Cnidian school, did not attach the same importance to theory as the Sicilian and the Coan.[23] Throughout its history the Cnidian school remained closer to popular practical medicine, in the sense that it focussed on detailed description of symptoms and possible cures, instead of seeking unifying explanations of disease.[24] The survival of a number of works of Cnidian medicine in the Hippocratic Corpus provides us with a more realistic insight into a different brand of medical practice, one that did not rely on theory or philosophical interpretations of the natural world, but on hands-on experience with patients and experimentation with practical treatments.

This sort of medical practice must be closer to the type of medicine actually practised by a large number of practitioners, who did not have the intellectual background, education or abstract mind of the great masters of Greek medicine whose works have survived to us. This type of some-times self-acclaimed medical man or woman, whom O. Temkin calls 'a leech',[25] might be a popular figure, enjoying respect and trust in the community, and perhaps perfectly capable of dealing with a number of conditions. Temkin (p. 219) describes his/her potential as follows: 'The leech can recognise diseases and symptoms and has remedies for them, partly drugs, partly simple dietetic measures; possibly he has also learned to take into consideration the strength, age, and sex of his patient. He treats internal as well as surgical complaints, relying on some anatomical knowledge, and an accumulated store of manual skills. This knowledge is passed on from teacher to pupil; it can be increased by contact with other physicians or by accidental observations.' Temkin also describes the short-comings of this type of practitioner: 'The limitations are those of any technique without theory. The leech may know very much, but his knowl-edge will always consist of a certain number of skills. Beyond this number he cannot go, that is to say he cannot deal with what is unfamiliar to him and he cannot individualise his treatment.' Undoubtedly this description fits a large number of medical practitioners throughout the Greek world.[26]

However, many leeches would not even reach the standard described above by Temkin. Surely a substantial number of charlatans and self-made medics claiming to be able to heal all sorts of conditions were practising around the ancient world. The fact that huge differences could exist from doctor to doctor is acknowledged by the author of *Ancient medicine* (1,572 = *VM* 1) when he writes about the practitioners of the art of medicine: 'there are some bad craftsmen, and some very different (i.e. very good)'. Serious practitioners were worried that those hopeless crafts-men gave medicine a bad name, since the layman might not be able to distinguish between a genuinely good doctor and a charlatan. The author of *Regimen in acute diseases* writes:

Yet the art as a whole has a very bad name among laymen, so that there is thought to be no art of medicine at all. Accordingly, since among practitio-ners there will prove to be so much difference of opinion about acute diseases that the remedies which one physician gives in the belief that they are the

best are considered by a second to be bad, laymen are likely to object to such
that their art resembles divination.[27]

Serious physicians tried to distance themselves from the bad craftsmen
wandering around the Greek world. *On the art* is a defence of good practice
against the bad name given to medicine by irresponsible charlatans, while
the inexorable polemic of Galen against bad practitioners before and
during his time is present throughout his voluminous work.[28]

Galen thought that a doctor could never be too careful, as laymen would
be quick to blame the physician if things went wrong, but rather slow to
attribute the recovery of a patient to his skills (6,154-6 = *San.* 1,8).
However, this is a rather bitter remark: in general the Greeks trusted
their medicine. This confidence in the art of medicine is captured by the
author of *Ancient medicine* (1,572 = *VM* 1) when he writes 'this is an art
that all men use on the most important occasions, and give the greatest
honours to the good craftsmen and practitioners in it'. Statements like this
suggest that many responsible persons were practising the art of medicine, with varying degrees of knowledge and ability, but certainly with a
deep sense of duty towards their patients. The ordinary practitioner might
not have the precise anatomical knowledge of Herophilus or Erasistratus,
the shrewd judgement of Soranus, or the tremendous intellectual ability
of Galen, but he would have a substantial amount of experience and
practical knowledge, and often some theoretical background too, provided
by the sect or school of medicine to which he subscribed. And, above all he
would have the almost mythical figure of the great Hippocrates as a role
model. He would have the moral guidance of the man whom the ancient
world acknowledged as the founder of rational medicine, a man who,
according to the tales told about his life, declined wealth and power and
with a deep sense of philanthropy travelled around the Greek world
tending the sick and unveiling the tightly kept secrets of nature concerning disease and treatment.[29] A number of studies offering ethical advice to
doctors have survived under the name of Hippocrates, and these served as
a source of reference concerning medical ethics for all doctors who wished
or felt obliged to practice their art in accordance with high ethical standards in subsequent centuries.

ii. Ancient Greek medical ethics

Perhaps the most important function of modern professional bodies for
medical practitioners is to provide ethical work-related guidance for their
members. Yet the absence of such bodies in the ancient world, as well as
the absence of uniform standards of practice, did not mean that doctors
were totally deprived of direction and moral objectives.[30] As was the case
with many offices in the Greek world, an oath could provide this kind of
direction, to a certain extent, by setting out a constitutional framework
and outlining the main duties involved.[31] An oath outlining the main

duties of a doctor and setting out moral standards of professional conduct
has survived under the name of Hippocrates. In later antiquity and
subsequent centuries this text has come to be treated as a document of
enormous ethical weight. The importance as well as the difficulties of this
document will be discussed separately in the next section. It is possible
that other oaths, similar in function but established on different principles, were administered to members of various sects or schools, but none
of these has survived. What has been preserved for us is a number of
studies, such as *The sacred disease, The art, Decorum, Physician*, and
several more preserved among Galen's works, like the study *Whether the
doctor should be a philosopher*, or the two treatises *On the therapeutic
method*, intended to offer ethical and practical guidance to medical practitioners. The advice found in these texts, combined with references in other
medical and non-medical literature, allows us to form a picture of the
ethical standards that ancient doctors were expected to meet. These
suggestions were not obligatory, and undoubtedly many practitioners fell
short of these standards. However, any doctor who wished to protect his
reputation as a serious, humane and dignified physician, and avoid conflict
with his conscience, would try to harmonise the exercise of his duties with
these suggestions, at least to a certain extent. Much depended on the
individual and the tradition within which he operated, and much was a
matter of personal interpretation, but guidelines existed and many, if not
most, doctors made an effort to adhere to them.

The most fundamental principle upon which the entire perception and
exercise of medicine was, and still is, based is *philanthropy*. The author of
Precepts says:

Where there is love for man (*philanthropiê*) there is also love for the art
(*philotechniê*).[32]

Philanthropy is also an indispensable quality of the ideal (*kalos kagathos*)
doctor in the study *Physician* (Hip. *Med.* 9,204 = 1), while the lack of feeling
and compassion towards the patient is identified as misanthropy, a quality
incompatible with the nature of medicine. In both studies mentioned above
it is suggested that a physician motivated by love for man would exhibit
the moral qualities required for the exercise of the art, while a physician
not motivated by philanthropy has entered the profession for the wrong
reasons. Galen, in his usual critical spirit, complains that philanthropy
characterised only a small minority of doctors in his time and that most
were motivated by money. He echoes the discussion in Plato's *Republic* and
refers to the cynical comment of Thrasymachus in his discussion with
Socrates that the shepherds will look after their own interest, not that of
the sheep or the cows.[33] With a touch of cold pragmatism he summarises
his overall impression of the reasons why people practise medicine as
following:

Some practise medicine for profit, some because they are by law relieved
from liturgies, but a few motivated by philanthropy, whereas others do it for
glory or honours. ... Thus the motivation of a doctor could be glory or profit
(*endoxon ê porimon*), as Menodotus the Empiric wrote. But this is the opinion
of Menodotus, not that of Diocles, or Hippocrates, or Empedocles, or many
other doctors of the past, who treated people motivated by philanthropy.[34]

This criticism of Galen leads us to an area that has been one of the most
serious concerns in medical ethics from antiquity to the present day,
namely the need to find a balance between the doctor's financial interests
and the patient's right to effective treatment without exploitation. This
thorny issue, which has acquired new urgency in recent years, has been
addressed throughout the centuries with the creation of centres where the
poorest members of society could receive free treatment, with structures
allowing the state or health insurance to pay for these costs, and often with
appeals to the doctor's conscience and sense of duty. Ancient literature on
medical ethics suggests that this issue was perceived as one of great
importance. Appeals to the doctor's conscience and calls condemning
avarice and greed as incompatible with good medical practice are abun-
dant. A primary moral duty of the doctor was not to undertake hopeless
cases motivated by money. It would be more appropriate to refuse treatment than prolong the suffering of the patient in order to extract fees.[35]
The author of *Diseases* (6,140-2 = Hip. *Morb.* 1,1) advises that a doctor
should not say or do, or even contemplate impossible things. On the other
hand, when treatment was possible and appropriate but the patient could
not meet the doctor's financial demands, it would be a highly moral act for
the doctor if he could sometimes offer his services free. The author of
Precepts advises:

> Sometimes give your services for nothing, recalling a previous benefaction
> or present satisfaction. And if there be an opportunity of serving one who is
> a stranger in financial straits, give full assistance to all such.[36]

And in a more practical spirit the same author instructs doctors to discuss
payment only after treatment:

> If you start negotiating about payment you might give the impression that
> you are going to leave the patient in pain or that you will neglect him, if he
> does not agree to your demands .... It is better to chase a patient who has
> been cured than try to squeeze money out of someone who is on the verge of
> death.[37]

Similarly, the ideal philosopher-doctor in the study *Decorum* is someone
free from avarice, greed and extortion.[38]
    There were other means of tackling the need for health-care of the poor,
such as the offer of some practical health care in the temples of Asclepius,[39]
or the appointment of public physicians by various city-states. Herodotus
(3,131), for example, mentions the case of Democedes of Croton (late sixth

to early fifth century), who was employed as a public physician in Aegina on an annual salary of 1 talent, in Athens on 100 minae, and in Samos on 2 talents.[40] However, most physicians operated on a private basis and the exercise of their art was their main source of income. The temptation to overcharge, administer unnecessary but expensive treatments, and undertake the care of a wealthy patient, even though his chances of recovery were non-existent, was always present. This is why the discussion of the financial issue reflects the anxiety of serious medical practitioners to protect their reputation from accusations of extortion and immoral exploitation of their patients' suffering.

Trust and confidence in the doctor's skills were also very important issues in ancient medical ethics, perhaps more so at a time when many charlatans and quacks were going about the Greek world claiming to be doctors. Any serious physician would need to adopt a style that would distinguish him from the charlatans, and this would not only enhance his own reputation and career opportunities, but was also good for the patient's morale. The ideal doctor as described in *Physician* should pay attention to his appearance, because people would not trust someone who does not take care of himself to take care of them. The author advises:

He should look healthy, and as plump as nature intended him to be; for people consider those who are not of this excellent bodily condition to be unable to take care of others. Then he must be clean in person, well dressed and anointed with sweet-smelling unguents that are not in any way suspicious, because these are pleasant to the patients.[41]

His behaviour must also be pleasant and one that inspires trust and confidence. He should be gentle, dignified and humane. He should look thoughtful but not stern, so as not to appear unfeeling and misanthropic, but, on the other hand, he must not be loud and jocular, as this might look vulgar. A degree of self-control could ensure that he was relaxed and accessible, but not immodest.[42] He should look confident and sure, not spending much time contemplating over the patient's bed, but taking action, and he should do things quietly and carefully, without revealing too many details to the patient.[43] He should treat the patient gently avoiding demoralising remarks, like that of Callianax, a doctor criticised by Galen (13B,145 = *Hip. Epid.* 6,4,9) for saying to a patient, 'Patroclus also had to die, and he was much better than you' (a verse from the *Iliad*: 21,107), or to another patient who cried that he was going to die, 'Yes, unless Leto has given birth to you'.[44] The patient's morals were not recorded and should be the concern of the doctor only to the extent that the his/her lifestyle created health hazards. However, considering that ancient medicine was perceived as psychosomatic, perhaps to a larger extent than modern medical science, the doctor's investigation into the patient's lifestyle, diet, exercise and daily habits might be quite extensive, especially in some sects of medicine that did not draw strict lines between the health of the body and that of the soul.[45] As R. Flemming, who has reviewed the relevant literature, puts it, 'it has been argued both that classical society goes far beyond this basic necessity for care – that being healthy emerges here as positive ideal to a greater extent than elsewhere'. She then proceeds with her own sober analysis of the available evidence, and confirms the widely accepted view that ancient healthcare was to a large degree psychosomatic.[46] Galen gives a rather wide and comprehensive definition of health in the following passage:

> We call health this situation, where we are not in pain, and we are not prevented from performing the tasks of our daily lives.[47]

This definition would have been acceptable to most ancient doctors, and it would be easy to infer that the physician often considered it his duty to advise on a patient's way of life. Thus medicine exceeded the narrow limits of a science dealing with the body and was concerned with the soul too. As Galen puts it:

> One should not think that it is appropriate only for the philosopher to form the ethos of the soul; it is for another reason that his primary task is the health of the soul, while that of the doctor is to protect the body from easily giving in to disease.[48]

Advice about morals and lifestyle required the doctor himself to be a man of great moral calibre. Galen is very proud of his education and the virtues of justice, courage and prudence that have been acquired through it.[49] He wants the doctor to resemble a god:

> Unless the patient stands in awe as he would stand before a god, he may not be inclined to obey. So it is better neither to flatter to the point of becoming the object of contempt, nor to be rude and rough like Callianax.[50]

The author of *Physician* (Hip. 9,204-6 = *Med.* 1) requires a doctor to be 'a prudent man ... of a great regularity of life ... and a gentleman in character'. Particular attention is paid to sexual morality in a number of studies. The doctor should never take advantage of the considerable access he has to patients, or their relatives and other members of the household. In *Physician* we read:

> The intimacy between physician and patient is close. Patients in fact place themselves into the hands of their physician, and at every moment he meets women, maidens .... So towards all of them self-control must be exercised.[51]

In a similar spirit any doctor who took the *Hippocratic Oath* had to pledge the following:

> I will abstain from all intentional wrongdoing and harm, especially from abusing the bodies of man or woman, bond or free.

and before that he had to pledge:

I will keep pure and holy both my life and my art.

These stipulations are certainly in line with mainstream medical ethics, as these are illustrated in other sources. The ideal doctor in *Decorum* is a wise man who combines a number of virtues and is free from several defects that were considered incompatible with the practice of medicine. This presentation of the ideal philosopher-doctor summarises the most important points in mainstream Greek medical ethics:

One must transplant medicine into wisdom and wisdom into medicine, for a philosopher doctor is equal to a god. This is because there is little difference between these two, as things pertinent to wisdom can be found in medicine too: freedom from avarice, shyness, a reserved manner, good repute, good judgement, quiet disposition, clear answers, clarity, the ability to give an opinion, knowledge of all things useful and necessary for one's life, riddance of the unclean, lack of superstition, divine excellence. What they have, they have in opposition to intemperance, vulgarity, greed, improper desires, extortion, shamelessness.[52]

Most of the ethical and practical advice offered to ancient doctors in the aforementioned studies would nowadays be enshrined in statutes or understood as a basic principle of appropriate professional conduct. It does credit to the founders and pioneers of rational medicine that they were not only concerned with the establishment of the purely scientific principles of their discipline, but also paid much attention to the function of medicine as a service to humanity. They understood from the start that there are inherent dangers in the exercise of an art that places one human being in another's trust to such an extent. They were aware of human weakness and tried to address it, and they were also aware of the human capacity for compassion and positive action, and tried to build on them. By adhering to the principles mentioned above, the men and women who took themselves seriously as medical practitioners in the ancient world would be in the position to safeguard their reputation and differentiate themselves from the crooks who passed themselves off as doctors with a view to profit or fame. Undoubtedly a major part of ancient Greek medical ethics covers this particular aspect: it is intended to instruct doctors and safeguard their reputation. However, at the same time the patient is never out of the picture. Philanthropy is the most fundamental principle and the entire orientation of medical practice is in the direction of the patient's best interests. Even if many of the axioms and conclusions of Greek medicine have been questioned and discarded by scientists in subsequent centuries, the ethical guidelines that it established have always been an authoritative source of inspiration and direction, and remain firmly established as indispensable principles of ethical professional conduct for all medical practitioners up to the present day.

iii. The Hippocratic Oath

The importance of this document as a basic source of reference for medical ethics is manifested in the fact that it is still regarded as a functional text of considerable authority. Graduates of medical schools around the world take this oath, and prestigious bodies such as the Supreme Court of the United States have been prepared to consider the background and content of the Oath thoroughly in recent years.[53] Most of its stipulations are considered to be fundamental ethical requirements for all those wishing to practise medicine, to the extent that they have become law in many countries.

The attribution of the Oath to Hippocrates was not in dispute until the nineteenth century. The oldest witness to the Oath is a second-century BC inscription from Philadelphia in Lydia (*LSA* 20), if my suggestion that the inscription is based upon the Oath is correct (see Appendix 2). The oldest explicit reference to the Oath is found in the work of the Roman pharmacologist Scribonius Largus (first century AD), and Hippocrates unquestionably figures as the author. Other ancient authors writing about the Oath in later years were equally convinced that it was composed by Hippocrates.[54] It was not until the authorship of all the works surviving under the name of the father of medicine was called into question that the authorship of the Oath became the subject of scholarly debate.[55] The Hippocratic authorship of the Oath, along with that of every other study of the Corpus, came to be viewed with deep-rooted scepticism, and this long, inconclusive debate remains open. Until recently the overwhelming majority of scholars were not prepared to attribute the Oath to Hippocrates, with the notable exception of S. Nittis, who argued that it was indeed his work, composed in 421 BC.[56] But since 1943, when L. Edelstein published his influential study of the Oath,[57] its non-Hippocratic authorship has been so widely accepted that it has become scholarly orthodoxy. Edelstein examined the stipulations of the Oath closely and concluded that it must be a text of Pythagorean origin, composed in the second half of the fourth century BC. Many scholars, with a greater or lesser degree of certainty, have subscribed to this view. It was only recently that Edelstein's thesis was seriously questioned in a study by C. Lichtenthaeler published in 1984. Lichtenthaeler challenges the 'Pythagorisation' of the Oath by Edelstein on linguistic, historical and cultural grounds, and his views, like those he is trying to refute, merit closer consideration.[58]

Scholars investigating the authorship of the Oath have been confronted by a challenge set out by D. Amundsen as follows:[59] 'Some of the stipulations in the Oath are not consonant either with ethical precepts prevalent elsewhere in the Hippocratic Corpus and in other classical literature or with the realities of medical practice as revealed in the sources.' More specifically, those stipulations of the Oath that seem to be objections to suicide, euthanasia and abortion have been interpreted as a departure from contemporary medical practice and social attitudes. Edelstein, in an effort to explain what appears to be a discrepancy, searched for the origins of the Oath in areas outside the mainstream of Greek thought and concluded that it must be a text of Pythagorean authorship, on the grounds that the Pythagoreans alone held principles which would support such ethical precepts as those included in the Oath. Moreover he tried to present in a Pythagorean light even those stipulations which would be broadly acceptable to everyone, such as the prohibition on sexual harassment of patients and their relatives, or the ideal of purity in a doctor's practice and lifestyle.

Lichtenthaeler approached the issue from a diametrically opposite point of view, and to some degree reiterated the conclusions reached by Nittis half a century ago. He tried to find similarities, linguistic and ideological, between the Oath and other works of the Corpus, and concluded that such similarities exist and in fact suggest that the author of the Oath is the same as that of other ethical studies. This author, he thought, was probably Hippocrates himself. However, Lichtenthaeler was prepared to concede the point that some of the contentious stipulations in the Oath are at odds with the beliefs and ideas of contemporary Greek society, and he agreed with Edelstein that, as far as these points are concerned, the Oath betrays Pythagorean influence. Lichtenthaeler holds the view that although the Oath in its entirety is a genuine Hippocratic work, it may be influenced by Pythagorean principles in some areas. Before one can decide whether the Oath is a text that represents a minority view, it is necessary to take a closer look at those of the stipulations that have caused the most intense controversy and are relevant to the subject of this book:

> I will give no deadly medicine to anyone if asked, nor disseminate any such information; and likewise I will not give to a woman a pessary to procure an abortion.

The prohibition on issuing a lethal drug is undoubtedly linked with the prohibition on giving to a woman an abortifacient pessary. They are part of the same clause, and apparently served the same purpose as far as the author was concerned. But what was this purpose? The principle that the fundamental duty of a doctor is 'to help or at least to do no harm'[60] would probably be acceptable to the overwhelming majority of medical practitioners in the ancient world. Thus, it would be reasonable to assume that the author of the Oath too understood it as a doctor's fundamental duty to maintain rather than destroy human life, whatever the circumstances. However, if we look closer, the language of the Oath poses problems. Who is this 'anyone'? Is the author referring to the patient or another party? Scholars tend to agree that only the patient is implied here, because otherwise, if the doctor gave lethal poison to a third party against the patient's wishes, he would be an accomplice to murder.[61] Thus this prohibition is most commonly understood as an objection to euthanasia. The doctor should not assist a patient to commit suicide by administering a lethal drug. Assuming that the author of the Oath indeed had in mind an attack on euthanasia, this would automatically distance him from mainstream Greek thought and medical ethics, because neither suicide nor euthanasia were perceived as unquestionably wrong. As far as suicide was concerned, Greek audiences had been educated in the theatre since the fifth century with the positive example of many a tragic hero or heroine. The message that it could be honourable and right to terminate one's own misery, pain or shame by committing suicide had been eloquently conveyed. The suicide of Ajax on stage in front of the eyes of his audience is presented as perhaps the only honourable course of action available to the dishonoured and humiliated hero. And tragic audiences were expected to feel deep sympathy, if not admiration, for Antigone, Jocasta, Deianeira and many other heroines, who did what was appropriate under the circumstances by committing suicide.[62]

Passive euthanasia, namely not trying to prolong the life of a terminally ill patient in pain, was equally acceptable to doctors and mainstream Greek thought. *The Art* (6,46 = 3) and *Diseases* (7,72 = 2,48) state that a doctor should refuse to treat a terminally ill patient, because if he tries to treat someone in great pain with no hope of recovery, instead of helping, he actually does harm and may be placing profit before duty.[63] This is not to say that doctors should refuse difficult cases. On the contrary, any practitioner who would run away from responsibility and challenge would not be properly performing his duty, and this is made clear in a large number of medical and non-medical sources.[64] Celsus (*Med.* 5,26,1) clarifies the issue: the doctor should not undertake desperate cases, but when he takes on a difficult case he should sincerely explain to the relatives the gravity of the situation. These sources clearly object to the situation where a doctor might put himself in charge of a patient whom he cannot help because he wishes to make a profit, while his care and assistance simply prolong the patient's suffering. Society and the medical profession generally agreed that in such a case the best course of action would be to let the patient die in peace. A substantial number of non-medical sources corroborate the statement that this was generally perceived as morally correct and humane in Greek eyes.[65] Aristotle did not generally approve of suicide, but Amundsen is probably right when he says that the philosopher did not have in mind the terminally ill.[66] Plato (*Lg.* 873c) reluctantly accepted that suicide might be an option in cases of intolerable or inevitable misfortune, but generally condemned it. In a famous passage in the *Phaedo* (62b) he condemns suicide without qualifications, and this has prompted scholars to suspect that Socrates at this point is voicing Pythagorean views.[67] The Pythagoreans are the only clear representatives of a tradition that adopted a negative view of suicide under any circumstances.[68] In fact this particular sect went further than this. They objected to an irregular lifestyle, excess, or anything that could be harmful to one's health, thus denying the individual the right to harm his own body deliberately and put his life at risk, even if he wished to do so.[69] However, such views were in the minority.

When it comes to active euthanasia, namely killing someone who is suffering intolerably in an act of mercy, the picture is very different. I do not know of any case where a Greek or Roman doctor categorically states that he gave a terminally ill patient lethal poison at the patient's request, and I believe there is a good reason for this silence in the sources. Actively killing a person who had been accepted in the family was a crime not only against the victim and his/her family but primarily against the gods and brought pollution (*miasma*) upon the killer.[70] This perception of homicide extended even to slaves, who, it is noteworthy, were treated as human only in death. A doctor who actively killed a patient at the latter's request might or might not risk breaking human law; to my knowledge, the lack of evidence does not allow a conclusive answer. However, he certainly risked provoking the anger of the gods and becoming contaminated with the deadly pollution that fell upon a murderer. This was the kind of risk that no one would want to take. After all, this was not what medicine was about, and no financial reward could offer protection against the inexorable wrath of the offended gods.

Things were different with newborn babies not yet accepted in the family.[71] As far as the law was concerned, newborns could be actively killed by their family with no repercussions, especially if they were handicapped, and seemingly some people at least would not understand this act as homicide, and therefore offensive to the gods. But there are indications that for others the religious aspect of homicide could be extended even to newborn babies. For example, people might expose a severely handicapped baby instead of killing it immediately after birth, for fear of pollution. Even though legally they were immune from prosecution for a 'mercy killing' of this kind, usually people were reluctant to go ahead with it either because they did not have the heart, or because they feared that the gods would be offended. An individual's conscience, strength of religious feeling, and broad perception of human identity would be important factors in the decision over the fate of an unwanted infant. As P. Carrick has put it, 'the Greeks had no single view on the meaning of death. Rather they held a plurality of often conflicting views, just as we do in our own culture today.'[72] And if perceptions regarding the status of newborn babies were so subjective, an even greater degree of uncertainty regarding the status of the unborn should be expected. As I argue below (Chapters 5 and 6), the law did not command automatic respect of someone's right to life before this person was recognised as a member of the human race and given a place in the community, even if this place was as lowly as that of a slave (see also Chapter 5 §v). Thus the conclusion of Amundsen that 'human value is acquired rather than inherent' is certainly correct as far as the law was concerned, and might also reflect the views of many individuals in antiquity.[73] This realisation brings us back to some crucial questions: Did the author of the Oath recognise the unborn as a human being with an

indispensable right to life? When he prohibited the administration of
lethal drugs and abortifacient pessaries in the same clause, did the author
of the Oath intend to link these activities as two practices opposing the
value and sanctity of human life?

Edelstein understood that the author of the Oath had deliberately
linked abortion with suicide and euthanasia in this clause. This was
crucial for Edelstein's argument, because based on this he could establish
that the Oath ought to be Pythagorean. The Pythagoreans were not only
objecting to suicide, or the right wilfully to harm one's own body or health,
but, as stated in Chapter 2, they thought that the unborn acquired a soul,
and thus human identity, at the moment of conception. In Edelstein's
view, the Pythagorean author of the Oath banned both assistance to
suicide and abortion, because they contravened the belief of his sect in the
inherent value of human life from the moment of conception. From this
point Edelstein proceeded with a 'Pythagorisation' of the rest of the Oath,
trying to interpret every other clause in the light of the teachings of this
sect. Lichtenthaeler's first serious objection to the Pythagorisation of the
Oath rests precisely upon this point.[74] He argues that, with the exception
of this particular stipulation, and perhaps the one banning surgery to
remove a stone, the rest of the clauses of the Oath betray no kind of
influence that would have to be exclusively Pythagorean. The objection
raised by Lichtenthaeler, although not conclusive *per se*, is important
because it can pave the way for an alternative explanation of the Oath as
a whole. Even if one concedes that the clause banning the administration
of lethal drugs and abortifacient pessaries has been influenced by Pythagorean principles, as Lichtenthaeler is prepared to do, one need not
assume that the *whole* of the Oath is a Pythagorean document.

The format and style of this particular stipulation, and of the Oath as a
whole, have furnished important arguments concerning the date and
content of this document. Lichtenthaeler, as K. Dreichgräber had done
before him,[75] dates the oath in the late fifth century, instead of the second
half of the fourth century, on account of unmistakable influence of the
sophists, especially Gorgias. In addition, Lichtenthaeler succeeds in shed-
ding light upon some interesting details. He correctly points out that a
series of negatives (*ou doso … oude … oudeni … oude … homoios de
oude*) leaves no room for doubt that the ban on lethal drugs and abortifacient pessaries is a stern prohibition, rather than a suggestion. Those who
took the Oath were expected to abide by it, and not to treat it as a kind of
unrealistic or idealistic principle.

Now, having discussed the general context of this stipulation we need
to examine in greater detail its content, starting from the kind of items
included in the ban. First there was a prohibition of issuing any form of
lethal poison. In ancient pharmacology this might be an issue less
straightforward than it seems at first, as the same drug might be used for
different purposes, depending on the administration.[76] Thus what mattered was not the doctor's action but his intention, and the same surely

3. The Doctor's Dilemma

applied to those doctors who had taken this Oath. A doctor who issued a drug for therapeutic purposes could not be held responsible if this substance was misused. However, a doctor who had given someone a drug with the knowledge that it was going to be used as poison was abusing his art and breaking the Oath. As far as the author of the Oath was concerned, a doctor should not issue drugs or advice if he thought that they were going to be used to kill someone. The message conveyed here was clear: not only lethal drugs but also giving advice about such substances were explicitly prohibited. There was no excuse or bypass for a doctor who had sworn to abide by this Oath and took his conscience and duty seriously.

The wording, although equally firm, is genuinely more ambiguous when it comes to the prohibition of abortifacient substances. Only pessaries are mentioned, while there is no reference to oral drugs, surgical or mechanical means, or any other way of inducing an abortion. Should one take it as an indication that the author of the Oath intended to ban pessaries for some reason but allow abortions by other methods, or should one consider pessaries to be a *pars pro toto*, and understand that all methods of abortion are banned? The clause is certainly open to different interpretations and has been understood in different ways from antiquity to the present day. The first author to mention the Oath in antiquity, Scribonius Largus, understood this clause as a general ban on abortion. He writes:

> Hippocrates, the founder of our profession, drew the principles of our discipline from the oath, where it is stated that no drug, which might kill the foetus, should be given or recommended to a pregnant woman, educating thus the souls of future generations in humanity.[77]

Scribonius Largus evidently understood this prohibition to be dictated by moral considerations. Reflecting the spirit of his time, he considered that abortion was incompatible with the basic principle of humanity in medical practice, and perceived this prohibition to be an exercise *ad humanitatem*.[78] However, this interpretation was not universally accepted in the ancient world. Soranus reflects the diversity of opinion in a passage of invaluable importance for our understanding of the ethical dilemmas concerning abortion among ancient doctors:

> Some say that an expulsive is different from something that causes an abortion, others say that the difference lies between the refusal to use drugs, but acceptance of leaps and shakes, if it so happens, and this was the reason why Hippocrates abandoned abortifacient drugs, in the study *The nature of the child* (7,490ff. = 13), but adopted leaps with heels up to the buttocks, in order to induce an abortion. There is certainly a disagreement. Some object to abortifacient substances invoking the testimony of Hippocrates who says, 'I will not give anyone an abortifacient', and (claiming) that it is in the nature of medicine to preserve and save what nature has begotten. Others, however, follow this with qualifications, namely not when someone wishes to abort the conceptus because of adultery or in pursuit of beauty, but when there is a danger that it will be prevented from being born, because the womb is small ....[79]

Soranus reveals a division of opinions and loyalties among Greek doctors, which will be considered in greater detail below (§v). This passage makes clear that at least doctors of the imperial era, who were in no doubt that the Oath was written by Hippocrates, did not unanimously understand that the ban on pessaries stood as a *pars pro toto*. Some, like Scribonius Largus, interpreted this passage broadly as a general ban on abortion. Others understood it more literally as a ban on pessaries, or drugs altogether, but not mechanical means. A few went even further: although they could see that the Oath was banning pessaries for the purposes of inducing an abortion, they were not prepared to comply fully and unconditionally with this prohibition. They would go ahead with therapeutic abortions, and prescribe substances to this effect, conscious of the fact that they were defying the Oath. Those doctors thought that it was their duty to help their patient have an abortion, if letting a pregnancy come to term would put her life or health at risk. Soranus himself explicitly states that he sides with the latter group of doctors, and later lays down his complex, and perhaps efficient method of inducing an abortion. However, he first makes sure that his objections to abortions for aesthetic reasons or for the purposes of eliminating the fruit of an adulterous relationship are expressly noted.

The difference of opinion regarding this prohibition of the Oath persists to the present day. Most scholars understand that the author of the Oath intended to prohibit abortion altogether.[80] However, a learned scholar on the subject takes the opposite view: Riddle concedes that the original text could be understood in two ways, but he himself considers that the Oath did not prohibit abortion altogether; it banned only certain ways of doing it.[81] This is certainly a valid interpretation of the text as it stands, and the aforementioned testimony of Soranus makes clear that it was embraced by a number of doctors of the imperial era. But still, I would not be prepared to accept that the author of the Oath intended to ban only pessaries and allow other methods of abortion, on account of the context of this prohibition. Nardi points out that the prohibition on issuing an abortifacient pessary is linked together with the one banning the administration of lethal poison; the first is intended to safeguard life before birth and the second life after birth.[82] Unless one assumes that the author of the Oath had in mind a scheme which considered these prohibitions as two sides of the same coin, it is very difficult to explain why they were linked in the same article. However, whatever the intentions of the author, one must recognise the fact that the way this prohibition has been drafted leaves plenty of room for manoeuvre. A doctor could induce an abortion by means of oral drugs, mechanical means, or surgery, and still be able to protest his perfect adherence to the letter of the Oath. Thus one could argue that the doctor who advised the musician to induce an abortion in early pregnancy by means of vigorous leaps (Hip. 7,490ff. = 13) was not acting in violation of the principle set out in this clause of the Oath. As Soranus says, some doctors interpreted the case of the musician in exactly this manner. Moreover, a doctor who performed abortions on a regular basis could always claim, for the sake of his professional reputation, that he did not prescribe pessaries and only used other methods of abortion, as suggested in the Oath. Precisely because the drafting of this clause of the Oath allows more than one interpretation, much was left up to an individual's conscience. Those who wished to interpret it in a narrow literal sense could do so, and those who, for their own reasons, wanted to understand this prohibition in a broader sense could do so too.

One remaining question concerning the drafting of this prohibition is why the author of the Oath mentions pessaries only, if in truth what he had in mind was all methods of induced abortion. Lichtenthaeler's answer that pessaries were the most dangerous of all is not very convincing, because, as I explained in Chapter 1, oral drugs, mechanical means and surgery could be equally perilous. Concern for the woman's safety may have been one of the reasons, if we understand that the reference to pessaries stands as a *pars pro toto*, but this still does not explain why the author chose to mention only pessaries. There may be more truth in an additional reason proposed by Lichtenthaeler (in fact, by an unnamed student of his). Pessaries had to be administered through the genitalia and this would make them more of a taboo. So, it is possible that the author of the Oath singled out pessaries and used them as a *pars pro toto* precisely because of the connotations of this term. This sounds plausible, but I feel that a clear, convincing answer still eludes us. Whatever the case, I think that the ambiguity and confusion caused by the use of the word 'pessary', instead of a general term referring to all methods, was unintentional. If this wording was not unambiguously clear to future generations, it seems to me that it was perfectly clear to the author of the Oath: by 'abortifacient pessary' (*pesson phthorion*) those who swore to abide by this text were expected to abstain from inducing abortions by any means available.

The motive behind this stern but ambiguously stated prohibition remains the key point in the entire debate. Was it dictated by the Pythagorean belief in animation and acquisition of human identity from the moment of conception, as Edelstein has suggested? Was it dictated by an inherent belief in the value of human life, as Nardi and others have thought? Was it dictated by a strict sense of good professional conduct based on the belief that abortion was incompatible with the doctor's primary duty 'to help, or at least do no harm', as Lichtenthaeler and Dreichgräber understood?

At first sight the Pythagorisation of the Oath seems to be the easy way out. There is something ingenious in this suggestion, which accounts for its widespread and lasting appeal. However, as Lichtenthaeler has pointed out, this ingenuity may be misleading. There is not a single scrap of external evidence linking this document with Pythagorean medicine, and the combination of this fact with the other objections raised mainly by Lichtenthaeler are sufficient to compel one to consider alternative explanations. First, it is far from certain that the ban on lethal poison effectively amounts to the prohibition of euthanasia, or a blunt expression of hostile attitudes towards suicide. Nardi in his wisdom explains this term in just a few words. He does not question who the 'no one' (*oudeni*) is to whom lethal poison should be issued, and it seems to me that the author of the Oath did not consider this question either. 'No one' simply means 'no one': the doctor who swore to abide by this oath should not issue lethal poison to anyone for any reason at all. The doctor did not need to question the motives or purpose of the request for poison. Simply he should flatly refuse. Preparation and sale of poison might be carried on by various shady characters who knew some of the secrets of ancient pharmacology and moved very close to the edge of criminal activity, but these were not actions appropriate for the great Hippocrates and those inspired by him, nor for Galen's ideal philosopher-doctor. Even if this explicit prohibition had not been included in the Oath, such an action would still be incompatible with other stipulations, such as the one where the person who swears the Oath pledges to use his art 'for the benefit of the sick' or the one where he promises 'to abstain from any harm or wrongdoing'. Such stipulations are perfectly in agreement with the fundamental statement that the doctor's duty was 'to help or at least do no harm', and are inspired by the principle of philanthropy. As such they are very much mainstream. A doctor who was issuing a substance which he knew was not going to be used for any therapeutic purpose, but in order to kill, could not possibly claim that he was acting out of philanthropy, even if he sympathised with the idea that a terminally ill patient had the moral right to end his own life. Letting a terminally ill patient die in peace without painful or crude interventions which were bound to have little or no benefit was one thing, but actually killing a person with a dose of poison was another. Much of the debate arises from the failure to distinguish between such passive and active forms of euthanasia. Most Greek doctors might not have objected to the first, but perhaps few would have been happy to take part in an active form of euthanasia – kill someone and proudly boast that they had done so without any sense of restraint or any fear of punishment from the gods.

Placed against this background the prohibition on issuing drugs intended to kill does not really represent a minority view, as Edelstein thought. This principle would have been dictated by a fundamental sense of duty, the correct code of practice, and a profound recognition of the value of human life, without which the medical profession would be nothing more than a profitable exercise in butchery. The doctor as an individual could not violate this right of another man without the fear of repercussions from heaven and conflict with his own conscience. As a professional he could not breach his pledge to act within the frame of philanthropy and exercise his art for the benefit of the sick, rather than their destruction. And finally he could not afford a confrontation with the severe homicide laws of the Greek city states. He did not have to belong to some kind of sect, like the Pythagoreans, to be asked to pledge at the beginning of his career that he would refrain from intentionally killing someone by means of lethal poison.

It has already been stated that the form and content of this clause of the Oath compels us to consider the ban on abortifacients as an extension of the ban on lethal poisons. Therefore the conclusion that both prohibitions were dictated by the same motive and understood in the same spirit is inevitable. This motive can be none other than respect for human life in antenatal or postnatal form. Poison should not be given to kill a person, and an abortifacient pessary should not be given to kill a foetus. However, in the latter case there are some latent inconsistencies and contradictions. How can one speak about human life in the case of a foetus, if one is not entirely convinced that the foetus has human identity? Why should one refrain from killing a foetus, while the same person might not hesitate to let the same foetus die after it was born, if, let's say, it was severely deformed? How can one speak about respect for foetal life, when this life does not possess an inherent right to exist? How can one resolve the conflict of interests, when the life of the foetus endangers the life or well-being of the mother? These dilemmas are not easy to resolve and are met by various legal and ethical systems with measures that are not fully consistent. All societies have contradictory laws and moral standards. The author of the Oath may have been aware of these dilemmas and contradictions but chose not to confront them when he laid down a blanket ban on abortion motivated by general principles concerning the value of human life and ideals about a doctor's conduct and aspirations. One did not need to have a specific Pythagorean belief in the animation of the foetus at the moment of conception before laying down such a prohibition. A noble motivation and failure to consider some of the implications would be sufficient. According to the testimony of Soranus, many doctors in later centuries were prepared to subscribe to these principles and ideals but, unlike the author of the Oath, chose to confront these dilemmas and contradictions by inserting qualifications into this prohibition. The great physician and gynaecologist was unashamedly one of them.

The previous discussion suggests that the Oath does not have to be interpreted as a Pythagorean document. Its stipulations could be an expression of mainstream views in Greek medical ethics, even if contradictory, unclear, or confused to a certain extent. It is perfectly possible that the Oath was a well-known and influential document in the classical period, and its principles served as an inspiration and a source of moral guidance for many medical practitioners. If my suggestion that the inscription from Philadelphia (see Appendix 2) follows the Oath is correct, then we may safely conclude that this document had already had a serious impact upon attitudes towards abortion in the hellenistic period (second century BC). In the imperial era it was certainly established as a document of high moral authority and universally accepted as the words of the Father of Medicine.

The Oath surviving under the name of Hippocrates is such an authoritative document that many of its stipulations have long been enshrined in the legal systems of many countries. The author of this document set out to prepare a basic code of conduct for anyone who has in his hands the bodies and lives of others. Love of humanity, respect for human life, dignity and welfare, a tireless effort to do good service, and an ever alert conscience, which would stop a physician from abusing or misusing his skills, were some of the ideals that motivated the author of this text. Different historical periods and different individuals have applied their own interpretations to it, some literal, others broader. Like any other influential text in the history of human civilisation, the Oath has not stood frozen in time. It is continuously read, and its principles are constantly absorbed, re-evaluated and recast into the cultural parameters of each individual or social group that looks up to this text as a source of inspiration. Scholars may disagree on close interpretations of individual passages, most notably the passage on induced abortion, but the spirit of the Oath is certainly something much larger, and something that finds general acceptance. One might discard some sections as irrelevant today (such as the teacher-student clause intended to safeguard that only certain people will be admitted into the study of medicine), but still there is something far greater left in this text, something lasting, a source of inspiration for our civilisation. The universal respect and appeal that the Oath has enjoyed through the centuries, and still enjoys today, is predominantly due to the fact that most of its stipulations are such basic and essential guidelines that they can not be ignored by anyone who aspires to exercise medicine for the benefit of humanity. Moreover, there is a didactic element in this document that reaches beyond the limits of medical practice. The Oath offers a sense of direction and moral guidance to all who are ready to adopt its general spirit of humanity, selfless devotion to the good of others, and personal discipline and improvement. This is not a text for saints. It is a text meant to guide imperfect human beings towards personal and professional amelioration. It is not possible to tell for sure whether it is a work of the quasi-mythical figure of Hippocrates, but if we agree with more recent studies that the late fifth century is the most likely date of its composition, then it could have been written by him. But whether Hippocrates or not, one thing is certain: whoever wrote this text did not set out merely to define the limits of good medical practice. He was motivated by high ideals, and was able to place good medical practice on a higher philosophical and moral plane, in the words of Scribonius Largus, 'pre-forming the souls of future generations to accept humanity' (*longe praeformans animos discentium ad humanitatem*).

iv. The preservation of human life

The important passage of Soranus quoted in the previous section informs us that a number of doctors in the imperial era refused to procure an abortion on the ground that 'it is in the character of medicine to preserve and save what nature has begotten'. As suggested above, the author of the Hippocratic Oath was indeed motivated by this principle that attached value to human life, antenatal or postnatal, and for this reason he laid down a stern prohibition on abortion. Scribonius Largus, the first author to mention the Oath in antiquity, was one of those who invoked the moral authority of the Oath on this matter, and subscribed to the principle that 'medicine is the art of healing, not killing' (*scientia enim sanandi, non nocendi est medicina*). A similar cultural background can be detected behind the words of the doctor who appears as a character in the novel by Apuleius (*Metamorphoses* 10,11). In this passage a physician says:

> I do not believe that to become the cause of someone's death or extermination agrees with my discipline. I would subscribe to the view that medicine should be studied for the salvation of human beings.

Galen not only subscribes to the view that it is not a doctor's duty to issue substances which are harmful to human life, but, moreover, insists that even to write about them brings ignominy upon the author:

> I wonder what some people thought when they came to write about them. How could they possibly hope to gain glory after death by writing about things the knowledge of which would bring ignominy to them even while still alive? [83]

A few centuries later Priscianus maintains the same critical spirit when he invokes the testimony of Hippocrates and says:

> It is not permissible to give anyone an abortifacient, because as the oration of Hippocrates attests, it is not appropriate for the conscience of the doctors to soil an office destined to do no harm with such a grave offence. [84]

Priscianus and his predecessors represent a strong tradition in the medical profession that was hostile to abortion on the ground that it is incompatible with the most basic function of medicine, which they understood as the preservation of human life, not its destruction. This tradition was a very old one, almost as old as Greek rational medicine as an independent science, and, at least in later antiquity, drew moral authority from the ban on abortifacient pessaries in the Hippocratic Oath. We do not know for sure whether the Oath was widely known among doctors, philosophers and other laymen interested in the subject in the classical and hellenistic periods, but even a physician who had never read or taken the Oath might independently subscribe to this rather basic principle.

On the other hand, even though many doctors broadly accepted the principle that induced abortion is incompatible with the nature of medicine as the science of saving human lives, they performed abortions at least for therapeutic purposes. K. Hopkins says that of 26 medical authors 18 mention abortion and 15 give advice on it. [85] Do they knowingly defy the

Oath? Some cases are truly noteworthy in this respect. The appeal to the moral authority of the Oath by Scribonius Largus when he condemns abortion is only a prologue to a description of methods of induced abortion to be used when the woman's health demanded it. R. Flemming points out the difference between Dioscorides, who seems uninterested in the moral implications of references to abortifacient substances, and Pliny, who denounces all *abortiva* only to go ahead and mention a substantial number of them later on in his work.[86] Her explanation is that 'Dioscorides pursues a policy that may be described as pro-knowledge, ... Pliny pursues a pro-natalist policy'. But this does not alter the fact that we often learn much about abortifacient substances from sources that are supposedly critical of induced abortion. Galen too, though critical of people who give details about abortifacient substances in their books, does not hesitate to include numerous prescriptions in his own voluminous work, at least in theory to be used when the woman's health demanded it. Soranus is careful enough to distance himself from what might look as duplicity by simply reporting the views of the two opposing traditions, those who reject abortion entirely and those who are prepared to accept the need for it under certain circumstances. Then in a straightforward manner he expresses his opposition to abortion if it is used to eliminate the fruit of an adulterous relationship or to pander to a woman's vanity, and lays down his own method of abortion, to be used only for therapeutic purposes. Priscianus also places his condemnation of abortion as a prologue to a list of herbs and substances with abortifacient qualities.

Is this blatant hypocrisy? I think not. For a doctor to perceive that it is part of his duty to preserve rather than destroy human life sounds like an easily acceptable principle. But subscription to broad theoretical ideals is often different from everyday reality and practice. What if a pregnancy put a woman's life at risk? Then the doctor would need to decide whose life to preserve, and he might have to go ahead with a therapeutic abortion even if it was against his own principles to destroy life. It should come as no surprise to us to see that some of the prominent names among ancient medical authors subscribed to the principle of preserving human life, but at the same time were perfectly prepared to induce abortions for therapeutic purposes. At least as far as therapeutic abortion is concerned the attitude of most Greek doctors was probably favourable: the interests of the mother would have to come before the interests of the unborn.

v. The health of the woman

In a substantial number of medical texts we find that several gynaecological conditions might be considered adequate reasons to terminate a troublesome or potentially dangerous pregnancy. A narrow passage or a small uterus not allowing the foetus to come safely to term are sometimes mentioned as reasons for a therapeutic abortion.[87] A dead foetus urgently required the intervention of a doctor by all available means (drugs, mechanical methods, or surgery), if the woman's life were to be saved.[88] Various other conditions such as cracks, tumours, or inflammation of the passage and the womb are also mentioned as adequate reasons for proceeding with a therapeutic abortion.[89] Nothing much needs to be said here about such conditions. Many health problems which today are nothing more than minor complications, would have been seriously baffling to the ancient doctor. On many occasions the only sensible course of action was to try to terminate the pregnancy, and we read in our sources that many doctors did not hesitate to take this course of action under these circumstances.

Further evidence suggesting that ancient doctors often put the health and welfare of the mother, in its broadest sense, before ethical considerations on the morality of abortion comes from a very telling passage by the Hippocratic commentator John of Alexandria:

> I wonder at this point, because he (sc. Hippocrates) is the one who says in the Oath 'I will not give an abortifacient', how can he instruct the woman to kick her heels up to her buttocks? Many answers have been put forward for this question. One is that he did not administer an abortifacient pessary in order to abort a baby, but that he only destroyed the seed, not a child. However, if the seed had remained inside, it would have become a baby, and so he would have killed it like a baby. Another possibility is that he ordered the termination of this seed so as to be able to see it and inform us; for Galen too and Archigenes often dissected someone while he was still alive for the public benefit. Plato in the *Republic* orders that a courtesan should not participate in the state, just in case she conceives an illegitimate child and a darkling is born. Hippocrates took over this from Plato, because this is what he implies. He procured an abortion on this woman because she was a courtesan, so that she will not give birth to an illegitimate son. If Hippocrates had let the seed grow, the woman was going to hung herself as her beauty would be fading away, for courtesans prefer death to ugliness. So, Hippocrates thought that it would be better to destroy one soul, namely the seed, than two, and this is what he is implying.[90]

This passage certainly lacks the clarity, rationality, and comprehensive character of the aforementioned passage of Soranus discussing the apparent conflict between the Hippocratic Oath and Hippocratic practice, and the perceptions of these discrepancies in hellenistic and imperial times (see §iii above). However, John presents things from a very interesting perspective: Hippocrates here is not an almost divine figure from a remote past, but a practising physician who is confronted by a serious dilemma. He knows that if the conceptus were to be preserved, his patient's well-being and probably life itself might be at risk. This woman was a courtesan and her appearance was everything to her. If she lost her looks through a pregnancy she might kill herself. Making allowances for the usual jibe about courtesans and their vanity, we still have a situation where the physician is portrayed as an understanding figure, showing empathy for the woman's circumstances, appreciating the fact that an unwanted pregnancy might be devastating for his patient's mental health and overall well-being, considering the possibility that she could be led to suicide as a realistic one, and finally concluding that the preservation of his patient's life and health should be his primary concern. Thus he makes an informed decision to abort the conceptus. According to John's interpretation, the great Hippocrates is simply doing what any ordinary physician might do under a similar set of circumstances: he is faced with a difficult decision and, fully aware of the ethical implications, adopts the course of action he deems best for the preservation of the health and well-being of his patient.

Another issue that merits closer consideration at this point is that of self-inflicted injuries caused by the woman herself, or her unskilled aides, in an effort to terminate the pregnancy at home. From the time of Hippocrates doctors were aware that women tried to induce abortions at home following advice of questionable origin, and as a result often damaged themselves, sometimes seriously. The author of *Diseases of women* (8,140 = 1,67) is dismayed that women doctor themselves and sometimes cause grievous injury in the course of a self-induced abortion; further on (8,152 = 1,72) he reiterates the dangers of attempting to cause an abortion by means of drugs, pessaries, or any other. Galen also stresses the danger of pessaries (16,180, 19,456) and Soranus sends a clear warning that pessaries can be dangerous and that it is better to use contraception and avoid a pregnancy altogether, than to attempt an abortion (I 61,63).

At times doctors had to face the situation of a patient who had tried to induce an abortion, but in the process had been seriously injured (see for example the case of the wife of Simos quoted in Chapter 1 §i). The above-mentioned references to gynaecological conditions, which might constitute legitimate grounds for a therapeutic termination, include injuries that might result from an attempt to have an abortion at home. Faced with a situation like this, the doctor would not have much room for criticisms or dilemmas. He had to choose between refusing treatment, which might lead to the woman's death, or trying to save her life with a therapeutic abortion. The seriousness of this situation might have a strong impact upon a doctor's decision to attempt a termination of the pregnancy, whether he generally disapproved of abortions or not. Thus something that might start as an attempt to terminate a pregnancy for social or personal reasons, could end up as an imperative need for a therapeutic abortion.

The fact remains that, if one makes allowances for abortion on some grounds but not others, sooner or later the boundaries will be transgressed, and information intended only for therapeutic abortions will be used for abortions motivated by social or moral factors. We should be in no doubt that when Soranus, Galen and many other less illustrious practitioners gave advice on abortion, they were aware of the fact that this knowledge might be misused. Hypocrisy or duplicity may not be the right terms, but to assume that advice on abortions was always issued in good faith and for reasons of health would be naïve.

We can safely conclude that the boundaries between therapeutic abortions and abortions dictated by social, moral or economic reasons were not absolutely clear-cut. Most Greek doctors would be willing to perform an abortion if this was required for health reasons. They might not be very willing to go ahead with an undertaking that could be potentially lethal if there was no serious medical reason for it, but surely they understood that other colleagues might. Medical writers in particular would certainly realise that someone could use the information they provided for abortions not strictly related to health hazards. They simply resigned to the fact, and someone like Soranus could only trust in good faith that his colleagues, and the midwives for whose benefit he wrote his book, would follow the suggestion that termination should only take place if a serious health reason demanded it. Reluctance to perform abortions dictated by aesthetic or social considerations might often be nothing more than a sensible reaction to a very hazardous operation. However, sometimes it was more than that; it could be an expression of a moral or philosophical attitude. Doctors who subscribed to an intellectual tradition that human life began at conception would be hostile to abortion on ethical grounds. Equally, doctors who believed that the embryo acquires a soul and human identity before birth, but a while after conception, would be unwilling to terminate a foetus in more advanced stages of pregnancy. Doctors who did not believe that the embryo acquires human identity before birth might not have the same ethical dilemmas. However, this does not necessarily mean that they went ahead with abortions on demand. All medical practitioners have to consider the mother's well-being before they suggest a life-threatening undertaking. All doctors also have to measure the need for an abortion against the cultural background and ideals of society and their own moral perceptions. Doctors are men and women of their time, and contemporary cultural stereotypes leave their mark on their work and personality. However, in the ancient world they often were poor individuals struggling to make a living out of a messy and sometimes unsafe profession. A handsome fee for the prescription of a powerful abortifacient drug might be a temptation difficult to resist. To what extent their reaction would be aligned with principle and a sense of duty can only be answered after we consider further what kind of interests they had to look after.

vi. Morals and money

Doctors were generally immune from prosecution for lives lost in their care. This rule allowed medical practitioners to assist patients without risking a confrontation with the law if things went wrong. Foetal life was not exempt from this rule. To my knowledge, until the third century AD the law did not penalise a doctor for assisting a patient with an induced abortion (see also Chapter 6). The law was not a threat; the danger to their professional and personal prospects came from other quarters. At a time when most doctors were practising on a freelance basis reputations mat-

tered a lot. An excellent practitioner with high ethical standards but
incapable of marketing himself well and establishing a good reputation
might struggle in obscurity. On the other hand, a complete quack with
hardly any knowledge of medicine might become well established by
means of careful marketing strategies. Thus an ordinary physician probably could not afford to turn away too many patients with stern criticisms
of their morals. But he could not afford to appear too permissive either,
because then people might think he was nothing more than a *pharmakos*,
a shady character on a par with magicians and criminal elements operat-
ing on the margins of society. His predicament was to balance the needs
and demands of his patients against an ethical code of practice, his own
moral standards, and those of the society in which he operated. And in all
this he certainly could not afford to neglect his own financial interests.

Criticism of a patient's morals was the duty of a Greek doctor, to the
extent that these morals had an impact upon the patient's health.[91] Galen,
describing a series of situations that can be harmful for a pregnancy, says
that Hippocrates considered these situations to be suspicious, in the sense
that they might be intended to cause an abortion:

> The negligence of women during pregnancy was suspicious for Hippocrates,
> because most of it is their own fault, like intemperance and licentiousness in
> their entire lifestyle, sexual passions, great excesses of the soul, abrupt
> leaps, oral drugs and everything else, which creates the danger for the foetus
> to be rapidly destroyed.[92]

The list of situations potentially damaging to the pregnancy includes
items easily recognisable as such, such as violent movements and oral
drugs, evidently intended to induce an abortion, but also a series of social
habits, practices and moral qualities. However, the criticism of paying
customers could go only so far. We have seen that there are many loose
ends and uncertainties in the attitudes of Greek doctors towards abortion.
Ideals and principles probably mattered for most doctors to some degree,
but it would be naïve of us to see the entire issue as purely a question of
ethics and moral standards, disregarding economic factors. When the
doctor had to make a living out of his skill, his own financial needs were
bound to play an important role in his policy towards induced abortion.
One can picture a doctor tempted to leave aside his ethical or professional
reservations, and utter not a single word of criticism of the patient's
morals, when a generous reward was placed in his hand. And often the
furtive nature of the operation, as well as the possibility that a number of
doctors might be unwilling to go ahead with it, would raise the price of
those who were prepared to do it. Women wishing to avoid indignity,
divorce and severe penalties for adultery, would understandably meet the
high price of a doctor who was prepared to go ahead without asking too
many questions. The temptation was there and undoubtedly many doctors
yielded to it. E. Eyben believes that the rich were prime customers of

doctors for abortions, and this seems plausible.[93] A passage of Juvenal alludes to the promiscuity of high-class Roman women:

> But one rarely sees childbirth in gilded beds.
> Such are the skills, and so potent the drugs
> of the man who induces sterility and undertakes
> to have humans killed in the womb.[94]

The reason why they had abortions, as he explains further on, was that they were pregnant by their lovers, not their husbands, and they did not wish to be detected (see Chapter 4 §i, where this passage is further discussed in context). These rich Roman ladies could afford the services of skilful practitioners, and discretion was no doubt included in the fee. Poor women might not be able to afford a doctor with an efficient, sympathetic reputation. They had to resort to crude mechanical means or drugs blended from easily available herbs. On the other hand, the suggestion that abortion was a profitable business should not be pushed to extremes: there is no serious evidence that there was a black market in the ancient world. The wide availability of known or alleged abortifacient herbs, drugs and substances reduced the need for a medical practitioner at least as long as serious complications did not arise. The woman could obtain information about techniques and drugs from other women with more experience. This might not be as efficient or adequately tested as the advice given by an experienced physician, but if it had the desired effect and nothing serious happened a doctor would not be needed. If women knew quite a lot about such herbs and substances, as Riddle maintains, this would explain why there is no evidence of an abortion black market such as the one that flourished before the relaxation of the law in the 1960s.[95] Women knew enough to risk the undertaking without the supervision and advice of a doctor, and doctors knew too little to make their presence indispensable, unless things went seriously wrong. But certainly there was a market for drugs and techniques intended to induce an abortion, and those who had the knowledge and the skills could capitalise on it, personal and professional convictions permitting.

vii. The views of famous doctors of the ancient world

The personal views of the pioneers of medical science, whose work has been preserved for us, may be subjective and need not be representative of the period and intellectual tradition within which they operated. However, they merit closer consideration not least because they probably had considerable influence on the opinions of other less illustrious practitioners in antiquity and after. The dominant view in the classical period, that the foetus acquires human identity some time after conception but well before birth, is reflected in the Hippocratic Corpus where a substantial number of abortifacient drugs is mentioned and advice is offered on how to perform abortions by mechanical means shortly after a missed period. But the

Hippocratic Corpus is too diverse to allow us to tell for sure who believed what. Probably some of the authors did not even call the administration of such drugs in early pregnancy an 'abortion', and this is why they spoke rather of emmenagogues, purgatives and expulsives. Abortions in more advanced stages are certainly mentioned and explained, and a crude form of surgery is in use intended to deal with difficult, life-threatening situations. Philosophers of the classical period with an interest in the subject accept abortion as a reality, even though they are not necessarily sympathetic. Plato and Aristotle accept abortion as a means of population control. In the hellenistic period Chrysippus and the entire Stoic movement are criticised by Tertullian for denying the foetus human identity by insisting that animation takes place only after birth. If we accept the testimony of Tertullian, Herophilos had similar ideas, and, along with Erasistratus and Asclepiades, used a special instrument designed to kill and remove the foetus from the womb. Soranus declares sternly that he is not sympathetic to abortions performed for aesthetic reasons or in order to eliminate the fruit of adulterous relationships, but recognises the need for therapeutic abortions and offers a complex, seemingly efficient, method for inducing them. Galen, in his characteristically rhetorical manner, severely criticises women whose licentious lifestyle is the cause of risky abortions, but nevertheless incorporates in his voluminous work nearly all the advice on abortion that ancient pharmacology, dietetics and surgery had to offer. Priscianus, in a similar manner, invokes the Hippocratic Oath and criticises abortion on principle, but nevertheless offers plenty of information, theoretically to be used only for therapeutic abortions. Aetius also offers plenty of such information, and so does Oribasius in his sensible summary of Greek medical science. This quick glance allows the conclusion that the great doctors of the ancient world possessed information about abortions and evidently performed them, some according to more stringent criteria than others, but not with any expression of profound remorse or guilt. At any rate, no one felt the need to keep the act secret from his colleagues and readers.

viii. The medical woman and the midwife

A fair number of sources refer to female physicians in the ancient world (*iatrinai* or *iatreousai* in Greek; *medicae* in Latin).[96] The context is usually healthcare for women. The sources suggest that women cared for women, while male medical practitioners treated both sexes. In this respect it is not easy to draw a distinction between female medical practitioners and the traditional midwives (*maiai*), whose prominent role in women's healthcare is much better attested; indeed, I find the existing evidence insufficient to draw firm conclusions. It is likely that there was some kind of distinction between the two. As R. Flemming puts it, 'the key point is to recognize that titular distinctions may be meaningful whether or not they map very precisely onto distinctions of activity; and, therefore, to leave the *medicae* in the particular category they claimed for themselves and in which they achieved some acceptance'.[97] To say that the *iatrinai* and *medicae* had more training than midwives, or that they extended their range beyond typical gynaecological problems, and even beyond treatment of women, though not impossible, would be mere speculation. It may be significant that in the surviving literature when there is a need for a physician because there are serious complications in a gynaecological problem it is not an *iatrina* that is called in, but a male physician. Of course our sources could be biased and the role of the *iatrinai* not properly documented, but still, in such cases the male physician is more likely the figure that would inspire greater trust and represent that last hope of finding a treatment. The medical woman/midwife might have to work with the male doctor, but it is clear from Galen that this relationship was not between equals. He views female healthcare workers as his subordinates, and even when he praises the work of a certain midwife, it is as his assistant rather than his equal.[98] Whatever the case, terminology and distinctions among female healthcare workers are probably not important for the purposes of our study, for the simple reason that when a woman visited either an *iatrina* or a midwife in order to ask advice on abortion she would do so probably because she was hoping to find a more sympathetic ear than that of the male physician.

The midwife or the medical woman was probably a figure more familiar and less judgmental than a male doctor, and especially in smaller communities she may have been the most authoritative figure on gynaecological matters.[99] She had the ear of women, and she was probably trusted more easily with a sensitive matter such as a pregnancy that should not become public knowledge. Women would expect her to be more sympathetic to their plight, and even if she were not willing to give in to their request, at least the whole matter would be kept among women. The few available references to the role of the midwife in the community reveal that Greek midwives were well-respected figures with an important role to play as health advisers, and a daunting list of responsibilities. How seriously their role was taken can be seen by the fact that the most famous gynaecologist in the ancient world devoted two chapters of his book to the duties and ethical code of conduct of the midwife. Soranus' account (I 3-4) is a valuable source, because it explains in some detail what were their responsibilities, how they acquired their training, what qualities they should possess, what role they played as health practitioners and workers in the community, and what kind of ethical standards they were expected to observe.

There was a fundamental difference between the training of midwives and that of doctors in the ancient world. A good doctor was expected to have at least some knowledge of theory and an intellect capable of accommodating philosophy, and perhaps rhetoric and relevant disciplines, the study of which was the privilege of free-born males. As I mentioned earlier in this chapter, he was expected to rise above the crude essentials of his skill and view medicine in context as an exercise in wisdom. The training of the midwife was very different. Midwifery was a skill that encompassed the experience of many centuries and learned through practical training. In the words of Soranus, a midwife could learn and improve herself by observing her more experienced colleagues, who should become her role models. A certain physical ability was important for the proper perform-ance of the job, so a midwife should try to keep herself fit. She should take care that her hands did not become hardened by typical female household tasks such as spinning. Ideally she should have long fingers, and keep her nails short. But it was not so much physical characteristics that made a good midwife as adequate training and the qualities of her character.

Soranus, describing the tasks she should be able to perform, says that she should know how to diagnose a situation correctly, regulate a patient's diet, administer drugs and perform surgery. Certain qualities in her character and mental disposition could decisively assist the exercise of these duties. First of all she should be prudent and know her limitations, instead of assuming medical knowledge that she might not have. Then she ought to be free of superstition in order to be able to make the correct diagnosis on the basis of the symptoms, not of dreams and supernatural beliefs. She should not be affected by fear or panic in difficult situations, but administer the correct treatment with a cool head. Soranus places much emphasis upon her ability to communicate with the patient, adopt a sympathetic approach, and use soothing words to alleviate her suffering. Like the doctor in the Hippocratic Oath, she should have integrity and good character, as she would be entrusted to enter people's houses. She should also be incorruptible by money, so that she did not give an aborti-facient when there was no serious therapeutic need for one.

That midwives would be one of the main providers of information and drugs intended to induce an abortion needs no further explanation. How-ever, the wording of Soranus is interesting:

> She should be above money, so that she does not inappropriately (*kakôs*) administer an abortifacient for the sake of money.

He does not have any difficulty with the fact that a midwife might issue such a substance as a matter of principle. His objection has to do with the *inappropriate* administration of it for profit. Evidently he had in mind cases where women would go to the midwife and seek an abortifacient after they became pregnant in an adulterous relationship, or cases of women who wanted an abortion in order to keep their looks. As I have mentioned above, he disapproved of abortions for such reasons, and he knew that a midwife, like some doctors, might be tempted by money to offer advice and drugs. This he condemned and understood to be incom-patible with the duties of a responsible midwife.

In another much shorter but equally comprehensive account of a mid-wife's duties, from a Platonic dialogue, Socrates is presented as saying:

Midwives can start the labour by means of drugs and incantations, and they can make it gentler if they wish, and make women with difficult labour give birth, and induce abortions if they decide to do so, while the foetus is still immature.[100]

This is a valuable piece of evidence: it suggests that the tasks of the midwife had not really changed much from the classical period to the time of Soranus (second century AD). The midwife of Soranus may be more sophisticated and equipped with more skills, but the core of her duties remains the same as for the Socratic midwife.[101] The midwife of the classical period should be able to give the appropriate drugs, and perform difficult operations when necessary, and, like the ideal midwife of Soranus, she should have excellent communication skills and be able to offer solace to a patient in pain. The use of incantations, a traditional technique which was a survival from the days before the arrival of rational medicine, might still be in use by many midwives in the second century AD, but it would not be very much in the taste of a rational man like Soranus to recommend it. Yet the similarity which I find most striking is the attitude towards the role of a midwife in relation to induced abortions. Plato, like Soranus, does not condemn the performance of abortions on principle. On the contrary, he considers it to be a rather typical duty of the midwife, as typical as that of delivering women in labour, but with one qualification: the abortion was to take place while the foetus was still immature. Plato, in accordance with the dominant view in the classical period that the foetus acquires human identity while the pregnancy is in progress, does not object to abortion in the early stages, while the foetus is still unformed. Like Soranus, Plato is prepared to accept that abortion is one of the tasks that a midwife will be asked to perform, but it should be done only under the appropriate circumstances.

This evidence suggests that, unlike a doctor with good education, the midwife would not have to battle with great philosophical questions, such as animation or the value of human life. However, she certainly had her own dilemmas. She did not need a deep knowledge of philosophy and ethics in order to have a basic concept of the moral issues at stake. Like any male doctor, she carried certain cultural values and these influenced her judgement on a matter like abortion. For example, a Greek midwife or *iatrina* almost certainly would have been brought up to believe that adultery was an immoral and seriously inappropriate act for any self-respecting woman. The fact that she was a woman would not necessarily make her adopt a softer attitude towards an adulteress. Perhaps she might even adopt a harsher stance than a male doctor, if she thought that someone's behaviour was a disgrace for all prudent women. In a sense she might be more sympathetic than a man to the desperate plight of another woman, whose marriage and entire life would be in disarray if an illicit pregnancy were detected, but we cannot assume that she would be automatically prepared to condone all forms of illicit sexual relations of her patients, simply because she was a woman. Much depended on her own temperament and values, and the specific circumstances of her patient. Some midwives might be more stern, others more tolerant, but surely limits existed and moral issues were to be considered as part of the request for an abortion.

One additional factor that has to be seriously considered in the case of the *iatrina* or midwife is finance. Women of the better-off classes would consider it rather degrading than rewarding for a woman to go outdoors and practise a certain craft. Whether we are speaking about classical Athens or imperial Rome, the finance of the household was primarily the responsibility of the man, not the woman, and females who could afford to stay at home and look after their families and domestic duties would do so. This is why it is almost certain that midwives in the ancient world were recruited from the less well-off classes, and were women who learned the job because they needed the income in order to supplement the finances of their household. The average female healthcare worker did not enjoy the sponsorship and financial comfort that Democedes, Ctesias, Galen and many other male doctors had. She had to work hard for a living, and she needed the money. This is why the temptation to make a profit out of the inappropriate administration of abortifacient drugs and advice might be greater. It is perhaps this aspect that Soranus is trying to address when he stresses that a good midwife ought to have moral integrity and be in the position to refuse inappropriate exercise of her skills for profit.

The background and role of a midwife, as well as the challenges she had to face, might sometimes be different from those of a doctor, but whether a doctor or a midwife would decide to proceed with an abortion or not finally rested upon similar factors. Both had to balance their own financial interests, intellectual and cultural background, and personal temperament and choices, against the demands, needs and personal circumstances of their patients. The decision might not always be easy, but it was theirs to make.

Conclusions

The strength of Greek paganism as a cultural experience lies in the fact that it did not discourage diversity. Greek society could accommodate different strands of thought, practices and points of view without the need for assimilation. In such a society individuals could maintain their own views, ethical standards and perceptions, and in fact they were encouraged to think, to make up their own minds as to what would be their own course of action. This does not mean that Greek society did not have ideals, or did not ask its members to comply with widely acceptable morals and codes of practice. It simply means that it would allow more room for manoeuvre and permit wider freedom of choice. This general observation certainly applies to the field of medical ethics. Greek rational medicine required from its servants ideals, morals, and a highly ethical code of practice. From the outset the pioneers of this discipline established that scientific knowledge not motivated by ideals would be pointless, if not positively harmful. The quasi-mythical figure of Hippocrates, the Father of Medicine, stood as a source of inspiration and moral guidance for all doctors in subsequent centuries, ever reminding them that their goal was not only to unveil the mysteries of nature, but also to use this knowledge for the benefit of humanity. More significantly, ancient doctors did not perceive the latter as a mere by-product of their scientific training, but as a very important task, central to their role as medical practitioners. However, the practice of medicine remained a difficult and often danger-ous task. Doctors would have to work hard to create and maintain a good reputation, keep their clientele satisfied, and make an adequate living. These conditions, combined with the needs of patients from very different backgrounds and circumstances, would often create ethical dilemmas and potential conflicts with one's personal and professional conscience. Greek doctors had to resolve these dilemmas by trying to balance all these factors and they were allowed, if not compelled, to think, use their judgement, and come up with their own personal answers.

Few issues have been so divisive, and few have created such conflict and given rise to so much debate as abortion has, from antiquity to the present day. The response of Greek medical ethics to this difficult issue was motivated by high ideals, but at the same time allowed plenty of room for personal decision and consideration of the circumstances. Ideally Greek doctors were motivated by the call of duty to help or at least do no harm, by integrity and dignity, by respect for human life, and by their obligation to look after the physical, and sometimes mental and spiritual well-being of their patients. These ethical duties had to be considered along with the need to look after their own financial and professional interests and the circumstances in which a request for an induced abortion was made. And this is precisely the point where Greek paganism may differ from other cultures. While other cultures many a time in history have sought to impose a uniform response to the consideration of these factors, the Greeks left much to the judgement and consciousness of the individual doctor, medical woman or midwife. They had to think, trust their own judgement and conscience and make up their mind. The response of one doctor might be diametrically opposed to that of his colleague, but both were entitled to their views, and society was prepared to accommodate this diversity in expert opinion and practice. Doctors who practised within the frame of strict sects or guilds might be more restricted, but they were in the minority. Greek doctors did not have binding guidelines to obey, nor a golden rule to follow. They had to use their judgement and for this a good training in philosophy might prove valuable.

4

The Woman's Point of View

Abortion in a Greek village:
an anthropological parallel

To introduce this chapter I quote a striking passage from a twentieth-century Greek novel. In Stratis Myrivilis' controversial *Life in the Tomb*, banned in Greece for a number of years for its pacifist celebration of life amid the dehumanisation and horror of World War I, there is an abortion scene set in a village on Lesbos in 1913. Belios returns from the war, and Stylianoula, his wife, who is pregnant as a result of an affair during his absence, is attempting secretly to have an abortion, with the connivance of *his* mother. The two women are determined to keep the matter to themselves, but Belios instinctively feels that something has changed in his household. Another woman, supposedly with knowledge of abortifacient drugs, gives his wife a potion but things go badly wrong and he finds out. What was at stake? What was so important as to make the woman put her life at risk, and moreover do so with the connivance of other women, including her mother-in-law?

All this secretiveness was a worm of affliction devouring Belios's heart.
  One evening when he returned home somewhat earlier than usual he caught sight of an old woman leaving the house by the front door. She was tall, with a black wimple tied in a knot beneath her large chin. At the sight of him in the distance she could not suppress a tiny movement that betrayed a certain fright. Going hastily around the first corner, she disappeared. Something told him that this curious visit portended some indefinable evil for his household. Quickening his pace, he flew up the steps three at a time, the stairway creaking behind him.
  'Who was that?' he demanded of his mother in a rage. 'I saw her ugly puss coming out the front door just now. Tell me who she is. I've never noticed the likes of her around here before.'
  'Oh ... you saw her?' said the old mother, swallowing hard. 'Well, she's from Aivaly. An old neighbor of Stylianoula's. Came to pay her a visit. She nursed her in her earliest years, before she was weaned.'
  Stylianoula, who had turned as yellow as sulfur, confirmed this with a nod.
  'She's a long-time friend of her late mother's,' continued the old lady. 'Her name is Urania. She tells fortunes by reading coffee-grounds, too.'
  'You keep those witches out of here,' yelled Belios, banging his fist on the

table. 'I don't like them, understand! If she sets foot in here again, she'll find some mighty bad coffee here, in my house!'

A little later that same evening, when they gathered around the dinner table with their customary bickering and began to eat, Stylianoula suddenly let out a scream with the first mouthful she took.

'Oooch! Oh mama! mama!'

A terrible pain was knifing through her stomach and abdomen, together with a nausea that made her retch the very lining of her guts. The old mother went berserk. Turning waxen yellow, she ran here, ran there, came back again, grabbed one thing, let go of another – and was of no use whatever.

The blacksmith became frightened in his own right.

'What's the matter, wife? I said: What's the matter?'

Finally, Stylianoula was able to blurt out in the midst of her throes:

'I'm poisoned! The old hag poisoned me. Oh god, oh god.'

She inhaled deeply. The shadow of death, passing over her eyes, made them dilate and bulge with dread.

Suddenly Belios caught on.

Seizing her hair and yanking it until he nearly lifted her off the ground, he brought her contorted and unrecognizable face close to his own at first, then dragged it next to the lamp that was hanging on the wall. In bringing it near to the light in this way, he apparently wished to read the truth in those terror-stricken eyes, for he stared into their depths with his face practically touching hers drove his gaze into her like a stiletto – until all at once, like a lightning bolt, the truth did flash through those glazed eyes that were goggling in paralyzed dismay. It was a truth that cast light for him, but at the same time burned him to the quick. 'Slut!' he howled. 'So you got yourself with child while I was away in the army, is that it? And you had that hag bring you an herb, and you took it to get rid of the bastard in your tummy? Right?'

Still clutching her by the hair, he knocked her head against the wall.

'Right, slut? And with my own mother as your bawd, eh? Viper! Whore! Lousy filthy whore!'

'Forgive me, forgive ..., forgive ...' whimpered his wife, who was dangling like a rag from his powerful fist, her body contracted like an injured snake's because of the repeated pangs that were slicing through her entrails.

'Tell me his name! Who was it? Who filled your belly for you? Whore! Bitch! Tell me his name! Tell me!'

Still pressing her against the wall, he began to kick her womb with the tip of his shoe and to slap her face while still banging her head against the plaster. Soon a wound opened in the back of her scalp and blood began to splatter the newly white-washed inglenook.

In due course she ceased to resist his blows any longer or to implore his forgiveness. Instead, she commenced to groan softly and continuously – unsilenceably. She sounded like an aggrieved child whining quietly in a corner. Eventually this muted wail died out as well, her body suddenly slumped inertly in his grasp, her arms thrashed limply this way and that as he pummeled her, the eyes rolled upward until only the whites were visible, then went glazed beneath drooping lids.

Belios felt a chill invade the roots of his hair and, after this, something shrink inside of him, shrink gradually into nothingness and vanish – as though his heart were suspended from a number of cotton threads that were slowly but inexorably being cut one by one. He released his grip on her hair. Blood and sweat had pasted some of the tresses to the wall. As her livid corpse subsided onto the patchwork rug that covered the floor, her forehead struck a corner of the hearth with the dry clack of one inanimate object hitting another. Belios stood rooted in place, gazing at her in dazed incomprehension.

'Criminal! You murdered her,' shrieked his mother. 'Dog! Filthy dog!' And she fell upon the lifeless body.

Only at that moment did Belios realize how much he had loved that exceedingly attractive and coquettish little girl and how indispensable she had been to his existence. He understood then that the drooping lids that had closed over those scintillating eyes had also lowered a dark, irremovable sorrow over the remainder of his days. He wept for her, mourned her, lamented – is still lamenting. They brought him to trial and acquitted him. 'Execute me,' he begged the jurors at the top of his lungs, and they voted for acquittal! His mother died soon afterwards with the same grievance on her lips. From that time onward a sepulchre formed inside Belios's breast, a tomb surmounted by an ever-vigilant cresset burning with a tiny red flame: the hope that one day he might be able to quench his wounded heart's thirst for revenge.[1]

This crude, realistic scene strikes me as timeless. What happened to these women in twentieth-century Lesbos, could have happened in fifth-century BC Lesbos or Athens. An affair while the husband was away at war, an unwanted pregnancy as a result, a women's conspiracy to keep it secret, the complications and detection, the violent reaction of the shaken husband, all these could happen anywhere in the ancient world, and are attested in our sources.

Whether legal or illegal, abortion has been a widespread practice in most societies. Social sanctions, severe penalties, financial cost, the unpleasant character of the whole operation, considerations of health, or even danger of death have proved inadequate deterrents. It is evident that what has motivated women to seek abortions can be stronger than any deterrent that society, law or religion might seek to impose. This ineffectiveness of deterrents has been one of the main arguments in the debate that finally led to regulation replacing prohibition in many countries in the late twentieth century. At first sight this is a curious phenomenon considering that the legal systems of all civilisations are largely based on deterrence. This seems to work with almost every other aspect of human activity but apparently has proved totally inadequate in the case of induced abortion. I think this can be explained by means of a simple observation: one deterrent proves inadequate when an even stronger deterrent is placed against it. It can be argued that in many social settings the likely penalties or dangers of an induced abortion seem less important when set against what a woman has to lose if an unwanted pregnancy is allowed to come to term, and this undoubtedly encourages many to take the risk.

Whether the motives and fears of women were realistic or not is less important, because what may seem insignificant to a third party looking into a situation with sober logic may appear to be crucial for survival or future well-being to the person concerned. The emotional and mental disposition of the person directly concerned, in this case the pregnant woman, certainly has a very strong input into any decision over the pregnancy. And this input, combined with the woman's temperament and personality, her values and ideals, her background and past experience, and her expectations for the future, add up to a very personalised view. To stand outside and make statements about what one should or should not do may be logical, and sometimes constructive, but it is not the best guide to an understanding of the situation in all its dimensions and implications. In order to achieve that one needs to make an effort to identify with the emotions and motives of the subject and see things from her point of view. One needs to take into account her background, beliefs and aspirations as well as the social, economic and cultural context.

In trying to understand why women in all periods in history have been prepared to defy contemporary morality, danger, or impending legal sanctions and seek abortions, we must try to understand the pressures that urged them to do so. These pressures may look insignificant if we see things from our perspective or cultural background, but they can acquire tremendous significance if we see them from the subject's perspective and in their own social, economic and cultural setting. This is why we can never create an informed opinion unless we try to see the whole picture.

A number of recent studies on the motives of women seeking abortion underline the complexity and diversity of factors behind this request.[2] These studies are based on real cases and reflect the experience of modern medical practitioners with distressed patients seeking terminations for a wide variety of reasons. In this respect they allow a realistic insight into the motives of women and a more comprehensive understanding of the issues involved. In addition to these studies there is some anthropological research into a number of societies that offers an insight into the connection between the demand for induced abortions and social, economic and cultural factors. A brief presentation of these studies here will allow us to acquire a better understanding of the issues involved before we move back in time and try to understand the motives of women in an era documented almost exclusively through the eyes of men, for which the existing evidence is more subjective, less comprehensive and less 'scientific'.

H.L. Shapiro[3] in an anthropological study of abortion summarises the main motives of women as personal, cultural and economic. These factors are not mutually exclusive. For example, an unmarried woman who wishes to have a pregnancy terminated may need to consider not only the disapproval of society but also the financial burden of single motherhood and the serious affect on her chances of entering into a good marriage in future. So in this case one could say that there is a combination of all three factors. In fact, if we look closer we see that the pattern is quite complex. A study of abortion in modern Greece in the 1960s and 1970s seemed to show that abortions were induced almost exclusively for purposes of family planning.[4] But if we look at this case more thoroughly we see a combination of factors at work. Greek society in those years was trying to recover financially from the trauma of post-war poverty. That generation of women well remembered the starvation and deprivation they had suffered as children in large families with meagre resources. They were determined that the children they brought into the world would not have to go through the same traumatic experiences. They had aspirations for their existing children and wished to be able to provide for them better. Family planning was seen as a necessity, as a key to a more prosperous future, and the reasons for this were not purely economic. This was a society rapidly moving towards modernisation, a society in which women quietly but steadily had started to receive better education. In ever increasing numbers they had begun working, first in traditionally female professions such as teaching and nursing, but as this tacit revolution went on they entered into traditionally male dominated areas too, such as science or politics. These women no longer had the time, energy or disposition to bring up six or seven children. Family planning had become a necessity, inextricably linked with the modernisation of twentieth-century Greek society.

The same realities observed for modern Greece apply to many other Western societies. The dramatic changes in women's approved social roles in the second half of the twentieth century did not come without a price. The modern woman has much greater demands made upon her time and energies. She has more roles to fulfil, more aspirations to aim at, and certainly a greater degree of responsibility in all spheres of life. Pregnancy, childbirth and traditional motherhood now have to be fitted into a much more complex frame. Family planning and tighter control of reproductive patterns appear as necessities in modern life. Perhaps this is why more affluent and advanced societies have a higher rate of abortion:[5] what is expected of women in such societies often comes into direct confrontation with traditional motherhood duties, and they have to choose.

L. Thomson[6] sees abortion as a phenomenon related to norms governing sexual behaviour, patterns of reproductive motivation, life goals and approved social roles for women, rights of privacy, and demographic trends. That norms governing sexual behaviour have been responsible for most of the abortions performed throughout history is not be hard to believe. Motherhood outside marriage was absolutely unacceptable in most societies before the last quarter of the twentieth century. Women who conceived outside wedlock would be stigmatised, ostracised, rejected by family, friends and society as a whole, and sometimes even penalised and not allowed to keep their babies after birth. For example, a woman who became pregnant as a result of an ill-considered teenage escapade would be rejected and marginalised at the time. If she went ahead with the pregnancy her family might intervene and compel her to give the baby up for adoption at the time of the birth, thus trying to remove the shame brought upon the family. And as if all this suffering was not enough, if the woman lived in a small community where such acts could not go undetected, she would certainly find it difficult to start her life again. Most men in the community would not wish to marry a woman with such a reputation, and most women would not wish to be associated with her. With such deterrents set up by social norms related to sexual behaviour it is no wonder that any deterrent intended to stop induced abortion would seem inadequate. In comparison to such repercussions an abortion would appear the easy way out, and this is why many women were prepared go to great lengths in order to have a pregnancy terminated.

Economic reasons are probably the second most common cause of abortions throughout history. The example of modern Greece, mentioned above, unambiguously suggests that the parents' ability to 'afford' another child may have a decisive influence upon their decision to continue with the pregnancy or not. Moreover, in modern life the action of economic factors is not limited to domestic finances. It extends beyond the walls of the family home into the job market, the careers of the man and the woman involved, and their share of duties and responsibilities. In societies that did not offer women the same opportunities for career development the motive for an abortion on such grounds would be much less pressing. For women whose role was to stay at home and look after the family, an abortion for the purposes of personal ambition would be irrelevant. In fact, women in such social settings might proudly be mothers of several children, as this strengthened their role in the family and society, and motherhood was a source of prestige and dignity. But in societies where women are expected to participate as equals in the political and economic process, motherhood may not always be as straightforward an issue as nature intended it to be.

Finally, two studies, one by P.C. Olley and one by G. Howard,[7] on the mental state of women seeking abortions, point out the importance of this factor on many occasions. I know personally of two women who had no apparent reason for attempting an abortion – apparent, that is, to anyone judging the situation from a purely rational point of view – who yet went to great lengths in their efforts to have self-induced abortions. No one around them, including their husbands, could understand their reasons and motives. One of them had a history of psychiatric disorders, the other a faltering marriage. It is very difficult to understand such motives fully, as it is difficult to obtain an insight into an individual's mind and personal perspective on a situation. This, however, does not make the woman's reasons any less compelling.[8]

Clearly we must take account of women's personal circumstances in trying to understand their motives for seeking an abortion. However, the historical background, and the social, economic and cultural setting are also important factors, and by no means mutually exclusive. Understanding this background is easier for well documented periods, but much more difficult when it comes to the distant past.

Our information on the history, society and culture of the ancient world is not desperately poor, but it is not as good as we might like. Specific references to the personal situations of women who attempted abortion are rather sparse and often subservient to other purposes, literary or ideological. But if we place these references against the social, economic and cultural background of the ancient world (on which we are better informed) we may get an insight into their motivation. Our sources reveal a wide variety of personal, social and economic factors. Women were not a homogeneous group: they could be classed as citizens, aliens or slaves; they were rich, comfortably well-off, or poor; they could be quiet or forward, passive or strong, virtuous or licentious, prudish or open-minded. So it would be a methodological mistake to treat all women as one and the same, or understand that they all had the same standards of morality, attitudes, beliefs and aspirations. However, some parameters, such as laws or some core beliefs with universal appeal, were fixed. This allows us to create a number of settings within which we can explore the motives of women seeking abortions. In the following sections I separate women who might seek abortions into groups, and I explore their personal circumstances against the social, economic, and cultural circumstances of their society. I believe that the pictures that emerge provide adequate explanations as to why women were prepared to undertake considerable risks in their desire to have an unwanted pregnancy terminated.

i. The adulteress

The ancient Greek world before Alexander was divided into small political units, the *poleis* (city-states), which were independent and proud of their separate identity. Each *polis* had its own legal system, constitution and institutions designed to suit a small geographical area and a small population. This adult male citizen population, whose voice really mattered in the institutions of the state, would be a minority outnumbered by women, children, non-citizens and slaves, who did not have a voice in most areas of public life. Naturally this privileged minority would be very much concerned with two issues: one was to keep its purity, the other was to perpetuate itself. This is why, regardless of the actual political system that each Greek polis had adopted (democracy, oligarchy, tyranny), concepts such as the legitimacy of children and the continuation of the citizen stock were very important.[9] Public and private life were organised on the basis of family units, the *oikoi*, ensuring that the future citizens of the state would be legitimately born offspring of citizens.[10] Marriage and childbirth within wedlock were sanctioned by society, religion and the laws of individual city-states.[11] Despite local variations, succession by legitimate heirs and the continuation of the citizen stock were important goals of ancient Greek laws regulating family life and sexual activity, and these concepts were also important with regard to social attitudes concerning family life and sexuality. The prominent role of these concerns in the formation of social attitudes had created a remarkable coexistence of basically opposing points of view regarding sexual morality in the Greek world, something that scholars have called 'a double standard'. Perhaps no other culturally advanced society in the history of humanity has known such levels of sexual freedom as the Greek city-states.[12] The human body and sexuality were celebrated in literature, art and athletic competitions, and eroticism proudly and openly pervaded every aspect of public and private life, religion included. Yet, at the same time we see in operation a set of severe laws intended to curb sexual activity, and we hear much in ancient Greek literature about virtues such as modesty, virginal shyness, sexual fidelity, and the inclination to withdraw from the predatory eyes of potential suitors. How could such extremes be accommodated in the same social setting?

The answer I think lies in the observation that both legitimacy of children and the continuation of the citizen stock were all-important concepts in the Greek world. Sexual activity was unrestricted where the legitimacy of any offspring was not an issue. Men could have affairs with courtesans, common prostitutes, slaves, or even keep a concubine if they could afford it, and no one would object because any offspring of such unions would be by definition illegitimate, and in most cases excluded from the line of succession and citizenship. Homosexual relationships between men (and probably between women too), which sometimes reached a very deep emotional level, were not only acceptable but also considered an important step in one's personal and social development.[13] Slaves of both sexes could copulate as they pleased, unless their master thought that such activity was affecting their performance at work, or was likely to produce unwanted offspring, and on such grounds decided to chastise or curb it.[14] Women and men could practise all forms of prostitution, and their work was not only legal but also treated by some city states as a craft similar to that of joinery, metalwork, or medicine.[15] However, in all these forms of sexual activity the legitimacy of the offspring was not an issue, and as such there was no clear reason for the state to legislate against it, and for society to condemn it.

The picture was very different when it came to the sexual activity of females designated to become mothers of legitimate heirs and future citizens. Citizen women, first-degree relatives of citizens, i.e. a citizen's wife, mother, sister or daughter, did not have the same levels of sexual freedom. On the contrary their sexual activity was strictly confined within marriage. Such restriction was seen as necessary for the husband, so that he could be sure that any offspring were his, for the family, so that they could be sure about the legitimacy of the offspring who would inherit the *oikos* and continue the family line, and for the state, so that it could be sure that children presented as citizens were truly of citizen stock. These concepts of marriage and legitimacy of children were also adopted by families in social groups such as alien residents or liberated slaves, even though the concept of legitimacy would matter much less in such groups in terms of political rights.[16] To put it simply, in every respectable family, whether citizens or not, a woman was definitely expected to remain faithful to her husband, and if she was unmarried she had to wait until a husband was found for her. This sense of respectability and the duty to remain faithful to their partner extended even to concubines, even though in most Greek states their offspring would be illegitimate by definition. Older women might have more freedom of movement, but by the time they had reached that age their deeply ingrained sense of propriety would not allow most of them to go about having affairs with strange men. The idea that sexual activity ought to be regulated by law only when it really matters with regard to the status of the offspring is clearly reflected in a passage of Plato. In his ideal state, childbirth was strictly regulated along the following lines:

> I said that a woman should give birth to children for the city between the ages of twenty and forty, and a man after he has reached his peak. From this point he should father children for the city until the age of fifty-five ... And when women and men are beyond the age of childbirth, we should let them free to go with whoever they wish.[17]

Perceptions such as these were common in the ancient world even outside the Greek city-states.[18] Whatever the place or the social setting, extramarital relationships were not tolerated for women whose purpose in life was to give birth to legitimate offspring, and in extension for all women who were placed under the authority and legal guardianship of a man (see below). Such relationships, whenever they materialised, were treated as a grave criminal offence by the laws of the state, and brought great shame and indignity upon the woman who had engaged in them, the woman's *kyrios* (namely the man under whose legal guardianship the woman had been placed), and her family as a whole.

In the Greek world the term *moecheia* was employed to indicate any illicit relationship of this type. Modern scholars translate it into English as either 'adultery' or 'seduction'. Both terms are inadequate, as neither can render the complexity and character of the Greek word. The English word 'seduction' renders well the intention of the parties involved: *moecheia* had been committed when both the man and the woman involved had consented to the relationship. But 'seduction' fails to encapsulate the technical character of *moecheia*, with all its legal and moral connotations. 'Adultery' encapsulates these aspects, but its usage in English is confined to breach of the marital bond. *Moecheia*, on the other hand, was employed to render any form of illicit sexual relationship, performed with any woman who belonged to a man and was under his authority and legal protection, and not only his wife. It was not an offence against any abstract idea (e.g. fidelity) or institution (e.g. marriage), but an offence by one man against another man's authority and masculinity, and posed a threat to the latter's family line and the legitimacy of his offspring. This is why it was so severely treated that in many places the killing of the adulterer was considered to be justified homicide. The Athenian homicide law of Dracon (seventh century BC), explaining the circumstances under which homicide

is justified, at the same time defined the groups of women with whom
adultery could be committed:

> If one kills someone unintentionally in an athletic contest, or overcoming
> him in a fight on the highway, or unwittingly in battle, or in intercourse with
> his wife, or mother, or sister, or daughter, or concubine maintained with a
> view to the birth of free children, the killer should not be convicted on such
> grounds.[19]

Other penalties imposed upon the adulterer included severe fines (in the
law of Gortyn in Crete), bodily humiliations (Athens, Rome), and public
humiliation (Crete).[20] All were imposed upon the man, the seducer, who,
at least as far as the law was concerned, was the prime instigator of this
crime against another man. They were designed to curb the activities and
sexual desires of men involving free females who belonged to other men.
And while in several states the law dealt severely with the man, it did not
bother to punish the woman; this was left to the family. In Athens we know
that the law did not punish the woman until the fifth century BC. However,
in 451 BC a law introduced by Pericles set down that only the offspring of
two citizens could be citizens.[21] With this law the woman ceased to be a
mere biological accessory to the process of childbirth. Her role was recognised by law, and this is why stricter precautions were introduced,
designed to protect the legitimacy of the children and keep illicitly conceived offspring out of the citizen body. The state decided to intervene and
order the husband of the adulteress to divorce her, on penalty of disfranchisement if he refused. The same law imposed severe sanctions upon the
woman herself: she was no longer to be admitted to the public temples, and
she was not allowed to wear jewellery. A quotation from this law is
preserved in an Attic law-court speech:

> After he catches the adulterer, the man who caught him shall not be
> permitted to continue living with the woman in marriage. If he continues
> living with her in marriage he is to be disfranchised. And the woman with
> whom an adulterer has been caught shall not be permitted to enter the
> public temples. If she enters, she is to suffer whatever she suffers, except
> death, with impunity.[22]

A contemporary orator paraphrases the text of this law as following:

> (The law) does not allow the woman with whom an adulterer has been
> caught to dress up and wear jewellery, or enter the public temples .... And if
> she enters or dresses up and wears jewellery, it allows anyone who wishes
> to tear her clothes, and remove the jewellery, and hit her, short of death of
> permanent injury.[23]

The clear intention of this law is to exclude the woman caught committing
adultery from public life, and from all activities that would be a source of
pride and dignity (such as marriage, outings in style, dressing up, wearing

jewellery). The exclusion from the public temples amounted to virtual isolation at home, since religion was the main area of public life in which women were active participants. Exclusion from the temples thus meant exclusion from public life, and in the case of the adulteress this exclusion was permanent. If she dared to ignore this law she made herself liable to a level of indignity and shame that no one dared to inflict upon any other woman in Athens, not even a lowly slave. There are some references to even stricter punishments in some cities. Two passages from Aelian's *On animals* clearly suggest that the adulteress at least deserved to share the guilt of her sexual partner and be treated with equal severity. In the first of these passages an elephant kills the adulterous wife of his master and her boyfriend, leaving the two of them lying on the mattress where the adultery was committed, so that her husband would understand what she had been up to.[24] In another story from the same book a stork blinds the wife of his master when he sees her committing adultery with one of the servants of the household.[25] A law in Lokroi allowed the killing of the woman too, if she was caught committing adultery.[26] Moreover, an important (and difficult to interpret) passage in Chariton's novel *Chaireas and Callirhoe* seems to imply that if a husband caught his wife committing adultery and in a rage killed her, he might be able to claim in his defence that she was an adulteress and thus that the killing was justified (as it would have been if he had killed the man caught with her). I have argued elsewhere that Chariton echoes here the narrative of Lysias' speech *On the murder of Eratosthenes*, where Euphiletos kills Eratosthenes, the man whom he allegedly caught committing adultery with his wife.[27] Thus it is difficult to tell whether the novel reflects reality or simply adjusts the narrative of a fourth-century law-court speech in a manner suitable for the plot. Whatever the case, one can not exclude at least the theoretical possibility that an ancient jury might accept the argument that since the law allowed the killing of the adulterer, his accessory to the crime should be treated equally severely.

In addition to any punishments and sanctions that the laws of the state might have in store for the adulteress, surely the family would have its own ways of punishing the woman who had brought indignity and shame upon the entire family. Two later epigrams mention a good thrashing and throwing the woman naked into the street,[28] and there is no good reason to doubt that such forms of punishment were imposed by the family. Mistrust, contempt, verbal and psychological abuse, and social ostracism would probably be realities in the life of a woman caught committing adultery for many years after the incident.

The evidence concerning the Roman laws on adultery in the republican period is not very clear. However, the practice seemed to be widespread among the upper classes, and, in the words of C. Edwards, 'for Roman writers, adultery among the elite was a telling symptom of disease in the body politic'.[29] Perhaps it was a social phenomenon of this kind that a series of laws on marriage and adultery introduced under Augustus in 18

BC was expected to correct. Two laws, the *lex Iulia de adulteriis* and the *lex Iulia de maritandis ordinibus* (the latter modified nine years later by the *lex Papia Poppaea*), introduced in 18 BC, were intended to put in order the marriage and adultery laws of Rome, seeking to discourage immorality among the Roman elite and safeguard the survival of the Roman family as an institution in a rapidly changing world. Under the new laws a woman caught committing adultery in her father's house could be killed together with her lover on the spot by her father, and sometimes by her husband too. If she survived the encounter, she ought to be divorced by her husband (or he would be subject to legal sanctions) and lose half her dowry and a third of her property. In future she was barred from wearing the *stola* (the dress of a respectable Roman matron), and could not remarry a free-born Roman.[30] Thus it may not be far off the mark to say that Augustus introduced legislation governing family life and sexual morality that bears remarkable similarities to the fierce laws that had been in operation for centuries in Greek cities. Roman law was much more technical and precise than the laws of the Greek city-states, but its spirit was the same: properly born women should not have sexual relations with any other man than their husband, and if they did, they should be treated as social outcasts and penalised by the law, because they were considered primarily responsible for the break-down of the family bond. The impact of this legislation is a disputed issue, and the laws were repealed by Constantine in the years after 315 AD.[31] Sources suggest that adultery among the Roman elite continued to be commonplace and the repeated efforts by Roman emperors to stimulate family life would rather suggest that the impact of this legislation was limited.[32] However, this does not alter the fact that Roman women, especially after 18 BC, had much to lose if they were caught having an affair, and thus had strong reasons to try to hide any illicit liaison by whatever means necessary.

Is it surprising that with such deterrents set up by society and the law, women who had conceived as a result of an extramarital affair would go to great lengths to have the foetus aborted? Such deterrents might appear to the woman's eyes as stronger than the potential dangers and pains of an induced abortion, and such social attitudes would make the dilemma over the morality of an induced abortion sound totally academic. Plutarch tells this story about a Spartan girl who became pregnant before she was married:

> Someone who lost her virginity and had the foetus aborted endured the ordeal in such a manner that she did not make a sound, so that neither her father nor anyone else around her noticed that she had been pregnant and had an abortion. Thus decency overpowered the strength of the pains brought upon her by her previous indignity.[33]

Anyone who has read Plutarch's *Life of Lycurgus*[34] can not fail to notice the unmistakable similarity with the story of a Spartan boy who had stolen a fox and hidden it under his garment so as not to be detected. The fox started eating his flesh, yet the boy would rather endure the excruciating pain of this than be caught stealing. Finally the fox ate her way through his guts and the boy died. The Spartans mentioned this story as an example of true Spartan virtue. Boys took pride in stealing, but they should not be caught, because if they did they were punished, and this conduct was encouraged by Sparta as part of the boys' military training.[35] The boy in the story endured excruciating pain until he died because the honour and virtue of a Spartan should come before personal suffering. The girl who endured the pains of an abortion in silence was motivated by the same sense of honour and virtue. Keeping her honour was as important for a Spartan woman as military valour was for a Spartan man.

This story is characteristic of the impact of social values and ideals upon attitudes surrounding induced abortion and its dangers. To start with, these social values, namely what Spartan society considered appropriate for a citizen woman, were the motivation for having the abortion. Not only had she to go ahead with the undertaking, but she also had to remain undetected. If she had been caught having the abortion this would have defeated the purpose of the entire operation, because it would have revealed her as a woman who had shamed herself and her family. Plutarch alludes to the indignity that this action would bring upon her father. So her father and everyone else around should not notice what had happened. In this respect the pressure of social norms and rules acquired a much more concrete form in the shape of the fear of her father and immediate family. This fear, combined with the strong sense of respect for social values and virtues that Spartan citizens, male and female alike, were reputed to possess, created a driving force strong enough to overpower not only any reservation or doubt that the woman might have, but, according to our story, even the pain of the abortion.

Similar elements and attitudes are well attested in a number of sources. Aeschines tells us how in early Athens a young woman who had sex before marriage was punished by her father. He shut her into a house together with a horse, sure in the knowledge that she would be killed by the horse at some stage. The orator says that the place where the house had stood was still called 'the place of the horse and the girl' up to his own time.[36] Other similar stories were probably in circulation and they certainly reflect a social morality that strongly opposed premarital relations for women. In archaic Athens a law of Solon permitted the father to sell into slavery a daughter of his who had intercourse before marriage, but MacDowell correctly says that this law was no longer valid in the fifth and fourth century.[37] In classical Athens the woman's father did not have the legal right to put her to death or sell her as a slave. However, an unmarried woman who had intercourse would certainly be classed as an adulteress (*hê gunê eph' hê an moichos halô*[38]), and she was subject to the disabilities imposed by the law upon women caught committing adultery. In addition, besides any legal sanctions, surely the woman's father had enough power in his hands to humiliate her on a daily basis and make her life unbear-

able, and enough authority as a man and head of his household to make
her tremble with fear at the thought that he would find out. And if such
deterrents were not sufficient the woman would normally have enough
respect and affection for her father so as not to wish to shame him publicly.
The fear of one's parents as the leading motive behind the decision to have
an abortion is also mentioned explicitly in the commentary of Zonaras on
St Basil's letter to Amphilochios:

> Some women conceive illicitly by corrupting themselves with men. Then
> perhaps because of fear of their parents, or masters, or someone else, they
> contemplate the expulsion of the embryo by means of some orally adminis-
> tered drugs, or even by other means, and destroy the foetus.[39]

The same idea appears in another Byzantine canonical commentary by
Blastares on canon 91 of the Synod *in Trullo*.[40] This canon is probably
inspired by Basil's views on the subject. A slightly different approach to
the subject is taken by Tertullian,[41] who says that a forced virginity is
responsible for abortions, because women who stray would go to great
lengths to conceal the fact that they had become 'mothers' (*ne etiam mater
detegatur*). The only effective answer he can provide is voluntary virginity
inspired by Christian ideals.

Whatever the source of the fear might be, from parents, family, society,
the law, scandal, indignity, one thing is certain: this fear could be intense
enough to cause serious emotional disturbance and mental confusion. The
state of mind of a frightened woman desperately trying to procure an
abortion in order to avoid being caught having a prohibited relationship is
captured by Ovid in one of the fictitious letters of his *Heroides* (11, 37-44).
Canace relates how she was feeling when all her attempts to have the
pregnancy by her brother Macareus terminated failed:

> Already the weight of the injured womb was increasing
> And the secret load burdened the sickened limbs
> Was there any herb or drug that my nurse did not bring
> And herself insert with a steady hand,
> So that the load growing inside our womb be killed?
> (this thing alone we kept secret from you).
> Ah! This strong baby resisted all administered drugs
> And defied the disguised enemy.

In this case the fear of detection of a premarital sexual relationship, and
moreover an incestuous one, led the heroine and her trusted nurse to try
in vain all kinds of herbs, drugs and pessaries. In despair they watched as
every available method failed to produce the desired effect. Canace speaks
of the marked deterioration of her own physical health as a result of this
situation (*vitiati ventris / aegraque membra*), and points out the frustrated
determination of her nurse, who went so far as to insert the vaginal
pessaries herself with 'a steady hand' (*audaci supposuitque manu*). Literary scholars have argued intensely over the interpretation of this passage.

Some have perceived Canace as an 'innocent mother', others as a type characterised by 'banality' and 'inflexible lack of moral tension'.[42] I do not wish to engage in such controversy; however, I find this passage intriguing as a literary presentation of the fearful, confused and desperate state of mind of the unmarried woman who is prepared to go to any lengths to have an abortion in order to avoid being detected having an incestuous affair.

Greek law did not even differentiate between an unmarried and a married woman who had an affair; the laws on *moecheia* would apply in both cases. Roman law differentiated between *adulterium* (an affair with a married woman) and *stuprum* (an affair with an unmarried woman), but imposed penalties on both. Thus unmarried women, including widows or divorcees, were in a similar position as far as the law and sexual morality were concerned, and similar pressures to those applying for married women would be in force in their lives too. To give one striking example, several Roman authors refer to the tragic incident involving Julia, the widow of Flavius Sabinus, and daughter of the emperor Titus.[43] Her uncle Domitian, who later became emperor after the death of her father, was offered her hand while they were both still unmarried, but he refused because he was in love with his future wife Domitia. However, after Julia was given in marriage to Flavius Sabinus an illicit liaison started between the two. The relationship lasted for a long time and continued even after the death of both her father and her husband. Now Domitian as emperor lavished his attentions on the young widow. However, at the same time the Emperor was campaigning for traditional morality and passing laws against adultery. Juvenal does not miss the chance to ridicule Domitian's hypocritical morals:

> Such was the case, not so long since, when you-know-who
> was busy reviving those stern decrees against
> adultery: even Mars and Venus blushed. But all
> the while he himself was flouting the law – and spiced
> his crime with a dash of incest, in the proper tragic tradition.
> his niece, a fertile creature, had her row of abortions,
> and every embryo lump was the living spit of Uncle.[44]

Domitian might be a hypocrite, but he was not prepared to be publicly exposed as one. This is why, when his widow niece became pregnant, he would not allow her to keep the child. Both Pliny and Suetonius categorically state that Domitian compelled her to have an abortion. But things went seriously wrong, and Julia died as a result.[45]

Married women who had become pregnant as a result of an illicit liaison could always claim that they were pregnant by their husband. D. Ogden, in his thorough study of bastardy in the Greek world, correctly points out that illegitimate offspring of adulterous liaisons were not easily detectable,[46] unless of course the father was of different racial origin. Juvenal makes a rather caustic remark on this:

But one rarely sees childbirth in gilded beds.
Such are the skills, and so potent the drugs
of the man who induces sterility and undertakes
to have humans killed in the womb.
Just be glad, you poor man, and give her the potion yourself,
for if she chose to let her womb swell,
vexed with the kicks of a child,
you might find yourself father of an Ethiopian.[47]

Juvenal implies that the wife had a love affair with an African slave and conceived as a result of this. If this pregnancy were allowed to come to term it would provide unambiguous proof of adultery, and it would be a great insult to the husband's masculinity. Aelian relates a story along the same lines: a woman in Sicily had a love affair with an African slave but the child was born white. However, the grandchild of the woman was born black, and thus her adulterous liaison was detected one generation later.[48] Aristaenetos also mentions a woman who had a love affair with a domestic slave.[49] Juvenal in another passage says that some women preferred to take eunuchs as lovers, not only for their smooth skin but also because there would be no need for an abortifacient.[50]

These of course are tales or general remarks, but there is no need to question the possibility that such cases really existed. We can easily understand why, in a society where arranged marriages, large age differences, and minimal emotional communication between husband and wife were commonplace, women would seek affection in the arms of their slaves.[51] Considering that most domestic slaves were brought into Greek or Roman cities from Africa (and called Ethiopians by the Greeks and Romans), or from around the Black Sea (slaves with names such as Xanthias [Blondie] or Pyrrhias [Redhead]),[52] conception of children with visibly different racial characteristics from those of the woman and her husband was a realistic possibility. And if the adulterous couple had so far succeeded in remaining undetected (not very difficult if the man was living in the same house as a domestic slave), the racial features of their offspring would reveal the illicit liaison. It is no wonder that women in this position went to great lengths to eliminate the most reliable witness to their infidelity.

Married women whose husbands were away for long periods were in a similar position, as they could not claim that the child was by their husband. Let us remember the scene from Myrivilis' novel, quoted above, where Styliano could not cover up her pregnancy and the affair since her husband had been away from Lesbos fighting in Macedonia and Thrace for the last couple of years. The absence of men for long periods of time, on military campaigns or business, was a regular occurrence in places such as Athens, especially during the years of the Athenian empire and the Peloponnesian war.[53] An adulteress who became pregnant during the lengthy absence of her husband would be in serious trouble.

Against this background even women who were seeking abortions for other reasons (with the exception of compelling medical conditions) could always be suspected of infidelity. Galen considers excessive lifestyle and lack of moderation during pregnancy to be suspicious, as it could be a deliberate tactic intended to induce an abortion, and consequently to conceal moral licentiousness.[54] Plutarch also considers such behaviour as typical of lustful women (*akolastoi gunaikes*), 'who use expulsives and abortifacients, so that they can fill themselves again with pleasures and hedonism'. Similar attitudes are expressed in the famous passage of Soranus, where he states that some doctors refused to perform abortions upon women seeking to eliminate the product of an adulterous relationship.[55] But perhaps most characteristic of all is a passage of Tacitus where it is said that Nero, who had fallen in love with Poppaea, succeeded in removing his wife Octavia after accusing her of intending to conceal an adulterous liaison by means of an abortion.[56]

Attitudes such as those mentioned above would put a woman seeking an abortion for whatever reason under suspicion of adultery. Such suspicions would often be perfectly justified. Abortion in the ancient world was a difficult and dangerous undertaking attempted by women in considerable distress and fear. The unwelcome consequences of a love affair in societies where extramarital relationships were considered absolutely unacceptable and inappropriate for properly brought up women would provide a powerful motive. What women had to lose if they were detected as a result of a pregnancy outside marriage was far too much to allow for prudent considerations concerning their health and the morality of their actions. With such powerful deterrents set up by the family, the state and society as a whole, an abortion may often have seemed the only way out. Women knew that it was risky and troublesome, and that success was not guaranteed. However, when compared to permanent stigma and indignity, social ostracism, exclusion from the temples and public life, almost guaranteed violence against their person if not an impending threat to their life, constant humiliations at home, a guaranteed divorce and probably permanent separation from their existing children if they were married, and no realistic hope of a future marriage, abortion definitely appeared the lesser of two evils. Many women were prepared to attempt it in the hope that they might succeed and get away with it.

ii. The prostitute

Prostitution was a widespread phenomenon in the ancient world, perhaps more so than today.[57] Not only was it perfectly legal, but it was also to some extent acceptable by religion and society as a fact of life and a necessary social practice. In the Greek world a number of festivals attracted courtesans,[58] and the sumptuous temple of their goddess protector Aphrodite in Corinth was famous for its riches. Athenian law recognised prostitution and in a sense tried to define it by not allowing accusations of adultery with any woman who was visibly practising any form of prostitution.[59] The state taxed the earnings of women established in brothels, set a ceiling price, and treated prostitution as one of the trades practised in the various workshops around the city.[60] Society was prepared to accept prostitution as a necessary outlet for the sexual appetites of men, which otherwise might be directed at decent women. Athenaeus praises Solon for his insight to establish women in brothels, for, he says, this way proper women were protected from the lust of young men. Male prostitution was as acceptable as female prostitution. However, the Athenians did not think it proper for male prostitutes to hold some offices closely connected with religion, such as the archonships, or advise to the Assembly.[61] The Greek cities were generally tolerant and broad-minded concerning matters of sexual morality, but at the same time resolutely determined to protect the family, legitimacy of offspring, and dignity of women destined for family life. This double standard created the ideal circumstances for prostitution to flourish. Slavery offered human resources in plenty, and limited job opportunities for women encouraged even some free-born females to take up prostitution as the obvious and least troublesome way to make a living. As men's access to properly brought up women was restricted, it is only to be expected that they would turn their attention to those who were willing or made by circumstances to offer sexual favours for profit. This was seen as a safety valve and thus prostitution was allowed to flourish in a large variety of forms, from common prostitutes established in brothels, to freelance street-walkers and expensive long-term companions. The last group in particular, the famous *hetairai* of the ancient world, was often associated with the rich and the powerful. Some of these women caught the imagination of authors and artists with their glamour, beauty, education and spirit, and have achieved a personal place in history, a dubious honour to which few respectable women could aspire.

In the Roman world, as the thorough study by T.A.J. McGinn has demonstrated, prostitution was equally widespread. Roman law, however, imposed stricter guidelines, clearly classed prostitutes in the lowest band of the social hierarchy, and was determined to prevent them from sneaking their way into the upper classes by means of marriage to the Roman elite. Throughout antiquity female prostitutes, whether free or slaves, high or low class, were entirely dependent upon their bodies for their livelihood. A pregnancy would disable them for several months, and it could have adverse effects upon their appearance. As a result they would lose their clientele, and along with this their only source of income. The more expensive courtesans might be forced thereafter to join the cheaper end of the market, with the consequent reduction in income, deterioration of their lifestyle, and the harder work that this entailed. A fictitious letter by Theophylact, a Byzantine author, which undoubtedly contains elements borrowed from classical authors,[62] offers a wonderfully vivid account of the prostitute's dilemma when it came to a decision between childbirth and abortion. It is a letter supposedly addressed by one courtesan to another, on the model of Alciphron's *Letters of courtesans*. The writer, a woman called Rhodine, is the good, unselfish courtesan[63] who prefers childbirth with all the cost to her appearance, because, as she says, it is safer and more humane than abortion. The addressee, a woman called Calliope, is the bad, selfish courtesan, who places her appearance first and induces an abortion every time she gets pregnant. Rhodine criticises her for her wickedness and inhumanity:

Rhodine to Calliope:
You slander and ridicule me to the lovers saying that I have gone all flabby and that my body has lost its firmness, while you think that you have succeeded in hiding your misdeeds because you expel the embryos prematurely, you evil woman, and you prefer abortion to childbirth destroying anything that is becoming alive in your womb with potent drugs, and you commit murders more cruel than the Colchian Medea. She was compelled to kill her children by her ungrateful husband, even though she was his benefactor and ally in his labours, while you are the maker of ten thousand evils, you whore. Stop then covering up your inhumanity and making fun of our piety, for childbirth is more humane for us than abortion. You must know as well that Justice is angry with you and it will not be long before you receive your punishment for the infanticide.[64]

Loss of one's figure and firmness, even if temporarily, was something no highly paid prostitute could afford. And those established in brothels would be in a worse situation, even though in their case looks were less important, since they were cheap to start with (only 1 obol according to the comedian Philemon);[65] pimps might not be prepared to pay for the maintenance of women who would be unproductive for months due to a pregnancy and for their offspring after childbirth. It is no wonder that we hear in a number of sources that prostitutes would do anything within their power to stop a pregnancy depriving them of their livelihood and ruining their lives.

Naturally the first resource would be contraceptive techniques and substances. It is a matter of common sense to realise that avoiding pregnancy altogether is a much better option than trying to terminate one at considerable risk, danger and pain. This certainly agreed with sound medical advice: Soranus does not hesitate to recommend contraception as an option greatly preferable to abortion:

Avoiding conception is much more advantageous than destroying what has been conceived. So one must watch the times that we have pointed out as the most suitable for conception, that is the beginning and the end of the period. And during sexual intercourse when the man is about to ejaculate, she must hold her breath and slightly pull back, so that the sperm is not ejected further into the cavity of the uterus. Immediately afterwards she must get up, and then squatting make herself sneeze, wipe thoroughly the vagina, or even drink something cold.[66]

Soranus then continues by providing a list of drugs with allegedly contraceptive qualities. This is a very significant passage. First, it shows that contraception was known, attempted, and for obvious reasons much preferred to abortion. Soranus mentions a kind of rhythm method, and a number of other mechanical techniques that, as he thought, might prevent conception. Further on in the same passage he mentions a number of contraceptive drugs and several blocking techniques intended to prevent the sperm of the man from mixing with that of the woman.[67] All contraceptive techniques thus far known to mankind were certainly known to the famous physician, and surely plenty of advice concerning various contraceptive techniques and substances circulated orally in the ancient world.

However, the actual efficiency of the contraceptive techniques and substances used in antiquity is very uncertain, and there is some disagreement in scholarly opinion on this issue. The difficulty originates with the ancient world's imperfect understanding of the reproductive process. As Dean-Jones has demonstrated in her lucid and informative account of the subject,[68] the Greeks empirically knew that both sexes contribute to conception, but what exactly this contribution was and how it worked was not well understood. Thus they did not know exactly how to protect themselves from unwelcome pregnancies. They had some knowledge of contraceptive techniques and drugs, but this knowledge was inconsistent and of doubtful efficiency. McLaren, in his thorough study of contraception in the ancient world, takes a rather cautious approach. He is prepared to concede that some of the mechanical techniques, especially some blockage techniques, may have been efficient, and that some of the drugs might sometimes work. However, his overall approach to the reliability of the methods employed by the ancient world seems to be rather sceptical. J. Riddle, on the other hand, in two intriguing studies published in recent years, is prepared to put more faith to the knowledge the ancient world claimed to have. On the basis of some pharmacological studies commissioned in recent years, he argues that some of the drugs that ancient medical authors class as contraceptives might in fact work. However, the author admits that these studies do not amount to proper clinical testing of these drugs, and a definite answer is still to be sought in further scientific analysis. Whatever the case, the fact is that the ancient world had some knowledge of contraception, but this knowledge was imperfect and its success rather sporadic.

If there was one group among the population who had a vested interest in the possession of accurate knowledge on contraception that group was the prostitutes. They must have shared advice on ways of preventing conception, but they knew very well that these were of only limited efficiency. It was therefore much safer to keep an eye on the early signs of a pregnancy so that they could immediately seek an abortion as soon as they felt that they might be pregnant. Certainly they knew that it would be easier and less troublesome to do it in the early months of the pregnancy. A Hippocratic passage confirms that they were well aware of the signs they should watch for:

The courtesans, the public women, who have a lot of experience of such things, when they go with a man, they know it every time they have conceived; then they have an abortion.[69]

The same idea, that a prostitute should always watch for the early signs of a pregnancy, is suggested by another Hippocratic passage. It is a medical record of a true incident involving a flute-player, one of those women who went to parties to entertain the guests by playing music and offering sexual favours.[70] The author describes how the musician, who was apparently a slave, was told by her mistress-procuress to watch for the early signs of pregnancy, and how he succeeded in having a pregnancy terminated at an early stage by asking her to jump vigorously and repeatedly:

A woman, an acquaintance of mine, owned a very costly musician, who associated with men. She had to avoid conceiving a child, so as not to become cheaper. This musician had heard the things that women tell each other, that once a woman is about to conceive the semen does not come out, but is withheld by nature. Listening to this, she put it into her mind and remembered what she was told. When she became aware of the fact and somehow realised that the semen was not coming out of her, she told her mistress and word came to me. And as soon as I heard, I advised her to kick her heels up to her buttocks, and she had already jumped seven times when the semen fell down.[71]

The story is repeated by the epistolographer Aristaenetus (1,19) almost word for word.[72] Among the differences only one is significant. The section of the Hippocratic passage that describes how the abortion was induced (by means of vigorous leaps in early pregnancy) is replaced in Aristaenetus by the vague phrase 'to do what I knew', and the phrase that makes clear that the pregnancy was successfully terminated is replaced in Aristaenetus by the euphemism 'I set her free from the expected hope'.[73] Evidently the epistolographer was intrigued by the story of the attentive, wise prostitute-musician and considered that it provided good material for his purposes. However, when he reaches the point describing the abortion he avoids the medical details as tactfully as he can, with euphemisms and vague vocabulary. Considering that Aristaenetus wrote in a period when abortion was widely condemned by Roman law, Christianity and probably large sections of contemporary society, it is not surprising that he felt so uptight about the subject.

However, precisely the element that embarrassed Aristaenetus is what makes this Hippocratic passage so valuable for us: its crude and honest simplicity. This is the medical record of a probably true incident and the author is not in a moralising mood. He simply narrates facts as they happened with the intention to describe what the product of the abortion looked like (an unclear and controversial description that does not concern us at this point[74]). In this respect he is somehow detached from moral issues and this makes his account all the more objective and reliable. First of all he describes briefly and with remarkable precision the circumstances of the patient: she was a slave, owned by a woman who procured her for a large amount of money. Evidently she was very attractive, and perhaps a talented musician too, and men were willing to pay dearly for her services. A pregnancy would make her cheaper, as it could spoil her figure, and this is why it was to be avoided at all costs. It was certainly in the interests of the mistress that the woman should not become pregnant, as the mistress was the main beneficiary of her earnings. The woman herself did not enjoy the profits of her trade, but she certainly enjoyed privileges such as associating with rich and influential men in lavish parties, probably personal presents, attention, and luxuries on a daily basis in the rich houses that she visited. Pregnancy and childbirth would remove her from the top end of the market, and her mistress might sell her to a pimp to become a common prostitute in a brothel. If this happened she would have to brace herself to endure wretchedness, exhausting hours, and squalor, and to serve the sexual needs of the lowest sections of society, including every slave and stranger in town. The prospect of being sold to a pimp and established in a brothel was certainly frightening.[75] Thus it was in the best interests of both the woman herself and her mistress that she should avoid becoming pregnant. However, she was well aware of the fact that there was no effective protection against pregnancy and this is why she relied mainly upon advice on the early signs of pregnancy that she had received from other women. The author clearly says that such advice was in circulation among women. Surely the purpose of watching for such symptoms would be to allow for an abortion at a very early stage, before the pregnancy became obvious, damaging to her appearance, and difficult to terminate. It seems to me that the sign that alerted the musician to the fact that she was pregnant was a missed period.[76] She had probably heard from other women that a missed period is a sign of pregnancy,[77] and she immediately told her mistress who asked for medical advice, and an abortion was successfully induced. This remarkable true-life story I think clearly delineates the pressures that urged prostitutes to seek abortions. Inescapable financial interests combined with poor understanding of contraception made abortion the only effective safeguard. The woman simply had too much to lose if she became a mother. This story had a profound influence upon later debates on induced abortion. Future physicians and moral philosophers discussed it in light of the Hippocratic Oath and tried to figure out why abortion was prohibited there but performed here. The answers were as diverse as the opinions of those involved in the debate.[78]

In the light of this discussion, its not surprising to hear from our sources that abortion was a phenomenon typically connected with prostitutes. Clement of Alexandria speaks of prostitution and adultery as the typical reasons behind the desire to have an abortion, as does Plutarch.[79] Plautus even dramatised the subject on stage. In his comedy *Truculentus* (vv. 201-2) Astaphium, the slave of the courtesan Phronesium (literally, 'Wise woman') relates to her mistress's lover that she (sc. Phronesium) was avoiding him because she was afraid that he might try to persuade her to have an abortion (but in reality Phronesium was lying; she was not pregnant by him). Similar to some extent is the approach of Corinna, the woman who has had an abortion in Ovid's *Amores* 13: she too concealed the pregnancy from her lover, but in this case no explanation of her reasons is provided. Corinna had an abortion and her lover found out about the entire affair only when things went badly wrong and her life was in serious risk as a result of *post eventu* complications (see also Chapter 5).

For courtesans and other kinds of prostitutes, abortion was a reality they might have to face on a routine basis. The fact that they often had to terminate unplanned and unwanted pregnancies was common knowledge – to such an extent that it had become a literary topos. Their bodies were their means of earning a living, and as a pregnancy posed a threat to their looks and might put them out of business for months at a time, naturally it was seen as a highly undesirable condition. Now, considering that the understanding of contraception in the ancient world was certainly imperfect, an abortion was often the only effective defence against nature's unpredictable and unwanted gifts. It is no wonder that prostitutes had the reputation of possessing the best possible knowledge of techniques that allowed them to diagnose a pregnancy in early stages and effectively terminate it. For those women such knowledge could be a matter of life and death.

iii. Abortion for the sake of beauty

Looks have always been important for women, perhaps more so than for men. Women use make-up, jewellery and cosmetics as much in the post-feminist world as they ever did, and this persistent cultural stereotype was as strong, if not even stronger, in antiquity. In the sources we encounter various statements about the importance of looks, while literature and art exalt beauty and provide evidence of numerous devices intended to improve physical appearance. The passage that comes instantly to mind is the dialogue of Lysistrata with the other women in the opening scene of Aristophanes' play:

> *Lys.* The salvation of the whole of Greece
> Is in the hands of women
> ....
> *Cal.* And what kind of wise or illustrious deed
> Could women accomplish? We are sitting all day dolled up
> Wearing make up and saffron dresses
> And Cimmerian tunics and fancy shoes!
> *Lys.* Precisely this is where I can see the source of our salvation,
> In the saffron dresses, and the perfumes, and the fancy shoes,
> And the rouge, and the see-through gowns.[80]

Passages like this (and there is ample evidence of women's vanity) very clearly suggest that looks were an important preoccupation for women; even the eternally beautiful, immortal goddesses of the Greek Pantheon were not exempt.[81] Personal grooming, including hair-removal,[82] cosmetics, perfumes and jewellery, was a necessity and to a certain extent a matter of status. A passage from the comedian Eubulus ridicules the excesses of Athenian wives when it comes to cosmetics:

> But, by Zeus, not plastered with rouge,
> Nor like you do when you dye your cheeks
> With mulberry juice. And if you go out in the summer,
> Two black streams are pouring down from your eyes,
> And the sweat from your cheeks leaves a red furrow
> On your neck, and any hair
> That touches your face, looks as if it has turned grey,
> For it is dipped in alcanet.[83]

A passage from Alexis contains detailed criticism of all the devices that courtesans used in order to enhance their looks, and provides us with an astonishing list of such devices.[84] Women were trying to impress their peers, and drew status and prestige from such items,[85] and this is why an adulteress was punished by not being allowed to wear jewellery or make-up.[86]

However, this adulation of cosmetics and good looks had its critics. A poem by Lycophronides suggests that good looks count for nothing if not accompanied by spiritual gifts such as reserve and modesty:

> Neither a boy's, nor a virgin's face
> nor the face of a woman deep-bosomed and adorned with gold
> looks beautiful, if it is not respectable,
> for modesty sows flowers.[87]

This ideal of beauty accompanied by modesty is amply represented in Greek art and wonderfully encapsulated in the words of the tragic poet Chairemon:

> The sight of her body was glowing,
> Shining with her pale skin and gleaming.
> Yet modesty added a light touch of red
> And tinted softly her bright colours,
> And the hair, like a wax-coloured statue's
> Moulded wholesome with its hair locks,
> Was waving loose into the fair winds.[88]

Spiritual qualities find expression in the redness caused by modesty in this powerful elevation of aesthetics into poetry. The two went hand in hand: good looks without modesty would be meretricious, and modesty without good looks probably uninspiring. This combination expresses an ideal that remained a strong cultural stereotype throughout Greek antiquity, and to a certain extent persists up to the present day. That one should come first, looks or personality, was an issue as divisive in the ancient world as it is today. Despite the assertions of the orators that priority should be given to spiritual qualities and virtues,[89] and the generally critical attitude of men towards cosmetics,[90] we can be sure that a woman's appearance and good looks were an asset even in a society that conducted marriages mainly with a view to childbirth and good household management.[91] The speaker in Lysias 19,15 assures the jury that many wealthy men wanted to marry his sisters without any dowry, obviously because they were very attractive, and that his father had married his mother without a dowry, it seems for the same reason. In Andocides 1,117-123 a massive argument between Andocides and Callias over a poor *epiklêros* (heiress) ends up in a bitter court-battle. Why would they fight if not, as MacDowell points out, because the woman was very attractive?[92] That it would be certainly easier for attractive women to find a husband is confirmed by a rather important reference in the speech *Against Neaira*: Here the orator says to the jury:

> At present, even if a woman does not have the means (sc. a dowry), the law supplies her with sufficient 'dowry', if only nature has created her with moderate looks.[93]

The orator argues that the law, by restricting lawful marriage to persons of the same status (citizen to citizen, alien to alien), protects Athenian women and endows them with a substantial advantage, even if they are rather unattractive. This is their citizen status. He implies that if mixed marriages were to be allowed men would rather marry more attractive or wealthy foreign women. The poor and the ugly would stand no chance of finding a husband. This passage is important for two reasons. It implies very clearly that in Athenian society, as in most other societies, good looks were an asset for the woman, as she could attract the attention of a man and make him want to marry her. However, the passage inserts another dimension: that marriage was a legal contract after all, conducted under certain conditions and with clearly specified purposes that were bound to have an effect upon a man's choice of a wife. It is widely accepted that this perception of marriage and the role of the wife in it was by far the most common in Athenian society. This perception of marriage, as a contract with a view to good household management and childbirth, does not necessarily exclude romantic love and a good sex life between husband and wife. However, this would only be considered as a bonus, an ideal state of affairs, not a prerequisite for a lasting and successful marriage.[94] Our sources are not hypocritical when they suggest that virtues such as good managerial skills, the ability to economise, the knowledge of how to cook well,[95] dignified and appropriate conduct, respectability, obedience to her husband and devotion to her family, were the most important qualities for a woman destined to become someone's wife. If she also happened to be beautiful, all the better! For her part, the wife would need to rely solely on her husband for sexual gratification, and this is why she might need to employ anything that would attract him and retain his sexual interest in her, from make-up to fancy clothes and jewellery. However, she should not overdo it, because, apart from appearing meretricious, it might also look suspicious. A fragment from an Attic speech says:

> It is right for a woman to adorn herself as she may please for her husband, but when she does so when going out, there is cause for concern, since this is not for her husband but for other men.[96]

The same idea is conveyed by Lysias 1,14 and 17: the first sign that makes Euphiletos suspicious of his wife (who was allegedly having a love affair) is trace of make-up on her face. Equally, Ischomachos strongly disapproves when one day he finds his wife made up. An underlying suspicion of her motives may be the reason behind his firm reprimand.[97]

Athenian women were not immune to vanity; they took care of their appearance and pride in their fine clothes and jewellery. However, they never lost sight of the fact that these were only secondary qualities. Their conduct and abilities as wives and mothers were far more important goals in their lives. In this respect married Athenian women had no serious motive to induce abortions for the sake of looks. They took pride in motherhood, and their position in the household could only become stronger if they gave birth to several children. Their role as child-bearers was far more important than their role as sexual partners. Quintilian uses a rather absurd parallel when he says that women should feel like other animals who lose sexual desire once they have conceived.[98] However, the ancient world was well aware of the fact that it does not work in the same way with humans. Athenian men and women did not make any effort to pretend that sex should only take place for the sake of procreation. Women's sexual desires were acknowledged to the point that various theoretical explanations (usually connected with the woman's role in reproduction) had been attempted in serious literature, and standard jokes about women's insatiable sexual appetite are frequent in comedy.[99] Greek women did not like the idea of losing their looks or appeal to the opposite sex. They were aware of the ill-effects of childbirth upon the body, and dreaded the consequences. A woman in one of the *Idylls* of Theocritus (27,30) says:

> I am terrified of childbirth, in case I waste the beauty of the body

Women knew that it would affect their looks and that their husbands' sexual interest in them might eventually diminish. But, like the woman in this poem, they were resigned to the fact. If a number of births gradually destroyed their looks, they would need to accept this as a fact of life, a price they had to pay for their position as dignified matrons in a respectable household. If we add to this the dangers of induced abortion and the often strong disapproval of this practice by husband and family, we can understand why few, if any, respectable Athenian women might attempt an abortion in order to retain their looks. There is no evidence anywhere in Greek literature from the classical period which unambiguously suggests that abortions took place for aesthetic reasons. The explanation for this might simply be that abortions were not generally attempted for such purposes. Surely the odd woman obsessed with vanity might be deeply disturbed by the consequences of a pregnancy and wish to have it terminated. I cannot categorically say that abortions never occurred for such purposes. What I'm saying is that society did not impose a strong motive upon Athenian women to risk their health and lives with an abortion for the sake of beauty. Any abortion performed on such grounds would be a rather personal choice related to the individual's emotional disposition and psychosynthesis, and not to a trend or fashion suggested by social and cultural stereotypes.

The position seems to have been very different in the imperial era. Several Greek and Roman sources state that in the Roman empire women attempted abortions in order to retain their looks. The impression we obtain from these sources is that those women had the self-assurance, leisure and means to enjoy the temptations of the world, and above all they had a degree of freedom that would be unimaginable for Greek women of the classical period.[100] Looks and image mattered a lot in this lifestyle, whereas childbirth would be nothing more than a nuisance. Juvenal suggests that this was a phenomenon particularly noticeable in the upper classes.[101] S. Dixon points out that, as with most affluent societies, small families and a dislike of childbirth and its responsibilities were common phenomena among the Roman upper classes.[102] And to make things worse, concerns about inheritance further limited the size of families and exacerbated what many saw as a serious social problem.[103] Repeatedly Roman emperors tried to address this perceived menace to the numbers of Roman citizens, and as such to Rome's best interests. The first and most striking reaction to Roman habits concerning childbirth is Augustus' aforementioned legislation on family life, the intention of which was to strengthen the Roman family and encourage childbirth.[104] Repeated further attempts by later administrations to encourage higher birth-rates and increase family size suggest that none of these measures was particularly effective.[105] We can detect in such measures a certain insecurity, if not frustration, on the part of the state, and a degree of paranoia that might be expected of an elite ruling a vast and diverse empire (see also Chapter 5). Moralists such as Seneca, and defenders of the allegedly traditional Roman ideal, such as some of the poets of the Augustan era, pick up this climate in their works and come forward with statements condemning women's reluctance to sacrifice their looks and lifestyle for the sake of childbirth.[106]

It is a historical fact that when compared with their Athenian counterparts, upper-class Roman women enjoyed much more freedom of purpose and movement. They could attend parties, keep lovers, and enjoy many pleasures in life that were well beyond the reach of any Athenian woman, if she wished to retain her respectability and place in the family and society. Childbirth, with all its responsibilities and unpleasant consequences for the body, was not really to the taste of these women. They did not wish, in the words of the Roman philosopher Favorinus, to see their flat, firm abdomen becoming loose and wrinkled by a pregnancy, and this is why they resorted to abortion:

> The foetuses conceived in their bodies are aborted, so that the flatness of the abdomen is not wrinkled, and it does not become loose by the weight of the burden and the labours of childbirth.[107]

Once they had done their duty to the family – that is, once they had produced an heir, those women no longer wished to spend their lives breeding.[108] Ovid speaks of this lack of enthusiasm for parenthood as a standard phenomenon of his times, and presents abortion as its typical symptom:

> Now a woman who wishes to be beautiful vitiates her womb and it's rare nowadays for someone to wish to become a parent[109]

These lines of Ovid, as much of his other literature dealing with abortion, were written against the background of the Augustan legislation intended to strengthen family life.[110] In this respect they can be seen as a reflection of a contemporary debate with voices rising in protest against this reluctance of women to become mothers and their resorting to abortion in order to keep their appearance. Ovid returned repeatedly to this subject. In another of his works (*Amores* 14) he raises the subject of the reluctance of young girls to become mothers and turns it into a literary topic. Abortion is the central theme running through the poem. *Amores* 13 and 14 have been interpreted as a criticism of abortions for aesthetic reasons, and to some extent I find this interpretation sound: the poet would not be concerned here with abortions performed for good medical reasons; he is annoyed by what he perceives to be a pointless and positively harmful exercise motivated by women's vanity.[111] (Ovid's views on abortion merit closer consideration, and I will return to this subject in more detail in Chapter 5.)

Another voice from the same century, that of Seneca, is raised in praise of his mother Helvia, who, unlike all those other vain women who were having abortions to keep their looks, preferred childbirth:

> Unlike others, who seek praise for nothing else except their beauty, you never concealed your growing womb like an ugly burden, and you never eliminated from your interior the conceived hopes of children.[112]

Helvia is presented as an exemplary mother for two reasons, first because she kept her children instead of attempting abortions, and second because she did so proudly, unconcerned with the consequences of successive pregnancies upon her looks. This passage actually implies that some Roman women were ashamed of their appearance when pregnant and tried to conceal with various means a swollen womb. This rather casual remark I find very significant, because it could explain why Roman women would go to such lengths to have abortions for aesthetic reasons. In circles where, it seems, looks were so important that a swollen womb would be viewed as nothing more than 'an ugly burden' (*indecens onus*), one would expect abortion to be a fact of life. This reluctance of Roman women to give birth may also be reflected in the story told by Ovid, and repeated by Plutarch, about the Roman matrons who obtained reversal of a law trying to stop them from using carriages by collectively refusing to give birth.[113]

S. Dixon is probably right when she advises caution in the consideration of this evidence.[114] It is true that these are moralistic statements of general character, not well-attested historical incidents, and one should beware of exaggeration. But, on the other hand, these statements would not make sense if they did not reflect an existing contemporary social practice, even if this practice was in fact more limited than Seneca, Ovid, and Juvenal wish us to believe. If abortions for aesthetic reasons did not take place in imperial Rome, there would have been no need to moralise against this practice. This is why I am inclined to believe that there was a certain degree of pressure upon upper-class Roman women to put image high in the list of their priorities. This pressure might sometimes result in an abortion, if the pregnancy was perceived as a threat to the lifestyle of these women and threatened to spoil their looks and make them undesirable. A. Rouselle[115] encapsulates perfectly the practice and the ideology behind it when she says: 'There was general agreement about the damage done to the mother's body by numerous pregnancies. But whereas Greek women simply noted the effects of pregnancy, Roman women refused to accept them.'

The moralists who objected to abortions for aesthetic reasons were certainly motivated by ethical, political or philosophical considerations. These men perceived that women who had abortions for such purposes were contravening the purpose of their nature as women and their role in society. But, on the other hand, the reasons of Soranus when he objects to abortions 'in pursuit of beauty' (*di' epitêdeusin hôraiotêtos*) might be different.[116] He was well aware of the dangers and probably did not consider beauty to be worth the risk. This, I think, is an important factor. Unlike the present day when the operation is safe and relatively painless, in those days it was a risky and painful undertaking. Was beauty worth it? This is where I think we find a clear cultural difference between the Greek and Roman worlds. While Greek women acquired status and prestige from their role in the family as mothers and leaders of the household, some Roman women, especially in the upper classes, were not be particularly concerned with these traditional roles and sought status and prestige in the image they projected as individuals in their society. Who they were, how they looked, what people thought about them as individuals mattered to those women a lot. This is why, I suppose, while Greek women thought generally that looks were not worth the risk of an induced abortion, some Roman women took a different approach. I think in this case the cultural values of each society are responsible for a drive in different directions. While Greek culture did not impose upon its women the need to risk everything for the sake of looks, Roman society had created a cultural climate that encouraged certain individuals to make their image and good looks an important priority. And if a pregnancy became an obstacle to these priorities, abortion was the answer despite the risks.

iv. Abortion for social and economic reasons

A considerable number of abortions in modern times are motivated by socio-economic factors, and these are the most controversial of all. Individuals and groups concerned with the issue may be willing to empathise with a woman seeking an abortion because the pregnancy presents a serious health risk, but far less sympathetic towards a woman seeking an abortion because the pregnancy is putting obstacles to her career advancement. This grading of abortions was clearly reflected in English law before the 1967 Act. The law allowed abortion if the pregnancy posed a serious risk to the woman's life, but not for any other reason. The 1967 reform did not allow abortion on demand, nor did it sanction abortion for socio-economic reasons. It permitted abortion only on grounds of health, but defined health in a very broad sense to include the mental health, balance, and well-being of the individual. The opponents of the 1967 Act objected on the grounds that such a wide definition of health allowed abortion on socio-economic grounds, and this they considered unacceptable. Those in favour of the Act were content that, with some safeguards, women could now seek abortions for a wide variety of reasons, since these reasons could arguably be related to their health and well-being in general. Thus allowance was made for abortions on socio-economic grounds and this was widely understood to be within the provisions of the 1967 Act, even though the Act itself did not include such terminology. What makes abortion for socio-economic reasons such an intensely contentious point is, in my opinion, its connection with the general issue of women's emancipation and equal access to all spheres of life. Defenders of equality for women demand for the woman the right to decide whether a pregnancy is desirable at this stage of her life. According to this point of view, if for whatever reason she thinks that the moment is inopportune, she must have the right to seek a termination. Defenders of a more traditional role for women which places motherhood very high on the list of priorities, argue against such liberties. What makes socio-economic abortion a controversial issue is the fact that it presupposes a woman's right to decide when, if at all, she wishes to become a mother. Women who seek abortions on socio-economic grounds may not do so because they resent motherhood altogether, or because they do not wish to have a child with this particular sexual partner at any stage. They may seek to terminate this particular pregnancy because it does not fit into the pattern of their lives *at this particular moment*. Many may have already given birth to children, and others may hope to do so at some point in the future. But motherhood at a certain point, under a certain set of adverse social/economic circumstances, is the problem and the real issue.

In this respect, and for the reasons mentioned above, socio-economic abortion is a sign of our times, and not something we would expect to find widely practised in the ancient world. It is not that ancient women invariably lacked ambition, or that they would not put this ambition before childbirth if need be. One such case is reported by Plutarch in the *Life of Lycurgus* (3): The widow of Lycurgus' brother, the queen of Sparta, wanted to have an abortion and remove her dead husband's heir from the succession, in order to marry Lycurgus, who was next in line to the throne of the Eurypontidai, and become his queen. Ambitious women like this surely existed in all parts of the ancient world. However, on the whole, the different less flexible roles prescribed for properly brought up women in ancient societies would make the demand for abortion on socio-economic grounds considerably smaller. In addition, the undoubtedly higher dangers and difficulties of induced abortion in antiquity, sufficient to make any woman think hard before taking the risk, would further discourage terminations on such grounds. This is why it is not surprising that the evidence concerning socio-economic abortions is rather limited. They did happen, but certainly to a much lesser extent than nowadays. The most significant piece of evidence concerning an abortion for social reasons comes from Chariton's novel *Chaireas and Callirhoe*,[117] and is described by R. Johne[118] as 'a unique passage in Greek literature'. In a sense this is correct: there is no other passage in ancient Greek fictional literature dealing with the subject to such an extent and in such depth. The heroine Callirhoe discovers that she is pregnant while in slavery, living far away from home and separated from her husband Chaireas. The father of the child is undoubtedly her distant husband, whom she loves very profoundly. The reason for their separation was that Chaireas was set up and made to believe that his wife had committed adultery. In a rage he kicked her, everyone thought that she was dead, and she was buried alive. The next day Chaireas discovered the plot and became prosecutor of himself in the trial for Callirhoe's death, but he was acquitted (as in the passage from Myrivilis quoted above) because the woman's father, the general Hermocrates, succeeded in persuading the jury that it was all a tragic mistake. Grave robbers opened her tomb to steal, found her, and took her away to be sold as a slave. At this point of the plot we find her in Persian territory, sold as a slave to the local potentate Dionysios. He has a crush on her, but since he does not wish to force her into a relationship, he asks his faithful servant Plangon to assist him in conquering Callirhoe's heart. Plangon gains the trust of Callirhoe and truly cares for her, but she also has in mind the interests of her master Dionysios:

> In the evening ... sitting on the bed (Plangon) said 'You should know, my child, that you are pregnant.' Callirhoe screaming and pulling her hair said, 'O Fortune, you have added even this to my troubles, to give birth to a slave.' And hitting her belly she said 'You wretched being, you have been to the grave even before you were born, and you were handed over to robbers.[119] What kind of life are you coming into? How am I going to carry you, what hope do I have for you, orphan, and alien, and slave? Experience death, before birth.' Plangon, however, restrained her hands, promising to assist her the next day to have an easier abortion.
> When each of the two women was left alone she was having her own thoughts ... Callirhoe, at first, wanted to have an abortion, saying to herself 'Am I going to give birth to the grandson of Hermocrates,[120] so that he will be the slave of our master, and bring into this world a child whose father no one has ever met? Some enemy will soon say "Callirhoe conceived on the boat of the robbers". It is enough for me to be in trouble. It is not to your benefit, my child, to come into a wretched life, from which you should try to escape, even if you were born. Go away free, without experiencing trouble. It will be better if you never hear your mother's story.' But, then again, she changed her mind, filled with pity for what she was carrying in her womb. 'Do you want to kill your child, you impious woman? Are Medea's[121] thoughts going through your head? But you will appear to be even more savage than the Scythian woman (sc. Medea), because her husband was her enemy, while you want to kill the child of Chaireas and erase every trace of the notorious marriage. And what if he is a son? What if he looks like his father? What if he turns out to be happier than me? Is his own mother going to kill someone who escaped the grave and the robbers? How many children of gods and kings we hear about, who were born in slavery, and then reinstated into their father's office, Zethus and Amphion and Cyrus![122] You too my child, you will sail to Sicily; you will look for your father and your grandfather, and tell them about your mother. A fleet will sail from there to help me. You will give both of us our parents, my child.' Troubled by such thoughts all night she fell asleep for a while. Then an image of Chaireas appeared in her dream, that looked exactly like him in everything: ... He stood there and said 'Wife, I entrust you with my son.' While he was still speaking, Callirhoe woke up wanting to embrace him. Considering that her husband had advised her to do so, she decided to keep the child.

The reasons that Callirhoe contemplates an abortion are social, related to the difficulties of her present circumstances. She is officially a slave of Dionysios and a foreigner in a land very far away from home. Her child would also be a slave of Dionysios and born in an alien land. The father of the child is an absent stranger in this part of the world, and Callirhoe, apart from the frightening prospect of having to bring up the child as a single mother in a hostile environment, is worried about possible rumours concerning the child's legitimacy. Moreover, her pride dissuades her from bringing into slavery the grandchild of the glorious general Hermocrates, the destroyer of the mighty Athenian fleet in Sicily. Callirhoe has serious reasons for going ahead with the abortion, but her emotions do not follow her logic, and the hope that she will give birth to a son, rescuer and avenger of his ill-fated mother, fires her true desire to keep the child. Her dilemma is a difficult one: her instinct and hope as a mother is battling against the wretchedness of her present situation. She cannot decide by herself. The determining factor is a dream where Chaireas appears and entrusts his son to her care. She interprets this dream as an expression of Chaireas' will to have the child and decides to keep it. Plangon, in her effort to persuade Callirhoe to marry Dionysios, realises that the dilemma of the latter offers a suitable opportunity for her to persuade the heroine to marry Dionysios. Plangon is aware of Callirhoe's conflicting emotions and thoughts and under the pretext that she will help her have a safer and easier abortion the next morning plays for time, confident that maternal instinct will triumph in the end. In this respect she is right: Callirhoe finally decides to go against her fears, sacrifice her feelings and the memory of her precious Chaireas, and instead marry Dionysios for the sake of the child.

The dilemma of Callirhoe is crucial for the plot. Chariton wants to present the heroine as totally faithful to the memory of her distant husband. She could not be persuaded by any other force or allurement to betray him and marry someone else. Only something higher and nobler, like securing the survival and then a promising future for the son of Chaireas, would be compelling enough to make her go against her feelings and convictions and agree to marry Dionysios, but even this does not happen without hesitation and lengthy deliberation. By presenting Callirhoe as seriously contemplating an abortion, Chariton stresses the integrity and high moral calibre of his heroine. Callirhoe emerges untainted by even the slightest suspicion of infidelity to the memory of her first husband. She has not compromised her love or dignity. The second marriage paradoxically is dictated and forced upon her by this love and dignity. By contemplating an abortion (but finally not going ahead with it) the heroine preserves her virtue and wins the sympathy and respect of the reader. In Callirhoe's dialogue with herself Chariton employs the powerful potential of this topic to advance the plot and illustrate the portrait of the heroine. Yet, one should keep in mind that abortion remains only a theoretical possibility that never materialises, and that, despite the frequent repetition of motives and topics in Greek novels, Chariton's experiment with this subject-matter was not followed up by any subsequent novelist.

The historical value of this passage is very significant. It seems to me that it recreates a seemingly realistic setting where we can see a woman contemplating an abortion of the child of her distant husband for social reasons. It offers us an insight into what social reasons could lead a married woman to attempt an abortion. It is true that, after all, this is fiction, and that some of the settings are exaggerated and subservient to the purposes of the novelist. But piracy, slavery, poverty, the predicament and insecurity of a single mother in a society where women were certainly in a vulnerable position, loss of status, loss of one's home in societies torn by war and mass population expulsions, large-scale atrocities such as the destruction of entire cities leaving streams of wretched refugees, economic pressure in societies that at best had an elementary system of social security and quite often none at all – all these were realities in the ancient world. The list of such factors, which at times created a very unstable and unsuitable environment for childbirth and family life, could go on for pages. Were women (and men) expected to ignore these realities of life? Should we expect that such pressures did not affect the mental state of individuals and urge them at least to consider abortion as a means of avoiding responsibilities which they might feel they could not handle under the present circumstances? In the next section where I analyse abortion as a political statement or a matter of policy, I discuss in greater detail a passage of Seneca the elder that presents abortion as a response to such pressures. In his *Controversiae* (2,5,2) he refers to a certain tyrant who raped and abused respectable women, married and unmarried alike (*matronae, virgines*). Women were absolutely terrified by this and some had abortions because they did not wish to bring children into this inhuman environment. In a sense abortion is presented here as a response to intense pressures in a dangerous and unjust world.

Pressures of this kind are bound to have an effect upon a woman's mental disposition. One of the arguments that has been widely accepted after the 1967 Abortion Act is that social and financial circumstances can have a profound effect upon someone's mental health and emotional balance as an individual. A pregnancy that comes at an inappropriate moment in one's life can put so much pressure upon a person that her health as a whole can seriously deteriorate. As I mentioned in the introduction to this chapter, modern medical literature offers ample evidence suggesting that the mother's mental state could play an important role upon her decision to seek a termination. Ancient medical literature was well aware of this fact too. Galen mentions a strong commotion of the soul, or a powerful emotion like fear, as some of the situations that could lead to an abortion.[123] Literature too assumes that a woman would be in a very disturbed state of mind before seeking an abortion. The fear of the Spartan woman was stronger than any physical pain she might feel (see above, p. 102), and the confusion and conflict of Callirhoe, or the obsessive frustration of Canace[124] are examples of how authors imagined the state of mind of a woman before she opted for an abortion. They suggest an awareness of the fact that her mental condition was an important factor in her decision. The sober-minded musician of the Hippocratic passage (see above, p. 111) is perhaps an exception. She treats abortion as a necessity of her trade, and one could say that she shows a professional attitude by not allowing herself to get too emotional over the issue.

When it comes to abortion motivated by purely financial pressures, we hear very little from the sources. Despite the fact that we have a considerable number of Attic law-court speeches dealing with inheritance disputes, there is absolutely no reference anywhere suggesting that abortion was ever used to manipulate the line of inheritance. Since legitimate descendants had priority over lateral relatives and, according to Athenian law, could not be disinherited,[125] relatives sometimes used various imaginative devices, such as trying to dispute the legitimacy of direct heirs,[126] yet attempts to eliminate such heirs by means of abortion are nowhere attested. It seems to me that the silence of the sources over this matter is significant. If we look closer at the status and role of women in the Athenian inheritance process we can understand why abortions for the purposes of manipulation of the inheritance line probably did not occur in classical Athens.

In normal circumstances women were not in the position to dispose of their property as they wished. A number of scholars, on the basis of a law quoted in Isaeus 10,10, take the view that women were legally disallowed from owning property. I have argued against this interpretation of the aforementioned law, but I maintain that women were nevertheless restricted by social morality.[127] Since they could not represent themselves in court, and could not go to the financial centres of Athens to perform transactions with strange men without compromising their dignity, they had to leave most financial affairs in the hands of their male relatives. They certainly inherited property, either directly from their father in the absence of a male heir, or indirectly in the form of a dowry, but this property was managed by the men nearest to them, that is husband, son, uncle, or legal guardian. In this context it would certainly seem meaningless for an Athenian widow to risk her own life with an abortion for the benefit of others. Since she could not really go about spending money for her pleasures, as some upper-class Roman women could do, why would she accept bribes and attempt an abortion, so that others could inherit her husband's estate? On the contrary, a widowed woman with child would probably find that it was in her best interests to continue with the pregnancy. According to Athenian law, the woman would need to return to her natal home after her husband's death if she was childless. However, if she claimed that she was pregnant she could stay in her husband's house in the hope that she would produce an heir (or heiress).[128] I imagine most Athenian women given the choice would rather stay in the marital home than return to their natal family, where they might be nothing more than a burden waiting to be disposed of by another marriage, preferably as soon as possible. Given the realities of life in classical Athens, it seems clear that the woman had nothing to gain by accepting bribes in order to have an abortion for the benefit of lateral relatives, and probably a lot to lose. This is why it is not surprising that we do not hear as much as mere allegation of such an incident in the Attic law-court speeches.

Abortion for the purposes of limiting the number of heirs, and thus avoiding fragmentation of the estate, is nowhere attested. In societies such as Sparta, where an inflexible inheritance system discouraged a large number of heirs, we might expect abortion to have been used for the purpose of keeping the number of heirs low.[129] Yet, although we hear a lot about the social problems created by this clumsy system, we never hear of such practices. In Athens, despite wider financial opportunities and a much more flexible economy, people sometimes tried to limit the number of their heirs and avoid fragmentation of their estate. However, in all attested cases this happens by other means, and not by a measure as drastic and dangerous as an abortion. One of the ways of limiting the number of heirs available to the father of a child was to refuse to acknowledge its legitimacy, which would automatically displace the child from the line of inheritance. In Demosthenes 40,8-15 Mantias refused to acknowledge the legitimacy of his sons by his former wife Plangon in favour of his son Mantitheos from his second marriage. By doing so, he had effectively disinherited his two older sons, until he was compelled later in life to acknowledge them, and thus restore them as his heirs. In Isaeus 6,22-4 a massive argument erupts between Euctemon and his adult son Philoctemon over the acknowledgement of the legitimacy of a second son of the former. By the act of acknowledgement the second son would become heir to his father on an equal footing with his older half-brother, and this was resisted fiercely at public and private level by Philoctemon, until he was blackmailed by his father and abandoned his opposition. In Andocides 1,125-7 Callias refuses at first to acknowledge the legitimacy of his second son by Chrysilla, surely because he did not wish this child to share the inheritance with his elder son Hipponicos. Incidents such as these indicate that if an Athenian man wished to limit the number of direct heirs to his estate he did not need to compel his wife to violate her body and risk her life. The law provided much safer alternatives. Certainly it would be difficult, unfair and socially unacceptable to deny a legitimately born child what by birthright was lawfully his or hers. But the possibility theoretically existed, and abortion was certainly a much less desirable method for such purposes. In addition to legal paths like those mentioned above, more extreme measures such as exposure or infanticide were available to Greek parents (see the discussion of these topics in Chapter 5). This is why families in the classical period probably did not have to resort to abortion for the purposes of manipulation of the inheritance line.

However, there is evidence that may suggest some change of heart towards later antiquity. Abortions for financial reasons are occasionally attested from the republican period onwards. Cicero reports one incident in which an abortion was induced for the sake of an inheritance:

> I remember a Milesian woman, when I was in Asia, who was sentenced to death, after accepting bribes from the alternative heirs and procuring a self-induced abortion by means of drugs.[130]

He then refers to a Roman woman who accepted bribes from the nephew of her husband, a certain Oppicianus, to procure an abortion, for the same reason, so that he would benefit from her husband's inheritance. In the orator's words 'she sold the hope entrusted in her womb by her husband'.[131] It is possible that changed roles for women in the Roman empire, with greater financial and personal freedom, made the option of an abortion for financial reasons seem more logical. Abortion for such purposes is certainly attested in other societies of the past. Nardi quotes a number of Byzantine legal and canonical texts that prescribe the death penalty for a woman who had an abortion, bribed by lateral relatives and alternative heirs.[132] These documents suggest that at least the possibility was real, or legal provisions would not have been designed to address this crime with such severity. L. Thomson reports that this phenomenon, namely using abortions in order to manipulate inheritance, was a standard practice on Fiji.[133] However, one should beware of anthropological parallels, because, as I implied above, the precise historical and cultural setting is likely to be a decisive factor.

In conclusion, abortions were attempted for socio-economic reasons in the ancient world, but the structure of ancient societies and the perilous nature of the undertaking restricted the demand. The ancient world did not impose upon women many of the demands of their expanded role in modern societies. Married women faithful to their husbands had fewer reasons for seeking an abortion than they might have nowadays. Moreover, since maternity would normally strengthen their role in the family, they would not need to worry about the increased responsibilities that childbirth would bring, simply because they would view such responsibilities as part of their role in society, as the primary duty that nature had bestowed upon women. At the same time most ancient societies had in place various ways of dealing with matters such as the financial implications of childbirth. We might consider practices such as the exposure of babies, infanticide or disinheritance of illegitimate children to be cruel and inhumane. But before we pass judgement on the ancient world we may first pause and consider how honest or ethical our own responses are to similar socio-economic problems and pressures. Then we need to consider some of the realities and parameters of ancient societies: it may be enough to mention constant warfare in an unstable world, financial insecurity caused by fragile agriculture and risky trade, limited health services, and in general the feeling that one's fortunes might change for the worse overnight, which is so vividly reflected in Greek mythology and literature. These parameters naturally created an environment that at times might affect quite seriously the emotional disposition and mental condition of mothers-to-be. Against these factors women had to weigh the perils of abortion, of which they were well aware. Their answers to these dilemmas were considerably different from ours. Some of the problems that may lead modern women to the abortion clinic were resolved in the ancient world by other means that did not require them to risk their health and life. However, a new-born baby was a *fait accompli*, a human being staring the mother in the eyes. Its disposal or exclusion from the family would have been as difficult then as exposure or adoption would be nowadays, and this factor must have weighed a lot on people's minds. Abortion has the definite advantage, if advantage is the right word, of allowing parents to avoid such inexorable dilemmas. This is why people sometimes attempted abortions for socio-economic reasons in the ancient world, too. The difference is that it probably happened far less often than today, and that the circumstances had to be absolutely compelling before a woman decided to take the risk.

v. Abortion as a political statement

Abortion is a political issue and has always been so. In the modern world one only needs to look at countries such as Ireland, where a prohibition on abortion is enshrined in the constitution, and the matter has been the subject of several referenda still exciting a passionate political debate. In the United States it has been a contested campaigning point before elections, and is often perceived as an issue that should extend well beyond the wishes of the individuals directly involved, a problem touching important aspects of public life. Thus it has been very much of a political issue there too, and as a matter of fact one that touches a raw nerve in American public opinion on both sides of the argument. The active participation of women in politics in the twentieth century has certainly played its role in the high profile politicisation of the issue, and has probably resulted in the liberalisation of the abortion laws in many countries. However, this has made the issue no less divisive, not least because women are as split over the ethics of induced abortion as men ever were, and perhaps understandably more vocal. The politics of induced abortion extend beyond the divide of the sexes and over the span of time. From antiquity to the present day it has been an important political issue because it is tied up with some of the most fundamental questions of public life, such as a person's right to life, self-determination, health and well-being, freedom of choice, the contrast between the interests of the individual and those of the community, the roles of the sexes in society, and so on. The numerous references to abortion in surviving literature from the ancient world unambiguously suggest that men were concerned about it, precisely for the reasons mentioned above, that is, its implications for important areas of public life. Their views and reactions I discuss in Chapter 5. Here, however, I explore some references that suggest that for ancient women too abortion could be a political issue.

The most famous of these references is the story told by Ovid, and repeated by Plutarch, of the Roman matrons who obtained reversal of a law trying to stop them from using carriages by collectively refusing to give birth.

> There is a story that women were barred by the council from using chariots;
> so they agreed among themselves neither to become pregnant nor to give

birth, and this was their defence against the men, until the latter changed their mind and gave in.[134]

Ovid, unlike Plutarch, who is reluctant to explain exactly how they would avoid giving birth, explicitly says that abortion was the means employed.[135] This is a very telling story. Both authors present abortion and the refusal to become mothers as an efficient weapon in the hands of women. In the political setting of an ancient society where the men are in control of the state and its institutions, they have the power and authority to take measures that are greatly disadvantageous to women. In this case the action taken by the men is perceived as designed to deprive dignified matrons of their privileges. Ovid uses the word *honor* to describe what the women had been deprived of. Women are not prepared to tolerate the insult inflicted upon their pride by their 'ungrateful men'. They decide to fight back. Plutarch uses vocabulary that would be suitable for the battlefield (*amunomenai tous andras*). But how can they fight against the institutionalised power and authority of men? Women were excluded from politics; they did not have a voice in male institutions like the council, the assembly or the Senate, and they did not have the power of voting either. Their position and authority in the institutions of the state was pretty much defined by their role as mothers, and this is the weapon they chose in order to fight back. A general 'strike' in motherhood by means of abortion, if other measures to prevent a pregnancy had failed, is what forces men to the negotiating table and finally defeats them. If motherhood is a woman's power, abortion is her most effective weapon against male authoritarianism.

A similar attitude, perhaps less militant though equally drastic, is reflected in a passage of Seneca the elder, who speaks about the effects of a tyrant's abuse of power over women:

> Matrons were dragged, virgins were raped; nothing was safe; no woman seemed happier than those who did not have children. Thus some women destroyed the foetuses that they had conceived, while others delayed their fertility.[136]

Abortion and contraception are the methods employed by women to fight against injustice, indignity and personal injury inflicted by an authoritarian state. If we try to read deeper into these stories we will find that through them run themes similar to those that make abortion a divisive political issue today. First of all comes the desire of women to be appreciated for their role in society, then their determination to control their bodies, and finally the conflict caused by men's attempts to expand their control over these areas of women's lives, and the reaction of women to male authority. These aspects play an important part in the modern politics of abortion. Ancient women did not have voting rights or access to an arena where an issue such as abortion could be brought forward and become part of a public debate in which women might have a say. However,

stories like these suggest that there was a certain degree of awareness of
the complex politics of induced abortion. Undoubtedly ancient women
were aware of the fact that, as motherhood was one of their main functions
in society, abortion could represent a rebellion against male authority and
an expressed desire for self-determination.

Conclusions

Assessing the point of view of women who sought abortions in antiquity is
a difficult task. We never hear directly from them; we have to rely on
sources written by men, quite often for very different purposes. We need
to beware of sexist bias, exaggerations and moralistic statements. We need
to use our judgement, and sometimes even our imagination, cautiously.
And above all, we need to be constantly aware of the nature of the source,
the purposes of the author, the place and the time. However, the shortcomings of our sources notwithstanding, we are not in complete darkness.
There is no good reason why we should doubt the authority of our sources
when they suggest that most abortions in the ancient world were procured
by women who had conceived as a result of an extra-marital affair, or by
prostitutes. We know enough about perceptions concerning premarital sex
and extramarital affairs to allow us to understand why the risks and pains
of induced abortion would seem lesser to many women compared to the
sanctions they would face if the pregnancy became noticed by family and
society. We can confidently say that the consequences of a pregnancy from
an extramarital relationship would be so devastating to the woman's life
that abortion inevitably seemed the only serious alternative. The same
applied to prostitutes: they also had very little choice. For those at the top
end of the scale the market was very competitive. Slavery, as well as
limited job opportunities for free women, provided human resources in
plenty. New recruits, younger and fresher, were constantly pouring on to
the market seeking to establish themselves and create their own clientele.
Pregnancies for those who were already established would undoubtedly
result in the loss of some of their clientele. Could they ever hope to get it
back, and could they take such a risk? As I have suggested above, a
pregnancy might push a prostitute down towards the cheaper end of the
market, and in that end conditions were much harsher. Pimps were not
prepared to cater for women who were unproductive in terms of income.
Prostitutes working in brothels could find themselves starved, sold, or on
the streets. The necessity imposed upon prostitutes to eliminate an ill-
timed pregnancy would be absolutely compelling, sometimes literally a
matter of life and death. Placed against such necessity, an abortion would
certainly appear the lesser of two evils.

Our task is more complicated when it comes to the evaluation of these
sources that suggest that, at least in the Roman empire, women were
attempting abortions for aesthetic reasons. The evidence in our hands
concerning the value that the Greeks and the Romans attached to good

looks is somewhat confusing. However, we can probably say with confidence that in the Greek world, although aesthetics were important, the cultural climate did not encourage the risks of induced abortion for the sake of looks. Women were generally well protected within the family, motherhood ranked high on their list of priorities, their destinies were clearly prescribed, and opportunities to parade themselves as society *belles* were rather limited. This is why I am not surprised by the silence of the sources when it comes to abortion for aesthetic reasons in the Greek world. But if this silence is significant, it may also be significant that some authors actually mention abortion for aesthetic reasons in the Roman world. I find it difficult to believe that these references are nothing more than a literary topos, or moralistic scare-mongering. A literary topos that did not reflect an actual practice is unlikely to have persisted over a considerable span of time, and across literary genres. Moreover, the explanation of such references as a mere literary topos cannot account for the testimony of Soranus that abortions might be procured for such purposes. Here we have a medical source, and an author notorious for his sober-minded, rational and down-to-earth approach to gynaecological issues. Literary topics were not to Soranus' taste, but actual social practice certainly was his concern. This evidence suggests that for some women in the Roman empire looks were precious enough to compel them to risk an abortion, and through this to try to maintain their image, lifestyle, social circles, lovers and admirers – that is, perhaps all that mattered to them in this world. The sources point the finger at upper-class Roman women, and there is no good reason to doubt that such practices were an upper-class phenomenon, as women in the lower classes would have had much more urgent preoccupations than maintaining a slender waist. I do not wish to speculate about the percentage of women who attempted abortions for aesthetic reasons in the imperial era. But considering the risks and doubtful efficiency of much of the advice in circulation, I am inclined to think that it happened much less often than our sources suggest.

Abortions for socio-economic reasons other than adultery or prostitution also seem to have been a very limited practice. It is true that in a sense ancient women were under less pressure from some socio-economic factors that dominate the lives of modern women, such as personal ambition, career opportunities, and desires encouraged by the allurements and demands of a consumer society. On the other hand, the ancient world often lived with intense insecurity created by constant warfare, a vulnerable agricultural economy, pestilence, invasions and looming instability. So it is fair to say that socio-economic factors acted as deterrents to motherhood and child-rearing in the ancient world too, even though from a different perspective than today. The main difference between the ancient and modern world is that while abortions nowadays are safe and relatively painless, in those days the procedure was too perilous and agonising to be viewed as an easy way out. On the other hand, the legal and social structures of the ancient world allowed alternatives such as adoption, exposure, or infanticide, which were certainly safer for the mother. Similar alternatives still exist: many religious and secular groups who oppose abortion see adoption as by far the best solution to an unwanted pregnancy, and occasionally incidents of abandoned babies make the headlines. What makes such alternatives undesirable today is the emotional attachment between the parents and the new-born, a bond that is normally very difficult to break without repercussions for the mental and emotional health of the natural parents. The same problem faced parents in antiquity, of course, but unlike their modern counterparts they did not have a choice between a quick resolution while the foetus was still in the womb or the more painstaking separation from a born child. Their choice was between the pain of being separated from a new-born baby and a perilous undertaking known for its grave risks and doubtful efficiency. Abortion was a truly drastic step, and it was generally carried out only by those who could see no easier way out of a serious crisis.

5

The Man's Point of View

Abortion is sometimes viewed as an issue that should exclusively concern women. Men are often presented as the opposition, trying to exercise illegitimate control, restrict women's rights to self-determination, and interfere with their bodies and civil liberties. The reader of militant feminist literature may get the impression that women unanimously as a group wish to have choice over the continuation of a pregnancy, while men oppose this right and try to restrict it by employing the powerful machinery of the state.[1] Women are presented as victims of a male-dominated state that wishes to extend control over their lives, while men are concerned only with issues such as population growth and reproduction, or simply presented as indifferent to the plight of women and their desire for reproductive freedom. Moreover, arguments suggesting that men as a whole have been greatly distressed by the sexual freedom recently afforded to women by means of safe contraceptives and abortions are quite frequently encountered.[2] Men have been presented as the 'enemy', against whom the thrust of the feminist offensive of liberation, with abortion as one of its central issues, should be directed.

There is some mythology in such views created by confrontational gender politics and blunt generalisations. First, we need to remember that the divide over the ethics of induced abortion is not a male versus female one. Many women oppose abortion while many men are pro-choice. Then, as I have stated repeatedly in this book, abortion is an issue inextricably connected with politics, law, religion, economics and ethics, and in this respect it does concern men too, since their lives are as directly affected by the influence of these factors as women's lives. Finally, concerns over ethical dilemmas, the reproductive process, population growth, inheritance and succession by one's biological offspring are as much a man's legitimate concern as they are a woman's.[3]

Bearing this in mind, we need to make a genuine effort to understand male attitudes towards abortion outside popular mythology on gender relations and beyond the politics of confrontation. We need to place abortion against a background of issues that naturally concern men as individuals and as members of the community and try to understand their reactions against this background. Moreover we need to view men as parents and as human beings with emotions and powerful instincts. The emotional dimension in particular seems to me to be seriously underestimated in the secondary literature concerning abortion, with detrimental results. Failure to empathise both with the man and with the woman involved can only lead to serious misunderstanding of attitudes, reactions and motives. One could argue over the politics and ethics of induced abortion, produce solidly logical arguments, and elaborate theories on civil rights, yet one might fail to touch or convince an individual directly involved if such arguments do not take into account the emotions and instincts of that individual.

Besides, it is erroneous to assume that emotional reactions to an issue such as abortion will always be confined to the level of personal conversations or confrontations. A man who feels that he has been robbed of his child may be very angry, willing to go to great lengths to seek redress for what in his eyes is a grievous personal injury. One option might be direct legal action, like that taken by the Scottish man who made headlines a few years ago when he went to court seeking an injunction against his wife in order to prevent her from having an abortion. Another option could be political activism: an angry man who failed to stop his sexual partner from having an abortion, and thus, as he perceived it, from murdering his child, might understandably try to stop her and any other woman in future from doing the same thing by politicising the issue and trying to influence government decisions. He might engage in intense campaigning against abortion through the media, church organisations, or action groups, and further options could perhaps be pursued, depending on the circumstances. The point is that it should not surprise us to see an injured man prepared to go to great lengths to stop women doing what his sexual partner did to him.

Apart from emotional considerations, men also have to think of the consequences of rearing a child as much as women do. Particularly in societies which are increasingly based upon equal distribution of domestic and parental duties between the sexes, the man will be asked to sacrifice hours from his career or his hobbies and pleasures to look after his child. Can he afford this time and energy, and is he willing to allocate it to the duties of parenthood? At least he deserves to be asked before a decision on the continuation or termination of a pregnancy is taken. And if we think that these kinds of questions are the concern of the 'new man' alone, we are mistaken. Children have been a responsibility throughout history, and although the specifics of this responsibility may depend upon the structures of an individual society and the division of labour and spheres of influence between men and women, men are still expected to take part in one way or another in the upbringing of their offspring, and to ensure that they are raised according to contemporary specifications and educational standards. In addition, men in all periods of history have had to give consideration to issues such as the size of their family and the available resources. Family planning ought to be, and normally is, a joint decision. This inevitably gives men a say over the prospects for their wives' pregnancies. In fact, in the Graeco-Roman world serious decisions with regard to family planning might well rest with the man, since he was often the person who decided whether to accept a new-born or expose it. Demographic trends in different periods of history have been an important aspect of family planning, and these, at least in the past, have been a primarily male concern. The adult male citizens were the ones concerned with issues such as the constitution and safety of the state. Abortion cut through to the heart of these matters, and this, if nothing else, made it an issue of male concern, especially in political settings where a higher birth-rate mattered.

Thus abortion is not, and has never been, an exclusively female problem. The fact that it is inextricably linked with wider political, financial, ethical and cultural issues, and very much with personal and emotional settings, has made it a matter that concerns men too. Male concerns about abortion in the ancient world could hardly be more comprehensively presented than they are in a list provided by Cicero in his speech *Pro Cluentio*. In his often quoted story of the Milesian woman who was put to death after having an abortion he describes in a climax, which becomes ever wider as it moves from the private to the public sphere, what her husband had lost:

> She deprived her husband of the hope of becoming a father, the memory of his name, the successor to his generation, the heir to his family, and the city of a future citizen.[4]

In the following sections I use this list as a guide to the exploration of male attitudes towards abortion in the ancient world. I also examine the possible attitudes of the sexual partners of some groups of women who were more likely to seek an abortion, such as unmarried women and prostitutes, and my account concludes with a consideration of abortion as an alternative to adoption, exposure of babies and infanticide.

i. The hope of becoming a father

G. Raepsaet has studied Athenian attitudes towards parenthood in an extensive article.[5] He concludes that childbirth and parenthood were linked with important religious, legal, social, cultural and personal factors.[6] Athenian men and women expected their children to look after them in their old age, and in fact the law made it obligatory for an Athenian man to look after his old parents under threat of a lawsuit which could lead to disfranchisement and various civic disabilities, such as a ban from holding office, if he failed to do so.[7] However, the same law, as well as social morality, created obligations and duties for the parents too. Once they had accepted a child in the family (*oikos*), they had to bring it up properly, that is, teach it practical skills as well as moral values.[8] Those skills and values were different for each gender in accordance with the different expectations that family and society had of men and women. Yet a good upbringing was considered equally essential for boys and girls, and the responsibility for it rested to a very considerable extent upon the family (more so for girls than for boys). Fathers (and possibly mothers) who failed their duty to their children were to be deprived of 'the benefits of bearing children'.[9] A son procured by his father into prostitution was not obliged to provide food and shelter for him in his old age; however he still had to take care of the funeral rites after his father's death.[10] Funeral rites were an obligation of the son or the nearest existing relatives, and female relatives of the deceased played an important role in the mourning and subsequent rites for the dead.[11] In this respect children were viewed as a form of security for one's old age and a guarantee that the traditional rites to the dead and the gods would be observed. Moreover, as I explain in the next section, the continuation of the *oikos* was an important goal of Athenian inheritance law, and succession by legitimate heirs, preferably but not necessarily natural sons, guaranteed that one's family would continue and the *oikos* would not become extinct. In this legal, social and cultural context childlessness was viewed as a misfortune, which ought to be avoided if at all possible. If it could not be helped the law provided alternatives such as adoption.[12]

But was it all mercenary? Did the Athenians view children solely as a 'prudent investment'?[13] Golden and Strauss agree that the motives of the Athenians were not solely dictated by expediency.[14] In fact, Golden correctly points out that sentiment and expediency are not mutually exclusive. Musonius Rufus, when he praises legislators who allegedly had prohibited abortion, says that it would be both morally good and expedient (*kalon kai sumpheron*) to follow their ruling. The feeling that one day a parent will be dependent upon his/her children should increase, not diminish, the motive to lavish them with affection and care. Genuine manifestations of emotion, love and care by Athenian men and women towards their children of both sexes can be found everywhere in Greek literature and art, and deep sorrow at the loss of a child is often reflected in funeral inscriptions.[15]

Against this background we can easily imagine Athenian men filled with joy at the thought of parenthood, and furiously angry at an abortion procured against their consent, since it would have deprived them of their expectations and the delights of parenthood. A true incident in which a man reacted in this manner is the case of Antigenes, the husband who, according to the testimony of the rhetorician Sopater, was prepared to stretch Athenian homicide law to the limits by attempting to have his wife convicted for homicide for an abortion which she had induced without his consent.[16] The legal implications of this case, as well as its background, are discussed in detail in Chapter 6. At this point it is sufficient to mention that the motive of Antigenes, when he went to extraordinary lengths in pursuit of this case, was surely anger. A man who tries to have his (probably former) wife convicted for an offence which was not even recognised by Athenian law as such (namely abortion), by means of stretching homicide law to apply to this case, sounds like a very angry individual. He had nothing material to gain, since a successful prosecution for homicide brought no reward for the successful prosecutor, and moreover he had to go to great lengths in order to bring this case to court. As I argue in Chapter 6, first he had to persuade (or possibly even blackmail) the *basileus*, the magistrate in charge of homicide proceedings, to accept the lawsuit, and then he had to prove in court that the foetus ought to be considered as human. This unusual procedure required a lot of time, preparation, effort, mental energy and iron nerve. Only powerful motives such as unabated anger and an unrelenting desire for revenge for an act which he perceived as a grave personal injury could have induced him to put himself through all this. I can only understand the battle of Antigenes, first against the laws and institutions of his own city, and then against the woman with whom he had shared a part of his life, as the action of a heart-broken, frustrated and angry man, who believed that he had been deprived of a child and felt that he must avenge its death.

Similar concerns are expressed in another text from the classical period, but this time they come from the mouth of a female character. Andromache, the eponymous heroine of Euripides' play, says to Menelaus:

> For if I gave drugs to your daughter and made her womb abort,
> As she claims, I will not kneel before the altar,
> But willingly, rather than unwillingly,
> I will be punished by your son-in-law,
> To whom I am equally responsible,
> If I have deprived him of children.[17]

Andromache is answering previous accusations by Hermione, the daughter of Menelaus, that the latter has become barren because of drugs and magic, allegedly administered by Andromache (vv. 157-8). Hermione considers Andromache to be the cause of her sterility; however, here Andromache's reply is more specific: she speaks not about sterility in general but about an induced abortion. Andromache firmly denies that she had secretly drugged Hermione with abortifacient substances. M. Lloyd has tried to remove the discrepancy by translating 'If I am drugging your daughter and making her womb barren, as she asserts, I will not crouch at an altar'.[18] However, the wording of the original in Andromache's speech (v. 356 *nêdun exambloumen*) undoubtedly refers to induced abortion. The discrepancy is not really significant or important for the purposes of the dramatist. Either way, Hermione was still childless, allegedly because of Andromache's sinister devices, and this was the real point of contention. Andromache denies that she used any drugs to make Hermione have an abortion, but agrees that if she had done so, she would deserve to be punished, not only because she would have violated Hermione's body contrary to the wishes of the latter, but also because she would have deprived Hermione's husband of the privilege of becoming a father.

The most important thing to be said about this passage is that it is a reflection of fears with which the audience of Euripides in the late fifth century BC would be expected to identify. Emphasis is placed not upon the injury that Hermione would have received if her body had been violated by abortifacient drugs without her knowledge, or the premature extinction of her unborn children, but upon the injury that her husband would have received. He would have been deprived of the joy of fatherhood, and Andromache concedes that this would be an offence grave enough to deserve the most serious punishment. In fact she challenges Menelaus and promises to submit willingly to punishment if these allegations against her are proven. She agrees that depriving a man of his future children ought to be considered a very serious offence. Of course the play was written by a man, and was primarily directed at the male judges of the dramatic contest and maybe a predominantly male audience. This remark expresses a view which Euripides presumably felt that his audience would share, and it is a reflection of male Athenian attitudes towards abortion as a threat to fatherhood. In this context abortion was to be condemned and perceived as a crime against the man concerned.

Roman sentiments and attitudes concerning fatherhood were in general terms not very different from Athenian attitudes. Even though different legal and social structures gave Roman men a greater degree of control over their families, children were still viewed as an asset for the future and a source of joy and pride, as they were by Athenian men.[19] This is why it is not surprising to see very similar concerns to those mentioned above expressed by Cicero in the speech *Pro Cluentio*.[20] The orator mentions a number of incidents in which abortions had been procured by women contrary to their husbands' wishes, and while he directs severe criticism against these women, in the meantime he expresses sympathy for their husbands at being deprived of their children and the joy of fatherhood.

It is remarkable that in the above-mentioned passages it is the man, the father, who is presented as the injured party that deserves sympathy. He is the one viewed as the victim of an abhorrent action which has deprived him of the privilege of fatherhood. Not a word of sympathy or pity for the foetus whose life had been prematurely terminated! To my knowledge there is no passage in Greek or Roman literature before the time of Augustus which expresses sympathy for the unborn, and this is certainly significant, especially in the light of changes that occur from the time of Augustus. From the second half of the first century BC expressions of sympathy for the unborn become increasingly common. Ovid in his daring elevation of abortion into a subject suitable for poetry (*Amores* 13 and 14) expresses sympathy not only for the man, but also for the foetus, while he criticises severely the mother for the abortion. His contemporary Chariton does the same thing: in a passage from the novel *Chaireas and Callirhoe* (quoted in Chapter 4 §iv) Callirhoe while contemplating an abortion understands that she is about to deprive her absent husband of his child, and at the same time feels pity for her unborn. In later centuries sympathy and pity for the unborn, which would be robbed of the gift of life by its cruel mother, is commonplace among Christian authors, starting with Tertullian.[21]

That sympathy for the foetus went hand in hand with hostile attitudes towards abortion is perfectly understandable. What is truly remarkable, and certainly significant, is the fact that such expressions of sympathy are nowhere attested before the time of Augustus, even though hostile attitudes towards abortion are not uncommon in the classical, hellenistic and republican periods. Until then when sentiment was expressed it would be for the father, who had been deprived of his offspring. However, it seems that there was a considerable shift of attitudes from the time of Augustus. As I argue in §iv below, his legislation on the family reflects the insecurity of a Roman elite ruling a sea of diverse nations, and at the same time attempts to generate a demographic trend which places emphasis upon the desire for higher birth-rates among the Roman citizenry. In this climate the unborn becomes more valuable, and more readily recognisable as a future citizen and a human being in the making. Thus it deserves sympathy and pity in its own right, and such expressions of sentiment become more commonplace. In subsequent centuries, as Christian authors became increasingly willing to acknowledge that animation occurs at conception and therefore human life begins at that point, expressions of feelings for the prematurely terminated life became more frequent, and such authors capitalised on this sentiment in their condemnation of induced abortion.

The apparent lack of feeling for the unborn in the literature before the time of Augustus, especially when accompanied by copious expressions of sympathy for the father, is probably related to perceptions of foetal life in that period. As I argued in Chapter 2, from the time of Hippocrates people, and especially men, became more aware of the possibility that birth need not represent the beginning of human life. As closer observation and clearer description of the stages of pregnancy passed into the medical literature of the time, and through this to the layman interested in the subject, the view that life begins before birth became increasingly dominant in the classical period. However, to say that this realisation automatically resulted in greater respect and an outpouring of sympathy for foetal life would be misleading. Even those who were prepared to acknowledge the unborn child as a human being did not seem to feel expressly sorry for the foetus when an abortion had ended its life. The foetus represented nothing more than 'a hope',[22] an unspecified possibility, while the Greeks and early Romans were more inclined to feel sorry for the father who had been deprived of his hopes. Now, whether men like Antigenes felt more sorry for themselves or for the foetus is difficult to tell, and I think there is no clear line to be drawn between the two: it could be both. Yet against this background I am tempted to think that generally Athenian men felt more sad and angry at the frustration of their own expectations than sorry for this unknown being, the foetus itself.

ii. Name, succession and inheritance

Private and to some extent public life in classical Athens were organised around the family unit, the *oikos*. The Greek word is more encompassing than the term 'family', because an *oikos* included the members of the family, the house where the family lived, and any other property that it owned. Slaves belonged to the *oikos* but in a different sense from free persons: they were part of the assets of the *oikos*. As MacDowell has pointed out, the term was flexible and used sometimes for the persons comprising a family, sometimes for the property belonging to it, and sometimes comprehensively for persons and property.[23] Each *oikos* had its own family cults and tombs, and its members were expected to perform the traditional rites and transmit them to the next generation.[24] The *oikos* was headed by an adult male, the *kurios*. Women, children and slaves were legally dependent: the *kurios* had to represent them in public bodies such as the Assembly and the law-courts. Athenian law assumed that every person who was not in a position to be legally independent had been placed under the protection and guardianship of a *kurios*. Other adult males living in the house, such as the man's son or retired father, were legally independent, but naturally the man in charge of the property could force his will upon them, sometimes with considerable conflict.[25] The *kurios* was held responsible by society, and sometimes even by the law, for the maintenance of discipline and appropriate conduct among the members of his household. In this capacity he had the authority to chastise them, and was certainly expected to do so when he noticed unruly or inappropriate behaviour on the part of his wife, children or slaves. However, his authority had limitations. Unlike the Roman *pater familias*, who, at least theoretically, had the right of life and death over his family, the Athenian *kurios* could only inflict moderate punishments upon women and minors. He did not draw most of his authority from specific punitive powers or legal provisions. He was expected to command the respect of his dependants and inspire trust and obedience, and certainly to be in a position to oversee all the affairs of the family. However, in practical terms it was primarily his wife who was in charge of all domestic matters while he was out representing the *oikos* in public bodies, or defending and enhancing its fortunes. The two, husband and wife, functioned in a partnership within the *oikos*, ideally aimed at good household management, stability and prosperity.[26]

Aristotle argued that the *oikos* is the source of political order, friendship and justice, and that the *polis* cannot be good unless its *oikoi* are also good.[27] Even though the Athenians embraced political concepts that perceived each citizen as independent and responsible for his actions, they never reached an absolute degree of individualism. The *oikos* remained the foundation upon which many of the institutions of the state rested. In Aristotle's words, 'the entire city consists of *oikoi*', and this is why the integrity and continuation of the *oikos* were important concerns of the state, the law, and the community as a whole. When an Athenian man died his *oikos* was continued by his son. The latter inherited the property and was expected to continue the traditions and religious rites of the family. Illegitimate sons could not succeed their father. If a man had more than one legitimate son, each one of them was heir to his father on an equal basis, since the Athenians did not recognise primogeniture.[28] In this case the *oikoi* of the sons were seen as the continuation of the original *oikos* of their father. If a man had no natural legitimate sons he could adopt an Athenian citizen. If he died leaving behind only daughters, their children were perceived as his heirs. If the daughters had no children, either because they were unmarried or because they were still childless, they became *epiklêroi*, sole heiresses, and the nearest male relative of their father could marry them. It was hoped that the *epiklêros* would produce an heir to her father's *oikos*, and sometimes the woman and her husband went as far as posthumously adopting a child of theirs into the *oikos* of her deceased father, so that his *oikos* was continued.[29]

In the light of this we can see why succession by legitimately born heirs, hopefully male, or even female if need be, was a primary concern of Athenian men. Legitimate heirs were a guarantee that one's generation would continue and one's name would continue to be spoken (especially since the Athenians quite often named children after their grandparents), the traditional family duties to the gods, the dead, and the family tombs would not be neglected, one's *oikos* would not be deserted (*erêmousthai* is actually the word used for an *oikos* which has become extinct), and the property would not be scattered among lateral relatives and thus incorporated into other *oikoi*. In a society which had such firm and stringent regulations concerning succession and inheritance abortion understandably could represent a serious threat not only to the feelings of individuals, but also to religious, legal and cultural institutions, which, as far as fifth- and fourth-century Athenians were concerned, had been in place from time immemorial.

The argument that abortion is wrong because it interferes with succession and inheritance plays a major role in the diatribe attributed to Galen, *Whether what is in the womb is a human being*, studied in greater detail in Appendix 1.[30] An action that had deprived a man of the hope of an heir could logically be perceived as a violation of a man's *oikos* and the continuation of his generation. When Antigenes decided to employ the homicide law of the city in order to exact revenge upon his wife for the abortion, he might expect his compatriots to empathise with the plight of a man who was angry because he had been deprived of an heir and successor to his *oikos*. The same concept underlies Andromache's admission that she would deserve to be punished by Hermione's husband if she had deprived him of his successors. In both cases the feeling of loss and bereavement experienced by the fathers-to-be could only be exacerbated by the thought that at the same time they had been left without an heir. Damage to the prospects of succession is the primary concern in the polemic against abortion by Philo:

> So, the person who destroys the infant is undoubtedly a murderer, because the law is not concerned with age but with the damage upon one's generation (*genos*).[31]

Similar concerns are expressed by Cicero in the above mentioned passage, and by Ovid in *Amores* 2,14, where, in fact, the case is amplified, and killing one's children is equated to vengeance upon the husband. In the story about the Roman matrons who had abortions in order to blackmail men (see Chapter 4 §v) abortion is also presented as a weapon directed against men. As children are considered to be a blessing by a number of sources, for the man's family and consequently for the state,[32] abortion is considered the opposite, namely a threat to one's *oikos*, and consequently to the interests of the state.

As things were, one might expect that the *kurios* of the *oikos* would have a very considerable say over the decision to have an abortion. Yet such authority is nowhere attested in the sources. As I argue in Chapter 6, Athenian law seemingly did not deal with abortion at all, and there is no Athenian source suggesting that men had to make decisions over the continuation or interruption of a pregnancy. The reason for this silence is probably that Athenian men were rarely consulted over the fate of a pregnancy. I mentioned in the previous chapter that abortions were mostly procured by prostitutes and by women who had become pregnant as a result of an extramarital affair. Men would not be asked to give their opinion in either of these cases. The father of a prostitute's child would be nothing more than an unwilling and absent contributor, while the *kurios* of the adulteress should never find out about the pregnancy. Most abortions would be kept secret from the men, if women could get away with it. However, as serious complications were not uncommon, men were bound to find out when things had gone wrong (as Corinna's lover does in Ovid's *Amores* 2,13). At this stage much depended upon the situation. If the woman happened to be unmarried, widowed, or temporarily separated from her husband she was in serious trouble; she could no longer lie. But if she had a husband, it would be difficult to prove anything against her. Medical science did not have enough knowledge to be able to make a clear distinction between a deliberately induced abortion and a miscarriage due to some unpredictable cause or accident. A characteristic passage from the Hippocratic study *Epidemics* indicates that the doctor was in serious doubt as to the cause of the abortion:

> The wife of Simon: abortion on the thirtieth day. This happened to her after she took something (namely, deliberately), or it was spontaneous.[33]

On these grounds it would be fair to say that quite often, even when an abortion had taken place and the husband of a married woman found out about it, he could not know for certain whether his wife had set out to ignore his wishes or just suffered a miscarriage. This uncertainty effectively undermined the need to consult the *kurios*, and this might be one additional reason why men are not reported in the sources as participants in decisions over abortions. The occasions when a married couple came together and discussed the fate of a pregnancy, allowing the man the opportunity to decide, were probably rare. As I argue below in §iv, elective abortion was far too dangerous to be employed as a method of family planning on a regular basis. A decision over matters of family size and the rearing of one's offspring was usually postponed until the moment of birth, because this was much safer. At that point the fate of the new-born rested primarily with the *kurios* of the *oikos*, and this is universally agreed among scholars and well attested in the sources (see §iv).

In all ancient societies, from Achaemenid Persia to imperial Rome, despite differences in legal, social and cultural perceptions of the family unit and its function within the state, men were at the head of the household, and were primarily responsible for order, prosperity and the transmission of values to the next generation. Whatever the precise setting, the leading male would be by right the person upon whom decisions over family planning and the fate of any potential heirs ought to rest. In reality, however, men in antiquity, not only in Athens but everywhere, were seldom consulted over the possibility of an abortion. The reason was that abortion would normally be employed by women trying to escape the attention of the *kurios* or *pater familias*, as they had something to hide. And even when this was not the case, it would still be hard to shake off his suspicions concerning the motives of the woman. This is why women throughout antiquity would leave the head of their household out of such decisions if at all possible. Abortion, as far as they were concerned, was a women's issue, not a family issue. Men would not welcome this attitude, but in most cases there was very little they could do. Either they were left in total ignorance, or, by the time they found out, it was usually too late to do anything to prevent or stop it.

iii. The future citizen

Demographic trends can fluctuate dramatically under the influence of historical circumstances. Whether a high or low birth-rate is favoured, it is very much a sign of the times and depends on political, economic and cultural factors. We could summarise the basic patterns of demographic trends as follow:

1. Some societies look for safety in numbers or for prosperity in plentiful, cheap labour and favour high birth-rates.

2. Other societies do not put their trust, safety and prosperity in large numbers, but in lean structures, higher efficiency, and a more even

distribution of wealth and privilege. These societies prefer low birth-rates, because they allow things to be more manageable.

3. In some cases a phenomenon noticeable particularly among the members of a privileged elite is that although there is an official policy favouring high birth-rates with a view to safety in numbers, the individual members of this elite are reluctant to sacrifice their privileged lifestyle and immerse themselves in the responsibilities of parenthood. In this case a conflict might develop between official policy that tries to encourage larger families and the actual practice of small families.

All three trends are discernible in various parts of the ancient world. The Greek city-states mostly favoured a low birth-rate. Plato explains the rationale behind this trend as follows:

> Of land we need as much as is capable of supporting so many inhabitants of temperate habits, and we need no more; and as to population, we need a number such that they will be able to defend themselves against injury from adjoining peoples, and capable also of lending some aid to their neighbours when injured.[34]

The nature of the political, religious and cultural institutions of the Greek *polis* meant that they could not have functioned well with large numbers. In a geographical setting mostly consisting of islands and small valleys local communities developed a strong sense of identity. They saw themselves as self-defined, and ideally self-sufficient units, proud of their political independence – their 'liberty' (*eleutheria*), as they would say – and their religious, social and cultural institutions. Federal unions were not favoured, and those that existed (e.g. Boeotia) were usually imposed by a strong centre, to the dismay of some of the smaller states compelled to participate. Within the borders of their *polis* the citizens felt masters of their own affairs. Regardless of the constitutional form (democracy, oligarchy, tyranny), the citizens of a certain *polis* were proud of their identity. Perhaps with the exception of some dire tyrannies, the adult male citizens normally assembled to consider the most important issues of state. In democracies the Assembly was sovereign, in oligarchies its authority was limited, while in tyrannies it might be nothing more than a formality.[35] But, at any rate, a body of limited size was manageable and functional, while a very large body could not have participated in the *polis* under these terms. Sparta was unusually large, covering the entire area of Laconia and Messenia (until 369), but still it could hold its citizen group together because most Spartans lived in the valley of Eurotas. Athens and Syracuse were unusually populous (*c.* 30,000 adult male citizens), but again the majority of their citizens did not live at a great distance from the centre. Most of the other Greek *poleis* were considerably smaller.

Keeping things small and manageable was an ideal for all Greek city states. Conquest would not increase the *polis*; it would simply increase the number of its subject and dependent territories. In this climate a large citizen body was viewed as dysfunctional and unmanageable. In 451 Pericles proposed a law which laid down that only the children of two Athenian citizens could be citizens themselves. This law, which was introduced in the height of the Athenian empire, was obviously intended to limit the number of people entitled to citizenship. The explanation provided by Aristotle as to why this law came into force is intriguing: he says that Pericles proposed it because there were too many Athenian citizens, and he felt that the number of the citizen body ought to be reduced.[36] And this was not the only instance where a large citizen body was viewed as an obstacle to the smooth functioning of the state. In 411, under the pressure of the Peloponnesian war, the democratic constitution was abolished. In future not all citizens were to participate in the Assembly, but only a fixed number of 5,000 – 'those who could be useful, on account of their wealth or physical strength'.[37] The measure did not last; it was abolished about a year later, because the principles of equality of speech (*isegoria*) and equality before the law (*isonomia*) were far too strong among the Athenians. However, history was to repeat itself about a century later: Antipater, after the decisive defeat of Athens in the Lamian war (322) limited the political franchise to 9,000, on the basis of a qualification of wealth, expecting that the city would be better run by this limited number than by the entire citizen body (31,000 according to Diodorus).[38]

This kind of limitation may have been exceptional and temporary for Athens, but it was a matter of course for some Greek states. In Sparta, for example, the disfranchisement of citizens who could not contribute to the messes was standard procedure. Any such citizen was reduced to the group of the 'Inferiors' until he could pay his way back to the messes.[39] Sparta is a good example of a city where the demographic trend towards a low birth-rate manifested itself so intensely that it proved devastating for the state. Aristotle directs a sharp criticism against Sparta for this depopulation of the citizen body:

> So, although the land was sufficient to support 1,500 cavalry and 30,000 heavy infantry, the number fell to below 1,000. The sheer facts have shown that these arrangements were bad: one single blow [sc. the battle of Leuctra in 371 BC] was too much for Sparta, and she succumbed owing to the shortage of men.[40]

Even if the figure given by Aristotle is too low, it is an indisputable fact that Sparta was facing an ever-worsening shortage of manpower that eventually led to her demise. The depopulation of the ranks of Spartan citizens was not the result of official policy of the Spartan state. On the contrary, the state tried to encourage higher birth-rates, partly by imposing sanctions upon individuals who refused to marry, and partly by introducing privileges for those who had many children, especially sons.[41] The state had very good reasons to encourage a high birth-rate. First, the Spartan citizens were a minority ruling large populations of helots and *perioikoi*, and it was natural for the Spartans to feel uneasy and desire the birth of many more Spartans. Then, men would be needed in a city with aspirations to rule over the Peloponnese, and for a period of its history (early fourth century) over Greece and Asia too. But despite this official policy, the Spartans avoided large families, and the reason is obvious. Despite what the state desired, the individual Spartan with modest means needed to think twice before begetting more than one or two children. If he had one or two, he might be able to leave enough inheritance for them to remain enfranchised. But if he had ten children, it would be mathematically certain that most of them would end up in the ranks of the Inferiors. This contradiction between official policy and actual demographic trend was not just one more Spartan paradox. It proved the most detrimental factor in the history of the city, and one may find it astonishing that no serious measure was taken to address the problem before it was too late. The reasons for this reluctance to take appropriate measures were many, but certainly one of those is the fact that Sparta, like the rest of the Greek states, had a 'gut-feeling' against enfranchising large numbers of people.[42]

The case of Sparta, a city-state with manifest interests in a large citizen body, and yet unwilling to take effective measures to produce it, simply confirms the rule that the Greek *poleis* did not favour high birth-rates. They often did not hesitate to take measures that kept the numbers down, and did not necessarily view a large citizen body as a source of strength and prosperity. Despite constitutional and ideological variations, the fundamental idea that a *polis* ought to be rather small and manageable was common throughout the Greek world before the time of Alexander.

It is in this context that we should take a look at the utopian states of Plato and Aristotle. Both favour states of limited size, and both recommend, among other measures, abortion as a means of population control. In his *Republic* Plato states that the number of marriages should be fixed so that the city will be neither too large nor too small. He then suggests that offspring should be born only to those who are at the peak of their physical and mental condition. A woman should have children between her twentieth and fortieth year, a man until his fifty-fifth year. After childbearing age both sexes were to be left free 'to have sexual relations with whoever they wish', provided that no children were born from such unions. Inappropriately conceived children were to be destroyed before birth, and if any such baby was born it ought not to be reared.[43] Plato's eugenic policies have been the subject of a number of studies, and it is outside my purposes to discuss them in detail here.[44] It is sufficient to note that the goal in his ideal state was a tightly controlled and limited number of births. Transgressions in the process should be corrected by abortion if possible, and this is viewed as a perfectly acceptable practice for the purposes of population control. Plato finds nothing morally wrong with abortion; on the contrary, if it can be put into good service, he does not hesitate to recommend it without qualifications.

We do not know enough about Plato's ideas on the human identity of the unborn. Various indirect reports of his beliefs on this matter appear to contradict each other. Some sources report that he perceived the unborn as a living being (*zôon*), on the grounds that it moved in the womb and received food.[45] Tertullian, however, reports that, like the Stoics, he understood the soul as an external force (*anima extranea*) entering the infant immediately after birth (see the discussion in Chapter 2).[46] The Platonic ideas on the soul and reincarnation, as presented in the *Phaedo*, appear to be consistent with the concept of an external soul entering the body immediately after birth. On the other hand, the term *zôon* is far too vague to allow the firm conclusion that Plato understood the unborn as a human being in its own right (see the debate in Chapter 2). We can conclude that Plato probably did not consider the unborn to be fully human, even though he was prepared to accept that it is a living being. If this conclusion is correct, we can understand why he did not hesitate to recommend abortion without qualifications.

Aristotle is more reserved. In a famous passage from the *Politics* he also recommends abortion as a method of population control, but not without qualifications:

> With regard to the choice between abandoning an infant or rearing it, let there be a law that no cripple child be reared. But since the ordinance of custom forbids the exposure of infants on account of their numbers, there must be a limit to the production of children. If contrary to these arrangements copulation does take place and a child is conceived, an abortion must be induced before sense and life are instilled, because what is permissible and what is not will be defined on the basis of feeling and living.[47]

As I have argued in Chapter 2, Aristotle was the first to link Hippocratic views on foetal development and formation with concepts such as animation and sensation, and concluded that the unborn should be considered as human from the moment that sense and life begin. This is why he is prepared to condone abortion for the purposes of population control before that stage, but not after. Remarkably enough Aristotle condemns exposure of surplus babies (unless they are disabled[48]) in the same passage where he condones abortion. He cannot accept the abandonment of babies to their fate, but he can accept abortion in early pregnancy, simply because in the latter case he does not consider that a human being has being destroyed.

The views of Plato and Aristotle on population control in their utopian states are perfectly in line with the tendency of the Greek *poleis* to have populations of limited size rather than large, ever-expanding citizen bodies. If abortion served this general pattern well, then it should be employed to serve the common good. But how seriously we can take these statements of Plato and Aristotle as a mirror of contemporary views and attitudes? One might be tempted to argue that these views are eccentric statements of intellectuals, suitable for utopian political theories but detached from reality. Utopian constructions probably do not take into account many of the troublesome drawbacks and conflicts of real life, and as far as the issue under discussion is concerned this is certainly true. Neither of the two philosophers takes into account the fact that abortion was a painful and life-threatening undertaking, and that a man could not really ask his sexual partner to do it, if she did not wish the same thing herself. Both philosophers also ignore the difficult emotional and moral issues that abortion raises. They simply see abortion as expedient in the pattern of population control that they wish to establish, and do not hesitate to condone it. But on the other hand, we should not underestimate the extent to which political theory of this nature borrows from reality. As I have suggested, Plato and Aristotle reflect contemporary demographic trends when they suggest that a *polis* should not have a very large citizen body. And if we consider that Athenian society in general was not particularly keen in large families or populations, the conclusion that abortion was not viewed as a threat to the structures of the state is inevitable. The Athenians in the time of Plato and Aristotle would not feel that the safety of the state was at stake if women had abortions freely. Whether they condoned abortion as a matter of course, as the two philosophers do, is another matter. They did not use it regularly as a method of limiting the size of their families, because the dangers certainly outweighed any possible benefit, and many of them would not like to see such things happening in their household for moral, religious or personal reasons. But they did not consider it as a threat to the state, and this is confirmed by the limited amount of evidence concerning the reactions and attitudes of Athenian men. In all the passages mentioned above (§i), abortion is presented as a personal injury to the father or a threat to the family line, but not as a threat to the state. I think this silence is significant, especially when contrasted with Roman sources.

Abortion is presented as a threat to the structures and existence of the state in a text of the late republic (first century BC) for the first time. The passage of Cicero from the speech *Pro Cluentio* mentioned above[49] is the earliest reference that I know in Graeco-Roman literature where abortion ceases to be a matter that concerns only the family and those directly involved in a personal or professional capacity, and becomes a wider issue that threatens the state by depriving it of its future citizens. In subsequent centuries this becomes a standard theme. Under the empire abortion is increasingly viewed as a practice that cannot accord with the efforts of successive emperors to stimulate population growth among the Roman elite.[50] Not much later than this rather brief remark of Cicero, which appears in the end of a climactic passage, a poet writing under the influence of the Augustan legislation intended to stimulate family life among the Roman citizenry, especially among the senatorial and equestrian orders, amplifies the subject.[51] Ovid in *Amores* 14 presents abortion as a threat to the state of Rome itself and its institutions.[52] Abortions for women are compared with warfare for men. Both involve violence and destruction of the progeny, only in the case of abortion this happens insidiously and in an undignified manner. Although a quiet feeling of anger runs through the poem, these verses come not from the heart but from the mind. The person who speaks in the poem, the *amator*,[53] draws a parallel between the wounds that men receive at war and the self-inflicted wounds that women receive during abortion. He cannot reconcile himself to the idea that tender girls can inflict such horrendous wounds upon themselves, or that they can be as cruel towards their unborn children as famous mythological figures such as Medea and Procne[54] who killed their own offspring. Abortion is presented as an irrational and unjustifiable crime since even Medea and Procne had strong reasons when they killed their children, but future mothers who induce abortions have no justification and punishment is awaiting them. As M.K. Gamel correctly says, 'the *amator* is here taking on not only the role of *paterfamilias*, but that of the *curator morum et legum* (caretaker of morals and the laws)'. Here the foetus is treated as human, a potential child with an independent right to life, and, on the whole, the tone of this poem is critical. Disapproval of the killing of the unborn is unequivocally expressed, up to the point that death of the mother as a result of an abortion that went wrong would be considered by some to be a fair punishment. However, at this point the *amator* distances himself from such remarks and prays to the gods, asking them to forgive his lover this one time, and reserve punishment for future offences. The *amator* very clearly considers abortion to be morally wrong and an offence against the gods. He does not even attempt to justify his beloved's actions; he only begs for forgiveness on her behalf.

The views expressed here by Ovid are probably a reflection of a vivid contemporary debate on morality, sexual behaviour and the role of the family. Within the frame of the Augustan legislation on the family, the debate on abortion, its ethics and purpose in family and community life surely intensified and negative views towards abortion, not unknown before but not as strongly expressed, probably became more vocal. The *amator* in this poem resembles the Roman statesman, maybe even Aeneas or Augustus himself, as Gamel has suggested, voicing his concerns about a practice that would appear to be unjustifiable and out of place in the moral system he was trying to establish. This new male, although capable of compassion, takes the moral high ground and tries to define personal relations along lines that would require submission of the impulses of the individual to the interests of the state. Ovid captures here the pulse of a contemporary debate on social issues and incorporates it into his poetry with a rare degree of realism and boldness.[55]

The concerns raised by authors of the late republic and early empire are represented even more vociferously in a passage by the rhetorician Musonius Rufus in the first century AD:

> The legislators, whose main task is to seek and consider what is good for the city and what is bad, what benefits and what harms the common cause, unanimously considered the large size of individual families to be most beneficial for the cities, while they believed that population reduction is most harmful. They perceived childlessness, or small numbers of children to be harmful, while they thought that having many children was beneficial. For

that reason they forbade women to have abortions, and imposed penalties upon those who disobeyed. And while they forbade contraception and deliberate childlessness, on the other hand they set up privileges for men and women who had many children, and made childlessness unattractive. So, do we not commit an unjust and illegal act, if our laws go against the wishes of those divine men who were loved by the gods, for it is considered to be good and beneficial to follow them?[56]

The views of Musonius may be generally extreme and unusual, but here it seems to me that he encapsulates a growing anxiety over the demographic and political consequences of induced abortion in the Roman world, which eventually led to its prohibition.[57] This passage advances a policy of 'safety in numbers' and seeks to persuade the reader that such a policy is not only imperative for the well-being of the state, but also sanctioned by tradition, and in line with the wishes of the legislators and wise men of the past. Musonius is not in a position to quote any specific legal provision of the past banning contraception or abortion, nor can he name a single wise man who had defended this kind of demographic policy. The reason is simple: even though Musonius tries to assure his readers that such policies were traditional, in fact they were not. A demographic trend that favoured large populations, sought safety in numbers, and considered practices such as contraception or abortion as dangerous for the safety of the state, would have been an alien concept in the writings of the great philosophers and intellectuals of the past. In fact, we have seen that Plato and Aristotle advocated the opposite. As I have suggested above, this kind of demographic policy first appears in seminal form in authors of the late republic, is sanctioned by Augustus, and becomes official Roman policy in the imperial era. However, for all its historical inaccuracy the passage of Musonius is an important document, because it is the oldest text where we can see this new demographic trend perfectly shaped. This trend would become stronger in the following centuries, be shaped into law under Septimius and Caracalla, and take a central place in Christian doctrine.

The reason that official Roman policy is distinctly different from that of the Greek *poleis* has to do with historical circumstances. From the time of Cicero Rome was a leading power with many diverse nations under its control. Although the Romans were more generous with the bestowal of citizenship upon foreigners or offspring of mixed unions than most Greek *poleis* had been, they still regarded Roman citizenship as a privilege that ought to be carefully guarded. It was not until Rome started feeling the first tremors from the barbarian attacks which eventually led to her demise, that the *Constitutio Antoniana* (AD 212) abolished the distinction between Italians and provincials, and extended Roman citizenship to all inhabitants of the empire. For most of its history the citizens of Rome ruled over many nations. Power and wealth were the privilege of the upper classes within the Roman citizenry, especially the senatorial and to some degree the equestrian order. Scholars agree that these were the classes primarily targeted by the Augustan laws on family life and successive imperial decrees intended to stimulate a higher birth-rate and traditional family values. For them numbers mattered. A healthy birth-rate among the ruling Roman classes was seen as a matter of safety, and a guarantee that Rome and its traditions would not be overrun by alien armies and cultures. Practices that endangered the numbers of high-born Roman citizens were inevitably viewed as a threat to the supremacy of Rome and bound to invite hostility. The successive measures taken by a number of emperors to safeguard Roman family life are firm testimony to the fact that Rome felt insecure and wanted more Romans of good birth in order to protect her interests. These measures, however, can be interpreted from a different angle as a reflection of conflict between official Roman policy and actual practice. As I mentioned in Chapter 4 §iv, upper-class Roman men and, perhaps even more so, women, were not particularly keen to conform with a high birth-rate policy. The individual Roman had to consider many factors before complying with the request of his or her country, and perhaps this is why we find that in Rome, as in Sparta, there was a conflict between what the state wanted and what the individual was prepared to do. Although the ideology of the state increasingly viewed abortion as a threat, it was employed quite often by Roman women.

Similar historical factors probably affected the attitudes of the ruling nation of another great empire in the ancient world, and had similar effects. The Persians under the Achaemenid dynasty ruled a large constellation of nations from the plains of India to the sands of the Saharan desert.[58] They were a minority of Aryan decent surrounded by Semites, and intensely aware of their racial, linguistic, religious and cultural differences from their subjects. Yet this awareness never actually resulted in racism as we know it. The Persians from the time of Cyrus II followed a general policy of acceptance and tolerance towards the diverse customs, religions and political structures of their subject nations, unless for some reason these were perceived as antagonistic to the authority of the Great King. The Persian monarchs were willing to promote into high office persons of a different nationality who had served them well. Even the highest of honours, namely marriage into the royal family, was at times bestowed upon non-Persians. However, one must stress that high office was conferred upon foreigners as an exceptional honour, an expression of personal favour by the Great King or his representatives, not as a matter of course. The most important jobs in the court and the local government were normally reserved for the high-born members of the two Aryan peoples of the empire, the Persians and the Medes. Under these circumstances we should not be surprised to find that the Persians, like the Romans, wished to maintain a high birth-rate, and took appropriate measures to this effect. Those who could afford it kept harems with concubines destined to satisfy their sexual appetites and provide them with sons. Artaxerxes II reputedly had 104 sons, and the rest of the Persian kings did not fall that far behind. Each had a number of children from different women. Sons were needed for the purposes of succession, the administration of the empire, and the ranks of the King's armies, while daughters were needed in order to strengthen the ties of the family with other families through marriage. Herodotus describes Persian demographic trends and policies as follows:

> Each one of them marries many lawful wives, and they have even larger numbers of concubines. After valour in battle it is accounted noble to father the greatest number of sons: the king sends gifts yearly to him who gets most. *Strength, they believe, is in numbers.* They educate their boys from five to twenty years old, and teach them only three things: riding and archery and honesty. A boy is not seen by father before he is five years old, but lives with the women: the point of this is that, if the boy should die in the interval of his rearing, the father would suffer no grief. This is a law which I praise; and it is a praiseworthy law, too, which does not allow the king himself to slay any one for a single offence, or any other Persian to do incurable harm to one of his servants for one offence. Not until an accounting shows that the offender's wrongful acts are more and greater than his services may a man give rein to his anger. They say that no one has ever yet killed his father or mother. When such a thing has been done, it always turns out on inquest that the doer is shown to be a changeling or the fruit of adultery; for it is not to be believed that a son should kill his true parent.[59]

Anything that might threaten the numbers of Persians available to the service of the Great King was viewed as a threat to his interests and his empire. Abortion did not fit into this demographic pattern, and this is why Darius I brought in a particularly draconian law on abortion. In the early fifth century he introduced a law-code on the model of the code of Hammurabi, which probably remained in force throughout the Achaemenid period. The code does not survive, but A.T. Olmstead maintains that large sections of it have been incorporated, and thus preserved for us, in the Persian religious text *Videvdad* of the second century BC.[60] The stipulations concerning abortion can be summarised as following:

1. If a man seduces an (unmarried) woman she cannot have an abortion.
2. If she does, she and her father are responsible for deliberate homicide.
3. If she tells the seducer and he advises her to have an abortion, all three are guilty of deliberate homicide.
4. The seducer must support her until the child is born. No hint is made to the acknowledgement of the child, or marriage afterwards. This probably means that the man was not obliged to marry the woman or support the child after birth.
5. If he refuses to support her during pregnancy he is to be guilty of murder.

This law is prepared to go to any lengths to protect the life of the foetus. At some stage the law is prepared to claim three adult lives for the life of the unborn, those of the woman, her father and her sexual partner. The stipulation that makes her father responsible for the safety of the unborn is also fascinating. The lawgiver probably assumes that the woman's father will support her during pregnancy if her seducer cannot be brought to book, and probably afterwards, along with the child, and this is why he does not explicitly compel him to do so. He simply makes sure that an abortion is not contemplated by threatening both of them with the death penalty for deliberate homicide if the pregnancy is terminated. The treatment of the woman's sexual partner is even more severe. The law cannot take it for granted that the partner will be willing to support her, and this is why it explicitly compels him to do so until the child is safely born. Beyond that the law does not interfere. From the moment the child is born, it is a person protected by the same laws as anyone else; the lawgiver feels that his duty to protect the child's life through the anti-abortion law stops at this point. It is also interesting that the law explicitly mentions only a pregnancy which is the result of an extra-marital liaison. Should we understand that it permitted abortion within marriage? I think not. It would be illogical to suggest that a legislator prepared to go to such lengths in order to protect the life of an illegitimately conceived child, would be prepared to allow the destruction of a foetus conceived within marriage. The king-lawgiver probably did not even contemplate the possibility of a married woman seeking an abortion. In his understanding such things were done only by those who had conceived as a result of an illicit liaison, and this is why he introduced a law confined to such cases.

This discussion suggests that there is a clear link between demographic trends and attitudes to abortion. The Greek city-states never aimed at high birth-rates, and thus never perceived abortion as a threat to the institutions and safety of the state. Pioneers of political theory were even prepared to accept and condone the practice as a method of population control, while the legislative bodies of the Greek city-states never felt the need to legislate against abortion. As far as we know, no city-state ever penalised it, even though some schools of thought and some sections of the population undoubtedly felt that it was ethically wrong. Upper-class Romans, who for the most part of their history ruled a vast, multinational empire as a privileged elite, felt insecure over their numbers, and thus official policy was in favour of a higher birth-rate and against abortion. However, there was a clear conflict between official policy and actual demography, as individuals defied the calls of the state for more properly-born Roman children, and employed abortion when this was demanded by the circumstances, despite ethical dilemmas or official condemnation. The Persians were in a similar position to the Romans, as far as the political setting was concerned, but also acutely aware of their racial, religious and cultural differences from their Semitic neighbours and subjects. They felt more intensely that they were only a small minority among the population of their vast empire, and sought safety in numbers by adopting every possible measure that could increase the numbers of Persians, polygamy included. Understandably they perceived any practice which might threaten these numbers as a menace, and thus introduced perhaps the fiercest anti-abortion law that has ever existed.

iv. Abortion, adoption, exposure and infanticide

In Mary Renault's novel *The Last of the Wine*, set in the Peloponnesian war, Lysis, the main character, is asked to expose his newly born half-sister. The family is hard pressed by extreme poverty and famine during the siege of Athens by the Spartan army, after the catastrophe of the Athenian fleet at Aigospotamoi and before the surrender of the city to Lysander (405/4). The family is unable to feed one more mouth and hopes that if she is abandoned in a public place some childless woman might find and take her. Their action is motivated by pity and care for the fate of the new-born baby. Lysis wraps up the baby, takes her at night to an open place, and abandons her with his heart torn apart by her cries. He is only too well aware that her chances of being found and brought up are truly slim in those times of deprivation. If nothing else, she will need to compete for the affections of potential foster-parents with abandoned baby boys, who would naturally be given preference, and since the entire area sounds with the cries of abandoned babies every night, a baby girl has less of a chance.

The historically aware novelist has captured in this scene a number of truths or alleged truths concerning the exposure of babies in the ancient world. First of all, that babies could be exposed not because their families did not care about them, but because they could not rear them; secondly, that families compelled to expose their babies did so with considerable distress; and finally, that baby girls were more likely to be exposed than baby boys, and less likely to be rescued by someone else. Such views on the exposure of babies in the ancient world are firmly established in scholarly opinion. A number of studies has suggested that exposure of babies was a frequent occurrence in classical Athens. Modern scholars seem to be fascinated by this practice, as if it were a peculiarity of the ancient world related to the alleged indifference of pagan Graeco-Roman antiquity towards human life, especially that of female infants. The debate has been long and difficult and it is outside my purposes to explore it in detail. However, it is necessary to clarify to some extent the main aspects of the issue.[61] Abortion, exposure, infanticide and adoption have often served as measures intended to dispose of unwanted babies. Each of these measures has its own peculiar ways of effecting the desired end, and by considering these peculiarities we may be able to understand why each measure might be given preference under a certain set of circumstances.

Adoption among the Athenians was intended to compensate for the lack of natural heirs.[62] However, unlike today, it was not seen as a process aimed at fulfilment of the emotional needs of childless couples, or providing a loving family for children whose parents were absent or unwilling to bring them up. I do not mean to say that considerations of this kind were always absent.[63] A childless couple might love their adopted baby, as we are told Polybus and Merope did, the childless king and queen of Corinth who adopted baby Oedipus and brought him up with great affection and care.[64] Yet adoption was generally seen as a clearly defined legal process with very specific objectives. Its purpose was to provide an heir who would continue the *oikos*, inherit its property and preserve the family rites. This is why the adoptee ought to be a citizen,[65] was often an adult, usually male, and almost invariably someone whom the adopter already knew, namely a member of his wider family or a friend.[66] Foundlings or unwanted babies could, of course, be sneaked in by families longing for children and presented as their own natural offspring, but adoption as a legal and social practice was not designed with such cases in mind, nor would couples follow normal adoption procedures under these circumstances.[67]

Adoption is nowadays considered by many to be the most humane and morally acceptable alternative to abortion. In theory this alternative was open to families in the ancient world too. However, Athenian law did not allow men who already had legitimate sons to adopt, as this would compromise their inheritance rights. Thus adoption, even though safer, was not a realistic alternative to abortion in most cases, because it would be quite difficult to find persons legally eligible and willing to adopt the unwanted baby. The fact that adoption is not really mentioned in the sources as a possible alternative to abortion suggests that married couples could not really rely on the possibility of finding people willing to adopt. And if it was difficult to find new families for legitimately born babies, it was almost impossible to find families willing to take on illegitimate offspring of adulterous relationships. Such difficulties make the moral and emotional dilemma between abortion and adoption, which people face today, seem purely academic in the ancient world.

Abortion was perilous but adoption was difficult, so what was the alternative for poor families, women who had strayed, or single women in prostitution? For those sensible enough to be afraid of abortion but without resource to adoption there was another possibility, well attested in the sources. Exposure of unwanted babies was certainly practised by the Greeks and Romans, as it has been practised by every society that has ever existed, including the most affluent societies today. There is nothing surprising or unique in the fact that they did it, but how often the Greeks and the Romans exposed babies, for what reason, and with what kind of attitude, remain highly controversial issues. The frequency of references to the exposure of babies in classical literature is relatively high.[68] It has been argued that girls were more vulnerable than boys.[69] Scholars have been particularly intrigued by the famous letter of Hilarion, in which the absent husband advises his pregnant wife to keep the baby if it is a boy, but expose it if it is a girl.[70] In Gortyn the possibility of exposing a baby if the former husband of a divorced woman refuses to recognise it, is enshrined in the law:

If a wife who is separated (by divorce) should bear a child, (they) are to bring
it to the husband at his house in the presence of three witnesses; and if he
should not receive it, the child shall be in the mother's power either to rear
or expose; and the relatives and witnesses shall have preference in the oath
as to whether they brought it.[71]

A complete list of all known cases is provided by S. Milligan in the
thorough account of the subject included in her PhD thesis.[72] The volume
of this evidence has sparked a debate that started in the 1920s with a
substantial article by H. Bolkestein.[73] With sober judgement the author
concludes that 'no fact can be pointed out, nor an utterance cited, as
regards the fifth and fourth centuries BC which could be used as proof that
the exposure of infants by their parents was a common thing in Athens;
on the contrary, indications are to be found which justify the drawing of
the opposite conclusion'. Equally cautious was A. Cameron, who concluded
that exposure of babies and infanticide are attested practices, but one
should not overestimate the frequency of their occurrence.[74] A.W. Gomme
also thought that there is nothing to suggest that it was common, and the
same view was held by D. Engels in a more recent article.[75] Therefore it
seems clear that scholars for the most part of the twentieth century held
the view that although exposure and infanticide occasionally took place in
the ancient world, such incidents were not a matter of course, but rather
extraordinary events that took place under the pressure of unusual and
difficult circumstances.

Engels has made extensive use of demographic data before reaching
this conclusion, and this was the main point that M. Golden disputed in
an article published shortly after Engels' study. Golden was joined by W.V.
Harris in condemnation of the demographic methods of Engels.[76] Both
authors point out that these methods are fundamentally flawed, but while
Harris considers extensive infanticide as merely possible, Golden on the
basis of statistical and demographic observations concludes that exposure
of female infants could be as high as 10% or even more. Golden's thesis has
become something like a scholarly orthodoxy in the last two decades. S.B.
Pomeroy has supported this view with further data on infanticide in the
hellenistic period from inscriptions concerning mercenary soldiers. Such
views have infiltrated the study of E. Eyben on family planning in the
Graeco-Roman world, who is prepared to accept that girls were more likely
to be exposed than boys.[77] Eyben places much emphasis, too much in my
opinion, upon evidence mainly from New Comedy and mythology and
concludes that exposure of children for the purposes of family planning
was a regular occurrence in the ancient world. On the other hand, C.
Patterson takes a more restrained approach.[78] Although she is prepared
to accept that exposure of children might be an option in difficult circumstances, she maintains that the existing evidence does not suggest that
this was a widespread practice, nor that girls were exposed on a regular
basis.[79]

Before we attempt a synthesis of the arguments, we should include in the debate one particular case of institutionalised exposure that allegedly took place in ancient Sparta. The case of regular exposure of babies in Sparta was a legend in the ancient world. Plutarch in the *Life of Lycurgus* describes the custom as follows:

> The father did not have authority to rear the baby, but he took it to a place called a *leskhê*, where the eldest members of the tribes sat and inspected the child. If it was well-built and strong, they ordered him to rear it, allocating to it one of the 9,000 lots; but if it was ill-born and unshapely, they sent it away to the so-called *Apothetai*, a place like a pit near Taygetus, believing that it was better both for itself and for the city that it should not live if it was not well-formed for health and strength right from the start.[80]

Sparta was a society so much concerned with excellence in the battlefield that everything else in life played a subordinate role. The entire political and social structure of ancient Sparta was oriented towards creating efficient soldiers; weak or disabled babies did not fit in. This is why it is not inconceivable that such babies were sometimes exposed. However, how regular or imperative this exposure was is a matter of interpretation and speculation. Against evidence suggesting that disabled children were exposed as a matter of course there is a number of well-known cases of disabled Spartan citizens: the most famous among them being that towering personality in Spartan history, king Agiselaus, who was lame in one leg.[81] The elevation of Agesilaus to the throne under the auspices of Lysander (398 BC) did not go uncontested. His disability was put forward as a reason why he should not become king. However, this congenital disability did not stop him from going through the *agôgê*, the military training that Spartan boys underwent from the age of seven, and eventually from becoming king, perhaps the most influential figure in Spartan politics for half a century. To this if we add tales like that of the blind poet Tyrtaeus who excited the Spartans to victory over the Messenians with his enthusiastic verses, then perhaps the idea that disability was an entirely unacceptable condition in Sparta is nothing more than a tale. Some take the evidence of Plutarch as fact and speak of widespread and systematic exposure of disabled infants; others, with whom I am more inclined to agree, treat it as one of those legends about Sparta.[82]

One can understand why the state had vested interests in the rearing of healthy male babies, but whether it actively intervened and compelled parents to expose disabled babies, or left some discretion to the father, is difficult to tell. Our sources do not say what would happen if the father refused to expose a disabled baby. Would the state punish him, or remove the baby forcibly from its parents? The elders might refuse to grant the baby full citizenship, but no source mentions that they would actually compel the family to expose. I would not be surprised if the final decision rested with the father. A Spartan man might put pressure upon the elders to allow the rearing of a child with mild disabilities, such as Agesilaus; and if they refused, he had to consider the prospect of rearing it as a person deprived of 'the life of honour' (full citizenship), or exposing it. If I am right to suggest that the decision ultimately rested with the father (who might also consult the mother), this would bring Sparta perfectly in line with other Greek city-states, and Spartan men, like other Greek fathers, had to decide whether it was in the best interests of the baby, the family, and the community to bring it up. Where the Spartans may have differed was in the weight attached to the potential contribution of the child to the community, and in this respect they may have been more inclined than other Greek fathers to expose a baby who could not be a soldier for Sparta.

The case of Sparta, as I understand it, is in line with what I believe was the general pattern of exposure, namely that ultimately it was an individual decision which had to do with the particular circumstances of the case, and rested upon the father. This view has been championed by Patterson, who correctly rejects the flawed demographic methods adopted in previous studies. The fact that on the basis of the same sources Engels and Golden can reach diametrically different conclusions provides a rather clear indication of the very unsafe nature of such material and methodology. To put it simply, we do not have enough information from the classical period to be able to compile statistics. Reliable demographic tables could only be produced if we had full archives recording the number of births, deaths and other such data over a considerable period of time. So long as we do not possess such material, demographic statistics are bound to remain mere speculation. For this reason I do not think that we can find any answers in such casual and unsystematic material, which, in addition, often contains unreliable numerical references. If any answers can be provided these must be sought in the attitudes and beliefs of the Greeks, on which we are better informed.

In every case of exposure, mythological or factual, there is a very good reason why the baby has been exposed. It is worth quoting the passage from Euripides' *Ion* where Hermes relates how Creusa, who had been raped by Apollo, exposed baby Ion. She had given birth while still unmarried, after successfully hiding the pregnancy from her father under the auspices of the god. Having thus far escaped her father's attention she could not possibly keep the baby and was forced to expose it in a cave. Hermes relates how he took the baby and left it outside the steps of Apollo's sanctuary in Delphi, where he was found and brought up by the priestess:

> Here Apollo forced a union on Kreusa, the child of Erechtheus,
> where the rocks, turned to the north beneath the hill of Pallas' Athenian
> land, are called Makrai by the lords of Attica.
> Unknown to her father
> – such was the pleasure of the god –
> she bore the weight in her womb.
> When the time came, Kreusa gave birth in the house
> to a child, and brought the infant to the same cave
> where the god had bedded her, and there exposed him to die

in the round circle of a hollow cradle,
observant of the customs of her ancestors,
and of Erichthonios, the earth-born.
.... And Phoebus, as my brother,
asked me this: 'O brother, go to the native-born people
of glorious Athens, for you know the city
of the goddess; take the new-born baby
from the hollow rock, with his cradle and baby-clothes;
bring him to my shrine at Delphi,
and place him at the very entrance of my temple;
The rest – know that the child is mine –
will be my care.' To gratify my brother Loxias
I took up the woven basket
and brought it here, and placed
the boy at the base of this temple,
opening up the wreathed cradle,
so that the infant might be seen.
It happened that, as the sun rose, the priestess
entered the god's prophetic shrine; she saw the baby
and marvelled that some girl of Delphi had dared
to cast her illegitimate child into the house of the god;
she was eager to take it away from the shrine;
but she let the harsh intent give way to pity
– and the god worked with her, so the child might not be hurled
out of his house – she took up the child and raised it.
She did not know that Phoebus was the father,
nor who the mother was, nor did the child know
about his parents. When young he played round the shrine,
and was nourished there; but when he grew to manhood,
the Delphians made him guardian of the god's treasures,
a trusted steward of all; and here in the temple
of the god he has lived a holy life.[83]

This passage is significant because it probably reveals some realities of
contemporary practice in cases of exposure. The unmarried girl, pregnant
as a result of rape, successfully hides the pregnancy from her father (with
some help from the god), but she cannot possibly keep the baby once born
as it would be manifest proof of an inappropriate relationship. Her only
option is to expose it. The baby is found on the steps of the temple, and the
priestess thinks that some local girl has abandoned her 'illegitimate child'.
But she is overcome by pity (and the god helps again), and decides to adopt
the baby. Caves, or places in the wilderness, like the pits of mount
Taygetus or the heights of Cithairon (in the case of baby Oedipus), were
chosen as the place to abandon a baby when its survival was not a desired
option. But temples, baths and public places were chosen when the mother
hoped that someone would find and adopt it. In another famous exposure
case from tragedy, baby Oedipus was to be left on the mountain to die
because his father Laios was afraid of the oracle saying that this child
would kill him and marry his wife Jocasta.[84] But, again, the servant who
is asked to do the task does not have the nerve to abandon the baby and

gives him away to a shepherd, who in turn gives him for adoption to a childless couple, the king and queen of Corinth. The same pattern can be observed in the tale of Herodotus concerning the exposure of Cyrus. Astyages, the king of Media, orders one of his servants to kill the baby of his daughter Mandane after a series of threatening dreams foretelling that his grandson would seize his kingdom. The servant, out of pity for the baby, hands him over to a shepherd to expose him. The shepherd's wife, who has just had a stillborn baby, persuades her husband to expose the dead baby and rear Cyrus instead.[85] How much historical truth is contained in the account of Herodotus is another issue, but as a matter of fact the historian would need an explanation as to why baby Cyrus was exposed and provides this explanation in his truly vivid and imaginative account of the dreams of Astyages.[86] These examples are sufficient to illustrate my point, namely than even in mythology a truly strong reason had to exist before a baby was exposed.

The cases of institutionalised exposure mentioned above clearly point in the same direction. Spartan babies would not be exposed unless they were born with severe disabilities, and the family was unwilling to take the strain of bringing up a child with such problems. The case of the Gortyn law is even clearer. Here the divorced woman, whose former husband refuses to recognise the child and contribute to its upbringing, has the choice between trying to cope with the difficulties of rearing the baby on her own or exposing it. The law is prepared to show understanding if she shrinks from the responsibilities of single motherhood. In both cases exposure is seen as a desperate solution to an exceptionally tough situation, not a course of action callously taken for the most trivial reasons. To say that exposure of babies, boys or girls, was nothing more than a calculated policy of population control, as some of the above-mentioned studies would have us believe, takes human emotion out of the equation, and this amounts to committing a serious historical error. The evidence cited above, as well as almost any other attested case of exposure, would strongly argue against it, and common sense would do the same. To cast out a baby, to leave it in a place to die, or even abandon it in a public place with a vague hope that it might be rescued, would be an agonising decision taken under the pressure of enormous forces financial, social, or personal. Parents in antiquity were not emotionally more indifferent to their young than modern parents. They would agonise over such a decision, and if they opted for exposure they would do so because in this particular instance they felt that they had no other option.

Previous studies, despite their readiness to adopt sparse, shaky and unreliable numerical data from the ancient world, have ignored a much more reliable study of data by Bolkestein. In the final note of his article he provides the results of his research into the Amsterdam archives covering a period of 200 years. He summarises his results as following: 'There is absolutely no connection between the number of inhabitants and the number of foundlings; that of the latter rises to an alarming degree during economic depression caused by, and following the French supremacy and the Napoleonic wars' (from around 30 a year in times of prosperity to 600 a year in times of depression). The conclusion drawn from the Amsterdam archives is clear: the rate of exposure of infants is directly related to specific socio-economic circumstances, not to vague population control policies. This reasoning, if applied to the ancient world, would be very much in accordance with the ideology and attitudes expounded above. Parents in antiquity exposed their babies only when poverty or dire necessity forced them to do so.

The same reasoning also applies to infanticide. Several sources suggest that active infanticide was a possibility if the father decided not to rear the child. So long as he had not recognised it at the Amphidromia, that is, for a week or so after birth, the father (or mother) could kill the baby without fear of the law. Seneca suggests that this happened regularly in the case of severely disabled babies:

> We destroy the monstrous foetuses and also we drown children, if they are born weak and deformed, not out of anger, but because it is sensible to separate the useless from the healthy.[87]

It is difficult to evaluate such statements, but I do not doubt that these things occasionally happened in Greece as much as in Rome. Sometimes babies born with severe disabilities would not be reared. They might be exposed, or even actively killed ('drowned' in Seneca's words) in an act that would be perceived as 'mercy-killing'. But again, in such cases parents would be motivated by strong emotions. There would be strong reasons behind their decision, and the circumstances were exceptional. If we add possible religious taboos in certain places and situations, as well as the limited capacity of ancient medicine to provide effective assistance to persons with severe disabilities, we can understand why under such extreme circumstances some parents might feel that a 'mercy-killing' was for the best.

Parents in the ancient world were faced with similar dilemmas to modern parents, when they felt that they could not cope with the responsibility of rearing a child. As in modern times, adoption might seem the best solution, but it presented serious legal complications and the institution as a whole was not designed with such cases in mind. Moreover, adoption could only address the overcrowding and financial problems of citizen couples. It could not address the problems of single women, or prostitutes. This is why exposure, and occasional infanticide, seem to have been realistic alternatives. However, before a baby was exposed or killed at birth it would need to be carried to term. At least the immediate family of the woman and those around her would know about the pregnancy. But the last thing that someone who had conceived as a result of an extramarital affair wanted would be for her immediate family to know about it, and in most instances the last thing she could expect from them would be support and acceptance. For such women abortion was not just a possible, albeit drastic, alternative; it probably seemed a 'must'. But abortion was dangerous and agonising, physically as well as emotionally, and the result was uncertain. Those who could avoid it and find another alternative, might do so. But for some, unless like Creusa they had the assurance of Apollo that he would keep their pregnancy secret, an attempt to have an abortion might seem their only realistic chance of remaining undetected. And if the attempt failed, their only realistic hope for redemption in the years to come might be to abandon their baby at the stairs of the temple, as the priestess suspects that a Delphian woman has done in the case of Ion. Abortion was the most drastic step of all, but in the eyes of some women their situation could not be effectively addressed in any other way.

v. The accessory to the crime

Some ancient authors would have us believe that abortion was a conspiracy of women against men, and that men were instinctively opposed to it. This is a fallacy. Let us for a moment assume that Juvenal is right when he alleges that Julia, the daughter of emperor Titus, had numerous abortions acting under pressure from her lover, the emperor's brother Domitian.[88] All authors who speak about the love-affair let us understand that it was already happening while Titus was still alive. So, what would be the position of the emperor's daughter if she realised that she was pregnant by her uncle? Even worse, what would be the predicament of Domitian if his brother, the emperor, came to find out that he had seduced his daughter? The prospect of Domitian putting intense pressure upon his mistress to have an abortion sounds very real to me under these circumstances. Regardless of what might happen to the woman, her seducer was in very serious danger himself, and the possibility of the emperor's anger translating itself into death or exile was certainly present.

In the ancient world adultery was primarily seen as an offence of one man against another. The laws of the Greek city-states penalised the man before they penalised the woman, and allowed the killing of the adulterer under certain circumstances. The Augustan laws, in a similar spirit but under stricter regulations, also allowed the killing of the man if caught in the act.[89] And concrete and serious penalties, such as physical abuse or heavy compensation claims, awaited the accessory to the crime if he did not die on the same bed as the act had been committed. In ancient Persia the law-code of Darius made the male party explicitly responsible by compelling him to pay maintenance until the woman gave birth.[90] The legislator implicitly recognised that the man might wish to avoid the responsibility and urge his partner to have an abortion. This is why Darius' law ordered that, if she terminated the pregnancy with her partner's consent, the man would be as guilty as the woman, and ordered the death penalty for both of them. Moreover the law ordered the death penalty for the woman's father. This last provision illustrates further the motives of the legislator. He did not only intend to make the male party directly responsible for the survival of the foetus, but also wanted the men to keep an eye on the woman and minimise the possibility of a secret abortion initiated by her. In addition, the law wished to minimise the risk of an induced abortion being presented as an accident, a miscarriage. The parties involved would think twice before they risked a confrontation with a law as severe as this; an unconvincing attempt to evade it would cost them their lives.

The consequences of an unplanned pregnancy for the male party, especially if this was the result of an affair outside marriage, extended beyond possible legal sanctions. Fear of the responsibility, disapproval by other members of his family, and sometimes society as a whole, the potential for conflict with his partner, financial considerations and other similar factors might induce a man to urge his partner to have an abortion. This is the kind of reaction that the courtesan Phronesium in Plautus' *Truculentus* (vv. 201-2) was allegedly expecting from her lover (except that Phronesium was not really pregnant and the whole thing was a trick for the gullible lover). Her slave Astaphium tells the man:

> She was hiding, afraid that you might persuade her
> To have an abortion and kill the child.

Why should a courtesan expect that her lover might try to persuade her to have an abortion? Surely the reasons were not legal. No man would be expected to take on any form of legal responsibility for the offspring of a courtesan, unless he specifically wished to do so. And bringing a child into this world was a responsibility from which, under certain circumstances, not only women, but men too can shrink. If this child was to be a permanent reminder of a sexual relationship that was not sanctioned by family and society, then the legal, emotional, social and financial implications, and complications, for both parents might be serious. They would probably not welcome the birth of the child. But even when no inappropriate sexual relationship was involved, the responsibility would still be great. Sometimes people might not feel prepared for it. Abortion presented a solution for both partners. Naturally the most important factor would be the woman's attitude, since she was the one who would have to put her life at risk and endure the operation. However, her partner's reaction and wishes could play an important role in shaping her decision, and might increase or suppress her determination to have the pregnancy terminated.

Conclusions

Male concerns over abortion in the ancient world could be strong. At a personal level men might react emotionally in a positive or negative manner to the prospect of their partner having an abortion, depending on whether the pregnancy was wanted or not. We hear about strong negative reactions when they wanted to become fathers and their partner's action had deprived them of this joy and hope. But we also hear that some men would be happy for their partner to seek an abortion, and we can conclude that such reactions would not be uncommon in relationships outside lawful marriage.

Beyond emotional considerations we can see that men were concerned with the continuation of their family name, their *oikos*, and the traditional family cults, and within the frame of such concerns they could adopt a hostile attitude towards a practice that threatened this continuity. As citizens in whose hands rested the defence, administration and prosperity of the state, men could collectively hold intensely hostile attitudes towards abortion, if they perceived it as a threat to the interests of the state. In societies such as Rome and Persia, where, at least among the upper classes, strength in numbers was seen as important for the well-being of the state, hostile attitudes towards abortion would go hand in hand with the official policy favouring a high birth-rate. Sometimes this collective desire for a high birth-rate was in harmony with the wishes of individual men. In ancient Persia it seems that men sincerely wanted large families, and took a number of measures to ensure that sufficient numbers of well-bred Persians would be placed in the service of the Great King. Abortion did not fit into this demographic pattern and was severely penalised by the law. However, in other societies the collective desire for a high birth-rate was not in harmony with the wishes of individual citizens. In Rome there was a noticeable clash between official policy, which favoured a high birth-rate and was prepared go to great lengths to encourage it, and actual practice, which favoured small families. In this demographic pattern, although the collective will was anti-abortion, and was eventually translated into anti-abortion legislation, abortion was still common practice.

Other societies, such as the Greek city states, which favoured a low birth-rate because they felt that their safety and prosperity lay in lean, more efficient structures, did not have such dilemmas. The collective will of the citizens seems to have been rather indifferent to abortion, and no laws were introduced to regulate or ban it. Individual citizens might have their own concerns regarding this practice, and according to these they might accept or reject it. Intellectuals such as Plato and Aristotle might find it an expedient measure for the purposes of population control, and ordinary citizens might resort to it pressed by utmost necessity. Others might angrily repudiate the practice and those women who had employed it. Their reasons might be emotional, related to frustrated expectations and hopes, or based upon rational considerations of the future of their family line. But whatever their reactions at an individual and family level, the citizens of the Greek city-states do not seem to have perceived abortion as a threat to the institutions and well-being of the state, and this is why they did not think it a matter which needed to be addressed by legislation.

Abortion for the male citizens of the Greek *poleis* was a private family matter, or maybe a matter for philosophical discussion and an interesting topic for medical ethics, but certainly not a hot political or social issue.

To what extent Greek men were aware of the realities of induced abortion is a matter for speculation. We can extract from the sources that women did not involve the men in such decisions if they could avoid it, and it is possible that the men in the Greek *poleis* were not fully aware of the facts. In their minds abortion could be suspicious if procured by a married woman, but then again, in many instances nothing could be proved against the woman by the abortion alone, because the doctors of the time might not be able to state categorically whether the abortion had been deliberately induced. Abortion could be viewed as an act of rebellion against male authority, an action intended to hurt the man and his interests in the continuation of the *oikos*. As such an induced abortion could certainly trigger a strong emotional reaction and lead to recriminations within the family. If an abortion was procured by an unmarried woman this might, despite the misgivings of her family, ultimately be a relief – a way out of a difficult situation. An unmarried woman carrying an illegitimate child would certainly be an embarrassment for her father and brother, and whatever they might think of the practice of induced abortion, it could constitute an easy way out of long-lasting social humiliation, and as such be regarded as a necessary evil. The sexual partner of the unmarried woman had even stronger reasons to be favourably inclined towards such a solution. If his partner decided to have an abortion, preferably early in the pregnancy and in secret, he might be spared considerable expense, litigation, social condemnation and the severe penalties laid down by the laws on adultery. Understandably in these circumstances the news that his partner had successfully procured an abortion might be a relief.

Abortion and the Law

The laws of each society perform a twofold task: they reflect the attitudes and beliefs of the community, and at the same time influence and regulate those attitudes by defining the limits of what is permissible and what is not. One might argue that the extent to which the law reflects social practice varies from one society to another depending on the degree to which individual members have a say over the way they are governed. Accordingly, in a direct democracy like classical Athens one would expect the way people thought and lived to be quite closely translated into law, while in non-democratic societies the law would reflect the wishes of the ruling elite. This is broadly correct, but over-simplified. Factors connected with historical developments in the evolution of the legal system can have a quite dramatic effect upon its shape. This is particularly significant when one tries to understand the Athenian legal system: it was not the creation of one man or group, but an ever-changing and evolving mass of laws and decrees introduced over centuries by many different hands in many different historical circumstances. In the classical period the Athenians maintained the illusion that they upheld 'the laws of Solon and the institutions of Dracon'.[1] But, in practice, the changes and modifications of the laws were so frequent that some fourth-century orators felt uneasy about it.[2] Thus we find in the Athenian legal system of the classical period old laws, like those of Dracon introduced in the seventh century under the aristocratic state, side by side with laws of the radical democracy. The spirit and style of such laws varied substantially. While, for example, the laws of the radical democracy are formulated in standard forensic language, have a bureaucratic touch, a secular spirit, and evolve around clearly specified rights and obligations of individual citizens, the homicide laws of Dracon are constructed with powerful families in mind and are firmly connected with religion.

Religion can transform the legal system of a certain society in such a manner that certain aspects of it do not reflect actual social practice, for one simple reason: religion is not susceptible to rational argument. In religion some things *are so*, and disputing these things or arguing against them is lack of belief or heresy. That is why legal systems closely connected with the teachings of a dominant religious dogma often do not reflect actual practice. Instead, they try to regulate and control contemporary practice and make it comply with the will of the divine, as this is interpreted by his/her representatives on earth, namely, the holy men or women who are the entrusted guardians of the divine wisdom. This divine will may be irrational, may be oppressive, may be out of touch with contemporary norms and morals, and yet it stands apart as an eternal, incorruptible, and, above all, irrefutable truth, with which everyone is expected to comply, regardless of how they feel or what they think.

The link between religion and anti-abortion attitudes, often translated into law, is unmistakable. Ireland, the only country in the European Union still upholding a virtually general ban on abortion, is a good example. The ban on abortion is enshrined in the Irish constitution, and the Irish government, in order to prevent a reversal by the European Court of Human Rights, negotiated an opt-out clause in the Maastricht treaty. The Church was the prime instigator of this move by consolidating public opinion behind the anti-abortion lobby. Women in Ireland have sought abortions as much as women in any other country. What is different here is that religion interferes with the legal system to a greater extent than elsewhere, and transforms it so that it no longer reflects contemporary practice, but rather 'the truth' of the Catholic Church that abortion is wrong. Irish society remains strongly attached to religion, and Christian values and views are often translated into law. These values and views may not be universally respected, but once they become enshrined in law they have to be universally upheld.[3]

Ireland is only a striking example among many. I witnessed the battle over the legalisation of abortion in modern Greece in the early 1980s, with the Church on one side seeking to continue imposing its view upon the legal system of the country, and on the other side the newly elected socialist government of Andreas Papandreou seeking to establish a law free of such influence. What made the difference in the end was that Greek society, although deeply Christian as a whole, mostly sees the law of the state as something secular and its role as distinctly different from that of the Church. The latter, influential as it may be in shaping attitudes, is perceived as a primarily spiritual experience, but not as a chief player in legal and constitutional matters. The difference between Greek and Irish society does not lie in the depth or intensity of religious feeling, but in the perception of the role of religion in secular matters, the legal system and the institutions of the state.[4]

These examples suggest that religion has played a serious role in the discussion on abortion. Many of the arguments of the anti-abortion lobby have been supplied by religion, and, as we saw, these arguments have sometimes been translated into law. But to translate religious arguments into secular law is not a peculiarity of our times, or indeed the Christian era as a whole. Pagan antiquity allowed religion to interfere with the business of the state sometimes to a considerably larger extent than modern secular democracies. An offence against the gods represented a threat for the entire community, since the gods might exact revenge upon it for the offences of one individual. Therefore the community ought to be on its guard and not allow offences against the gods, even minor ones, to go unpunished. If the Greek or Roman gods were offended because an individual woman had had an abortion, they might not wait for her to die before punishing her for her actions. Instead, they might bring down pestilence, adversity, famine, or natural disasters upon her entire community, and they might do this right away, if they so wished. Thus a critical question arises, which we must answer before we try to determine legal provisions concerning abortion in the Graeco-Roman world (or the lack of them): did pagan antiquity perceive abortion as an act that offended the gods? After attempting to provide an answer to this, we should take a closer look at the legal provisions of the Greeks and the Romans and try to place them in their historical and cultural context. We need to understand how social norms affected legislation and how legislation affected social norms in relation to this particular issue. Therefore, the study of the law is expected to provide an insight into the beliefs and perceptions of the society that created it.

i. Religion, abortion and the law

'Abortion is murder' is one of the placards frequently seen in anti-abortion rallies, and this provides the justification for its condemnation. One of the main objections brought forward by the Christian Church is that man does not have the right to take a life created by God.[5] However, the idea that human life is a gift of God, and therefore sacred, is not exclusively Christian. Half a millennium before the Christian era the orator Antiphon[6] wrote these words:

> For when God was minded to create the human race and brought the first of us into being, he gave us the earth and sea to sustain and serve us, in order that we might not die for want of the necessaries of life before old age brought us our end. Such being the value placed upon our life by God, whoever unlawfully slays his fellow both sins against the gods and confounds the ordinances of man. For the victim, robbed of the gifts bestowed by God upon him, naturally leaves behind him the angry spirits of vengeance, God's instruments of punishment, spirits which they who prosecute and testify without giving heed to justice bring into their own homes, defiling them with the defilement of another, because they share in the sin of him who did the deed. And similarly, should we, the avengers of the dead, accuse innocent persons because of some private grudge, not only will our failure to avenge the murdered man cause us to be haunted by dread demons to whom the dead will turn for justice, but by wrongfully causing the death of the innocent we are liable to the penalties prescribed for murder, and because we have persuaded you to break the law, the responsibility for your mistake also becomes ours.[7]

The perception of homicide as an offence first and foremost against the gods, and only on a secondary level against the 'ordinances of man', was dominant in Athenian homicide law. The Athenians never changed the law of Dracon on homicide. The procedures that it had established were faithfully observed within the legal system of the classical period, even though by that time they must have seemed archaic and extraordinary. The connection of homicide law with religion certainly had a major role to play. The magistrate responsible for accepting and processing homicide cases was the *basileus*, namely the archon in charge of religious affairs. The entire process of a homicide prosecution was intensely coloured by religious undertones. While for any other offence it would be sufficient to submit a lawsuit to the appropriate magistrate, who would then arrange a preliminary hearing and the date of the trial, prosecutions for homicide were accompanied by formalities which make sense only in a religious context. The process began with three proclamations by the *basileus* asking the person accused of homicide to keep away from the temples and the agora. This was to prevent the pollution (*miasma*) carried by the killer from spreading. Then the trial was held in an open place, so that the members of the court would not be polluted. The trial itself contained curses and oaths, and was organised in a stricter format than ordinary trials before Athenian courts. The reason was obviously related to what Antiphon says in the passage quoted above: conviction of an innocent person would be murder, and it would bring pollution upon those responsible for the death of the innocent. More significantly, the traditional divisions between men and women, citizens and aliens, free persons and slaves, were less important in homicide cases. The blood of the victim demanded revenge, and society ought to satisfy this demand by punishing the killer, even if the victim was just an insignificant slave. Evidently the main concern here was not merely human justice with its distinctions along lines of gender, status and social class, but divine order and supernatural forces far more powerful than any human institution.[8]

Religion, killing and human law were interconnected in classical Athens perhaps to a greater degree than in any Christian society. So the background for a perception of abortion as an act that offended the gods, and therefore as a crime that ought to be dealt with severity by the law, if the whole society were to avoid the divine wrath, was certainly there. However, such a perception had not entered pagan thought, and abortion was never linked to homicide in mainstream Graeco-Roman religious culture. A number of important religious documents preserved in inscriptions unambiguously suggest that abortion was treated as a rather ordinary affair. The deadly *miasma* that fell upon a killer and would normally require his death in order to be expiated, did not befall a woman who had an abortion. All that was needed after an abortion was purification similar to that after childbirth, loss of one's virginity, menstruation, sexual intercourse, or a natural death in the house.

The relevant documents have been presented by Nardi in two independent studies, and briefly discussed in his book on abortion.[9] The oldest (331-326 BC) is an inscription containing a sacred law from Cyrene regulating purification after an abortion:

If a woman has an abortion,[10] if the foetus is large and clearly formed they are contaminated as with someone's death, but if it is not yet formed, the house is contaminated as with childbirth.[11]

This document does not draw any distinction between a spontaneous and an induced abortion. This is probably crucial, because by not making this distinction the sacred law of Cyrene falls short of introducing any concept of guilt or crime against the gods especially applicable to induced abortion. All that the law requires is routine purification procedures like those that deal with a birth or death in the house. Abortion does not carry the same type of *miasma* as homicide. If the foetus is large and formed, and therefore bearing the appearance of a human being, then it is to be treated like an ordinary death; if the foetus is unformed, then it is to be treated like an ordinary childbirth. Clearly this text does not suggest a link between abortion and homicide in sacred law.

Similar perceptions are reflected in an inscription of the same period from the island of Cos (the homeland of Hippocrates). It contains a list of various prohibitions which the priest of Zeus ought to observe, and among others we read:

And he is not to enter a house where someone has died for five days after the day the dead was carried, nor enter a house where a woman has given birth for three days after the day of birth, and five days after the day of an abortion.[12]

Abortion is treated as nothing more extraordinary than a natural death or childbirth, deserving only two extra days of purification from childbirth, and the same number of days as a death. The number of purification days which the priestess of Demeter in Cos has to observe, as attested in a third-century BC inscription, is marginally different:

She is not to enter a house where a woman has given birth or had an abortion for three days, nor enter a house where someone has died for five days after the day the dead was carried.[13]

Here abortion is treated on a par with childbirth, while death requires a slightly longer purification period. Another inscription from Cos from the second century BC also sets abortion on the same level as childbirth, but this time the purification period is ten days.[14]

A century later another purification law preserved on an inscription from Delos specifies different periods for childbirth and abortion for those entering the temple of Apollo:

They may enter ... three days after intercourse with a woman, seven days after childbirth, forty days after an abortion, and nine days after period.[15]

The duration of pollution as specified here is distinctly longer for an abortion than it would be for childbirth, but still not that long. A similar difference can be observed in an inscription from Eressos, where it is probably to be understood that a woman may not enter the temple for ten days after birth and forty days after an abortion.[16] Forty days is the purification period required after an abortion in an inscription from Ptolemais in Egypt too (*c.* first century BC).[17] A document from Smyrna (second century AD) imposes a ban of 40 days from the temple of Dionysos, but if seen in context this ban is relatively short:

> All those entering the sanctuary and temples of Bromios[18]
> Abstain for 40 days from the exposure of an infant,
> In order to avoid pollution, and the same number of days
> From a woman's abortion. And if death buries under the ground
> A close relative of a person, they are to abstain from the doorway
> For 3 months. And if miasma from someone else's oikos befalls
> Upon someone, they are to abstain for 3 days from the death.[19]

The period of purification for all kinds of pollution is longer than usual here. In proportion, however, abortion needs the same period of purification as exposure of an infant, but considerably less than the death of a close relative.

Forty days is the required purification period in an inscription from Lindos (second century AD). I find this document very revealing, because abortion is one of the items that cause pollution in a list that includes lentils, goat meat, and cheese:

> Good Fortune
> Among other things needed for appropriate
> entry to the sanctuary, first and foremost:
> They must be clean and healthy in their hands
> and minds, and not carry in their conscience
> anything terrible.
> And abstain from these:
> from lentils 3 days
> from goat meat 3 days
> from cheese 1 day
> from abortion 40 days
> from death of a close relative 40 days
> from lawful intercourse, they may enter
> on the same day, after being sprinkled and anointed
> with oil.
> From loss of virginity ....[20]

Abortion carries a longer purification period than goat's meat, cheese and lentils, but the same as death of a close relative. Another inscription from Lindos from the third century AD in a similar spirit lists abortion among many ordinary items that can cause impurity:

> From an abortion of a woman, or a dog, or a donkey 40 days
> From loss of virginity 41 days
> From death of a close relative 41 days[21]

Believers are to abstain from the temple of Athena if they had been near a (probably spontaneous) abortion not only of a human but also an animal. Far from being treated as homicide, from a religious point of view abortion here is no more significant in a human being than it would be in a dog or a donkey. It is interesting to see that an abortion is a less serious cause of impurity than loss of virginity, which requires the same period of purification as death.

The same concept of abortion as something explicitly and distinctly different from homicide is seen even more clearly in an inscription from Attica (second/third century AD). It also sets a purification period of forty days after an abortion and ten days after a death. However, this text is important because it explicitly imposes a permanent ban upon someone who has committed homicide. Abortion and homicide are placed side by side but treated in a very different manner. Abortion is more or less as serious a cause of impurity as menstruation, sexual intercourse, or a death in the house. On the other hand, killing is on a totally different scale. It is a grave offence that deserves permanent banishment from the temple.

> One is to purify him/herself for 10 days after a death,
> Seven days after menstruation,
> A killer is to go nowhere near the place,
> (One should abstain for) forty days from an abortion,
> While from (intercourse with) a woman, a man may enter
> On the same day, after washing his head.[22]

These documents unambiguously suggest that, with minor local variations, the purification period for an abortion was on the same level as that for natural events such as a birth, sexual intercourse or death. More importantly, none distinguishes between a spontaneous and an induced abortion, and none places abortion on par with homicide or other serious crimes against the gods. Parker has noticed that in later antiquity the purification period for abortion tends to be longer.[23] This surely has to do with increasingly hostile attitudes to it, as attested in texts from the late republic and the imperial era, becoming more widespread (see Chapter 5). However, it never comes near equating abortion to homicide or other serious offences against the gods, and if we contrast pagan sacred laws and the teachings of the Christian fathers we see the difference immediately. (There is one exception to this rule: on the inscription from Philadelphia in Lydia [*LSA* 20] abortion is treated as a very serious crime, but as I argue in Appendix 2, where I discuss this text in some detail, this document has probably been influenced by the Hippocratic Oath.)

Church laws and teachings from the Christian era are based on the assumption that induced abortion is a crime against God on a par with homicide, and impose severe penalties on the woman. Athenagoras provides the following explanation:

Why are we speaking about homicide when we say that those women who

use abortifacients are killers and will be accountable before God for the
abortion? Because it is the same thing to kill what is carried in the womb,
since it is considered to be a living being (*zôon*), as it is to kill one who has
already come to the world.[24]

A ruling of the Synod of Ancyra (clause 21) revises a previous life-long
period of confession and ban from Communion, and brings it down to ten
years, 'on the grounds of humanitarian considerations' (*philanthrôpoteron
de ti*), for 'those women who practise prostitution and kill what has been
created and are expert in making abortifacient drugs'. Basil in his letter
to Amphilochios accepts this ruling and comments that it is not the length
of time but the manner of the penance that should define the healing
process.[25] The Synod in Trullo returns to a stricter penance and rule 91
orders that 'the same penalty as for murder is to be imposed upon those
women who either accept or induce others to take drugs in order to have
an abortion'.

It is clear that the link between abortion and homicide made by Christian theologians, was never made in the sacred laws of pagan antiquity.
The reason probably is that, since the ancient world never came to an
agreement on the human status of the unborn, it could not really equate
its destruction to murder. Doctors, philosophers and intellectuals might
struggle to come to grips with concepts such as motion, formation or
animation, and some minority sects such as the Pythagoreans argued
strongly that human life is sacred from the moment of conception. However, for the ordinary person the conclusion that the destruction of
something which had not yet been born or seen should be equal to the
killing of a person, and as offensive to the gods as the murder of a man,
woman or child, was far from self-evident. Thus Greek religion did not
intervene into the debate on the ethics of induced abortion, and consequently secular institutions and legislative bodies in the Greek city-states
did not have to take firm religious attitudes into account when considering
their position on this matter. Whether they would legislate on it or not
depended on the consideration of human, not divine will.

ii. Was abortion a crime in the eyes of the law?

The view that abortion was illegal in antiquity, at least when it was
procured without the husband's consent, is widespread among scholars.[26]
The main sources invoked in support of this view are as follows:

1. Euripides *Andromache* 355-60. Here Andromache replies to Menelaus that she would willingly subject herself to punishment if it were
proven that she had secretly made his daughter Hermione have abortions
against the wishes of the latter. Andromache's words might be interpreted
as a reflection of Athenian legal practice: the reason she was going to be

punished was that abortion was illegal, especially as it would have happened against the wishes of Hermione's husband.

2. Lysias fragments 19-24 Carey: This speech was delivered during a trial concerning an induced abortion, and it has been interpreted by a number of scholars as an indication that abortion was illegal. On the basis of the fragments and testimonia from this speech, Caillemer, Harrison and others maintain that a woman who had an abortion could be prosecuted by anyone by means of a public prosecution (*graphê amblôseôs*). Harrison tries to refine the legal technicalities of the case, arguing that a public prosecution (*graphê*) was seen as appropriate because the injured party, namely the foetus, was no longer around. However, he is not sure that this was the case and proposes an alternative possibility, namely that a public prosecution was appropriate only when the father was dead, while if he was alive he could prosecute the woman privately through a *dikê*.

3. Further support for the view that abortion was illegal could be furnished by other statutes which suggest that Athenian law was prepared to acknowledge the human status of the unborn. One could mention the law that allowed a pregnant widow to stay in her husband's house in the hope that she would produce an heir.[27] Moreover, Attic inheritance laws did not permit the distribution of one's property to lateral relatives if he had left behind a pregnant wife. Thus the law established that an unborn child had the right to inherit. Laws motivated by a similar spirit are also attested in other parts of the ancient world. Diodorus for example mentions that in Egypt a pregnant woman sentenced to death was not executed before she gave birth, and in the *Digestae* (11,8,2) we read that a pregnant woman was not to be buried before checking that the foetus she was carrying was also dead.[28] In the *Digestae* alone there are 49 references to specific legal provisions concerning pregnant women, which can be taken as an indication that Roman law implicitly recognised the rights of unborn children.[29] Probably similar laws were in place in other parts of the ancient world. The logical inference from these statutes would be that the law implicitly recognised the unborn as a human being with an independent right to life.

4. Cicero *Pro Cluentio* 32: Cicero refers to a Milesian woman who was put to death after a trial over an induced abortion. She was convicted, we are told, because she had deprived her husband of the privilege of becoming a father, his family of an heir, and the city of a future citizen. The passage is commonly interpreted as proof that abortion could be punished by death.

5. Musonius Rufus, a first-century AD writer, speaks of past legislators who have criminalised abortion. This has been taken as evidence that he had in mind specific legal provisions prohibiting induced abortion. (The passage is quoted above, Chapter 5 §iii.)

6. Pseudo-Galen 19,179: Here it is stated that Solon in Athens and Lycurgus in Sparta had prohibited abortion. Arguably this piece of information might be corroborated by Plutarch *Lycurgus* 3, where we are told

that Lycurgus deceived the pregnant wife of his dead brother, and stopped her from having an abortion, because, in the author's words, he felt intense hatred for the woman's character, when she revealed to him her plan to have an abortion of the child of her dead husband. Could this suggest that he included a ban on abortion in his legislation since he opposed this practice?

7. Plutarch *Life of Romulus* 22,3: Here a law of Romulus is mentioned that declares abortion to be sufficient grounds for divorce.

8. *Digestae* 47,11,4, 48,8,8 and 48,19,39 clearly suggest that abortion was prohibited by Septimius Severus and Caracalla. The woman was to be exiled to the provinces for as long a period as the governor of the province deemed fit.

I will argue that a closer look at these sources clearly suggests the opposite, namely that abortion was not illegal in any part of the Graeco-Roman world before the third century AD, when the aforementioned law by Septimius and Caracalla criminalised it. This is not a new approach. As far as I know, C. Brecht was the first scholar who opposed the view commonly held in the nineteenth century that abortion was illegal in antiquity. In this century G. Glotz has presented a series of compelling arguments suggesting that there was no law against abortion in the classical, hellenistic and republican periods in any part of the Graeco-Roman world.[30] His views have been widely accepted in recent years.[31] However, many questions remain unanswered, and frequently the legal implications arising from the above-mentioned evidence are not well understood. For these reasons is necessary to consider these sources carefully and discuss their legal background.

Euripides' play *Andromache* refers to the reality of fifth-century BC Athens (the play was first staged in the early years of the Peloponnesian war). Here we find the heroine facing accusations of grave bodily harm against Hermione, the daughter of her master Menelaus. Andromache denies the accusations and offers to subject herself willingly to punishment if these accusations prove to be true. The underlying thought is that Andromache agrees with her accuser that these allegations are serious. She agrees that if a woman had made another woman have an abortion, against the wishes of the latter, then she would deserve to be punished. *blabên opheilô* could be interpreted as standard forensic terminology referring to an established legal procedure, perhaps a trial for an abortion, which should result in a fine (*blabên*) in the event of conviction. But the difficulties with such an interpretation of the passage would be serious. First of all, women in classical Athens could not be prosecuted with lawsuits punishable by fines, simply because they did not have sufficient legal control over their own finances to be able to pay them. Then, when Andromache says 'I will not kneel before the altar' (as a suppliant) she implies that her expected punishment would be immediate, not the punishment after a trial in court. The heroine does not expect to be tried for the abortion; she expects that, if Hermione's allegations are believed, she will be subjected to immediate punishment, probably physical torture. Thus, the word *blabên* should be understood not as implying a fine imposed by the court, but the immediate physical punishment which a slave would expect to receive from her master.

But what would Andromache be punished for? Was she going to be punished for the abortion, or for interfering with the womb of Hermione, and by means of poisonous drugs causing her grave bodily harm? If we were to consider this question from a modern legal perspective, even in a society where abortion was perfectly legal Andromache would still be liable for unlawful activities such as the administration of harmful drugs to someone without that person's knowledge, or interference with someone's reproductive cycle without that person's consent. According to our legal system we would judge such actions to have violated the body of the victim, and intentionally caused damage. Common sense suggests that the Athenians would think the same. Regardless of the legal status of abortion in classical Athens, violating a woman's body as Hermione's had allegedly been violated would have been perceived as serious criminal activity deserving punishment. The law on deliberate wounding of a person would probably apply in this case, and the penalty for such an offence was exile and confiscation of property.[32] So the legal data do not match; Andromache does not refer to a specific procedure, and this passage does not prove anything about the legal status of abortion in classical Athens.

The speech of Lysias 'On the Abortion' is undoubtedly a very important source, and has been treated as such by Brecht, Glotz, Harrison, Nardi, Eyben, Demand and all other studies that discuss the legal status of abortion in the ancient world. Unfortunately the speech does not survive in its entirety. We can try to reconstruct the content and context from sparse fragments and references to this text in ancient lexicographers and rhetoricians, but this is not an easy process. The available evidence is confusing and at first sight contradictory. The importance as well as the difficulties of this source require that the fragments and testimonia are discussed in considerable detail, and this I have done separately below (§iii). Here it will be sufficient to mention my conclusions: I argue that in early fourth-century Athens a woman known to us as 'the wife of Antigenes' was prosecuted by her former husband for an induced abortion. He brought homicide charges against her, evidently because he had no other means of redress for what he perceived to be a grave personal injury against him. A careful consideration of the testimonia leaves us in no doubt that this was a homicide trial, and this would be an unorthodox procedure *per se*. However, Antigenes was determined to bring his former wife to justice, and since he had no other means of doing so, because induced abortion was not illegal, he brought homicide charges and succeeded in putting this case through the Athenian legal system. In the trial before the Areopagus he argued that the foetus was formed when it was aborted, and this was why her action should be considered as homicide. He produced testimonies from doctors and midwives supporting the view that a formed foetus should be considered as a human being. His case rested heavily upon medical arguments, and he tried to convince the Areopagus that the Athenian homicide law of Dracon ought to apply in this case. However, the court for some reason that we cannot safely infer from our sources acquitted the defendant.

Even if one were to disagree with parts of my reconstruction of this case the fact remains that Antigenes would not have brought homicide charges against his former wife if there was an Athenian law especially designed to deal with cases of induced abortion, because then he should have prosecuted his wife in accordance with that law. However, the sources unanimously state that this was a homicide trial (see §iii below for the evidence and discussion). Antigenes would not have followed this path if an existing law prohibited abortion. Apart from the initial difficulty of bringing the homicide prosecution to court, during the trial he had the uphill task of trying to convince the judges not only that the defendant had had an abortion (which was not hard to prove), but also that homicide charges were appropriate and in accordance with the laws of the city. From the fragments and testimonia we can safely gather that this was the harder part of his task, and this is why the prosecutor concentrated much of his effort upon the legality of his case. The rhetorician Theon says that one of the main themes of the speech was the question whether women could have abortions without fear of legal repercussions (§iii below). The fact that the orator felt compelled to address this issue in considerable detail should be taken as an indication that there was no written law prohibiting abortion. The legal technicalities of this lawsuit only make sense if there was no anti-abortion law in Athens, and this is why it seems to me that this important source beyond reasonable doubt suggests that Athenian law did not criminalise abortion. Further corroboration may be provided by the treatment of the subject by Plato, Aristotle, and the Hippocratic corpus. Nowhere in these sources it is hinted or suggested that this was an illegal practice. If abortion was illegal Plato and Aristotle might have been expected to address this issue when they recommended it for the purposes of population control.

The information provided by Pseudo-Galen that Lycurgus in Sparta and Solon in Athens had prohibited abortion cannot be considered reliable.[33] The study in question, *Whether what is in the womb is a living being*, was written in later antiquity, and its general character does not suggest that the author has used reliable historical sources from the classical period for his account. The historical information provided by this study is vague and confined to nothing more than what a moderately educated individual of his time could know either from his general readings, or from oral tradition. The information that Solon and Lycurgus had criminalised abortion follows a sentence stating that Zeus had legislated for the Cretans, Apollo for the Spartans, and Athena for the Athenians. The context suggests that one is dealing with mythology, not accurate historical knowledge. But even if the context is mythological, why is it implausible that this author has accurate knowledge concerning the anti-abortion laws of Lycurgus and Solon? Two studies that have discussed this question in some detail come to the same conclusion, that Pseudo-Galen did not possess reliable information. Crahay points out that the connection of Lycurgus and Solon in the same line should make the reader instantly suspicious, and this view is also shared by Nardi.[34] I concur: the two famous legislators of the ancient world are both presented as opposed to abortion by Pseudo-Galen, yet no other source suggests that it was prohibited by either of them. Nardi considers the absence of any such information in the biographies of the two men by Plutarch as particularly significant, since Plutarch presents a detailed account of the Solonian laws concerning women, and mentions one incident when Lycurgus was involved in a case concerning an induced abortion. Would Plutarch have omitted to mention an anti-abortion law introduced by Solon or Lycurgus in any of these passages, if he had knowledge of such a law? Especially in the case of Lycurgus, the silence of Plutarch cannot be easily brushed aside. The biographer mentions that Lycurgus came to hate his brother's pregnant widow, when she wanted to have an abortion and remove her dead husband's heir from the line of succession in order to marry Lycurgus, who was next in line to the throne of the Eurypontidai, and become his queen. The incorruptible Lycurgus felt disgusted by this proposal but pretended to agree. He convinced the woman that an abortion was inadvisable because of the risks involved. He told her that it would be best to wait for the birth of the child and then secretly expose it. Through this trick he conned her into keeping the child, and when a male heir was born, he took the child under his protection and acted as a regent until the boy, named Charilaus, was old enough to be king. If Lycurgus in later years, when as regent for the young king he introduced his famous laws, had established a law prohibiting abortion, would Plutarch fail to mention it?

Nardi believes that Plutarch's reference to this particular incident was the main source of Pseudo-Galen. The latter misinterpreted this passage as a ban on abortion by Lycurgus, and then involved Solon too, Lycurgus' Athenian counterpart, in order to present this ban as a widespread practice in the ancient world. Even if we were prepared to cast aside the serious possibility that the Pseudo-Galenic treatise was actually written before Plutarch's works, this explanation of the passage would be unnecessary. Ancient authors had a tendency to relate to Lycurgus every single Spartan law and institution, and to Solon a large number of Athenian laws, even though some of those can certainly be identified as laws or decrees of the radical democracy (namely, introduced after 462 BC).[35] It seems likely to me that Pseudo-Galen is inventing: it is convenient for his argument to maintain that abortion was illegal, and for this purpose he first presents the gods as anti-abortion legislators, and then drops the names of the quasi-mythical lawgivers of Sparta and Athens in order to add authority to his statement.

The argument that abortion must have been illegal because the law recognised the human status of the unborn, implicitly if not explicitly, is an important argument in *Whether what is in the womb is a living being*, which is translated in its entirety in Appendix 1. I will not repeat all the arguments, but here are some crucial questions which the author asks:

> Who would exact revenge upon an obviously perfected human being on behalf of something that never was human in the womb, and had not come to life in the first place? And who would abandon an inheritance on the grounds that he does not know whether the embryo is a living being? How will you try to prove that what is in the womb is not a living being? Who appoints as his heir someone who is not believed to exist? Who will declare that one who is the object of doubt ought to be put in charge?[36]

The author draws attention to the universally observed legal provision that the unborn child is to be heir to his/her father, and the legal implications that this entails. On the basis of this Pseudo-Galen may justifiably argue that Athenian law by implication recognised the unborn as a human being. Consequently a ban on abortion would appear to be legally consistent with this perception of the unborn as a potential human being and heir. But do legal systems always exhibit this degree of consistency? Perhaps theoretically this should be the case; in practice, however, laws can be contradictory in spirit. Inconsistencies of this nature are not unknown in the legal systems of all civilised societies. This apparent contradiction is quite familiar to us, as the legal systems of most western democracies have laws protecting the rights of pregnant women and unborn children, while still allowing abortion. All available evidence suggests that the legal systems of the Greek city states, the hellenistic kingdoms, the Roman republic and the early Roman empire did so too. In the core of this contradiction lies the ambiguity over the human status of the foetus, which has been explored in greater detail in Chapter 2.

A historical example illustrating this ambiguity in relation to the status of an unborn heir is relevant at this point. Plutarch mentions in his *Life of Alexander* that after Alexander's death Roxane, his barbarian wife, was held in special esteem by the Macedonians because she was pregnant by the dead king.[37] Her child was expected to be the lawful heir to his father, and successor to the vast empire that Alexander had conquered. In the meeting held on the day after Alexander's death, Perdiccas, the general to whom Alexander had entrusted his ring on his deathbed, proposed that if Roxane's child proved to be a boy he should be king. However, the claim of the unborn child was resisted by a considerable part of the Macedonian army, and in a compromise solution it was decided that he should share the throne with a son of Philip II called Arrhidaeus, who was renamed Philip III. Roxane's child was a boy and succeeded his father as joint king Alexander IV.[38] This case seems to suggest that although Greek men could not really put too much faith in the succession by an heir who had not yet been seen, and perhaps could not even be recognised as a human being at that stage, they nonetheless hoped that an heir would come along to fill the vacuum. The status of the unborn heir was potential, not definite. It would be inaccurate to read in this expectation a definite recognition of the unborn as a human being with specific legal rights. This is why the argument that abortion must have been illegal in classical Athens because Athenian law in some instances implicitly recognised the human status of the unborn is fundamentally flawed.

Depriving the husband of an heir by means of an abortion seems to be the main reason that Cicero's Milesian woman was put to death. The details of this interesting trial greatly resemble those of the trial of Antigenes' wife in fourth-century Athens. It seems to me that the charge against the Milesian woman too was homicide. As I argue in §iv below, where the details of this trial are discussed, she could not have been sentenced to death in accordance with Roman law for two reasons: first because abortion was not yet illegal, and second because even when it was criminalised in the third century AD and subsequent centuries it never carried a capital sentence. A closer consideration of the legal formalities of this trial, as presented in §iv, confirms the conclusion that abortion was not illegal in Asia during the late republic, and that the prosecutors of the Milesian woman had to resort to homicide charges in order to punish her for her actions, as Antigenes did against his wife. However, unlike Antigenes' wife she did not escape conviction, and was put to death for killing her dead husband's child and heir.

Two centuries later (first century AD) Musonius Rufus in a much discussed passage mentions that past lawgivers had prohibited abortion. Like Pseudo-Galen he seeks corroboration for his view that abortion should be considered a crime in the authority of past legislators. However, unlike Pseudo-Galen he does not attribute anti-abortion laws to specific lawgivers. This suggests that he did not have any concrete evidence in his hands. Probably he did not know of any specific anti-abortion law or any lawgiver who had prohibited it and this is why he vaguely refers to 'the legislators of the past'. It serves the purposes of the rhetorician to suggest that large families, and hostile attitudes to anything that might threaten their size, have been enshrined in political wisdom from time immemorial. On the contrary, however, the political wisdom of the past rather favoured small populations. Moreover, one significant detail in the passage of Musonius unambiguously suggests that abortion was not illegal in his time. The last sentence of the passage only makes sense if abortion was permissible. He writes:

> So, do we not commit an unjust and unlawful act, if our laws go against the wishes of those divine men who were loved by the gods, for it is considered to be good and beneficial to follow them.[39]

This sentence implies that there was no law in his time that prohibited abortion. He objected to this lack of legal regulation of a practice he considered unjust and unacceptable, and sought further corroboration for his views in the authority of tradition. However, he was unable to quote any specific laws of the past condemning abortion, and this is why he simply came up with a generalisation stating that the great lawgivers of the past would surely have opposed to the practice.

Texts from the late republic, such as the above-mentioned passage of Cicero or Ovid's extraordinary abortion poems,[40] as well as texts from the early empire, such as the passage of Musonius, reveal an ever more vocal condemnation of abortion. Moreover, circumstantial evidence from that period points in the same direction: Parker, for example, noticed that the sanctions for abortion in the sacred laws of the Greek states (see §i above) become stiffer in later antiquity, even though they never went so far as to equate abortion with serious offences against the gods, such as impiety or homicide. Finally, sympathy for the foetus as a potential human being, whose life has been prematurely and maliciously interrupted, appears for the first time in texts of the late republic, such as Ovid and Chariton (see Chapter 5), while until then the rights of the foetus did not come into the picture; only those of the father did. Sympathy for the foetus becomes established as one of the main objections to abortion after that period, and finally occupies a central position in Christian anti-abortion arguments from the fourth century AD. The reason for this ever-increasing trend against abortion from the late republic onwards can be traced in increasing concern among the ruling Roman classes that they would be vastly outnumbered and their identity lost in the sea of cultures that surrounded them, if they did not make an effort to maintain those values enshrined in the traditional Roman family. Thus the prohibition of abortion by Septimius and Caracalla at the beginning of the third century (between AD 198 and 211) did not come out of the blue; it was not a surprising decision or a whim of the emperor. On the contrary, it was the culmination of a long process, and a true reflection of changing attitudes. Several jurists refer to this provision:

1. *Tryphoninus in Digestae 48,19,39*: Cicero wrote in the speech for Cluentius Habitus (32), that when he was in Asia a Milesian woman was condemned to death because she accepted bribes by the alternative heirs and procured an abortion by means of drugs. But if, after a divorce while she was pregnant, she had an abortion in order to avoid giving birth to the son of her estranged husband, she is to be punished with temporary exile, as ruled in the rescript of our excellent emperors.

2. *Ulpian in Digestae 48,8,8*: If a woman has violated her womb in order to procure an abortion, he ruled in response to an enquiry that the governor of the province is to exile her.

3. *Marcian in Digestae 47,11,4*: The divine Severus and Antoninus have ruled in response to an enquiry that the woman who deliberately procured an abortion is to be temporarily exiled by the governor; because it would seem intolerable if she could defraud her husband of children with impunity.

The provision of the law, as it emerges from these passages, was that a woman who deliberately procured an abortion was to be punished with temporary exile. Two of the jurists understand that this provision had to do with the rights of the woman's husband as a father. Her action had deprived him of children. Cicero's words about the loss of the husband of the Milesian woman come to mind, and in fact Tryphoninus relates the ruling of Severus-Caracalla to the Ciceronian passage. He sees the same intention behind the condemnation of the Milesian woman and the imperial rescript of Severus-Caracalla, namely the desire to safeguard the rights of the father. This may be true to some extent, but, as I have stated in greater detail in Chapter 5, the overall picture is much more complex. Probably there is no direct link between a homicide trial in a province in 79 BC, and an imperial rescript of the third century AD. The verdict in the trial of the Milesian woman was an exceptional and isolated incident, in fact so remarkable that Cicero thought it worthwhile to refer to it thirteen years later in a trial held in Rome. The rescript of Severus-Caracalla had binding force and affected the lives of millions who were governed under Roman law at that time. The fact that the ruling of Severus-Caracalla is a rescript may be significant. A rescript was a ruling in response to a written enquiry submitted to the emperor either by an individual or by a judicial magistrate. So the mere fact that the enquiry was made can indicate two things: either there was confusion in an existing anti-abortion law, which the person who made the enquiry was seeking to clarify, or there was no law at all on the issue of induced abortion. I prefer the latter on account of the corroborating evidence cited above, which suggests that no such law had previously existed, and the actual wording of the jurists. This wording does not indicate clarification of a certain aspect of an existing law; it establishes a new ruling, one simple provision, that abortion was to be punished by temporary exile. So in this case the rescript is intended to close a gap in the law that allowed women to defy their husbands and procure abortions without punishment.

On the basis of the evidence of the jurists it does not seem that abortion became illegal only under certain circumstances. A number of scholars have suggested that the abortion would be illegal only if it happened without the husband's consent.[41] Ulpian, however, who appears to keep closely to the wording of the rescript, says nothing about conditions or particular circumstances. The references to the interests of the husband appear to be personal interpretations of Tryphoninus and Marcian, not stated intentions of the law. The wording of Marcian provides significant support for my understanding of the legal provisions: he uses indirect discourse in order to describe what exactly the letter of the law said, namely that a woman who had an abortion was to be punished with temporary exile (*eam ... dandam*), but then changes into direct discourse in order to express his own view on the reason behind this legal provision, namely that it was intended to protect a father's right (*indignum ...*

fraudasse). The syntax here provides strong evidence that the husband
was out of the picture in the actual wording of the law. It seems that the
ruling made no specific reference to the interests of the husband, or to his
consent as a legal condition. Abortion was criminalised, and that was it.
How the law was applied in practice is another matter. It is reasonable to
assume that if a married woman had an abortion with the consent of
her husband, she did not need to worry about legal consequences,
because the matter would remain private and the magistrates would
not be involved. However, if she did so against his wishes then he could
prosecute her and demand her exile. So, in practical terms, the husband's consent would be a very important factor even if it was not
enshrined as a condition in the letter of the law. In the case of unmarried women one can reasonably assume that their family would be
inclined to keep the matter private and avoid scandal, and thus that
probably very few, if any, cases involving unmarried women ever
reached the courts.

If we recall the Persian law of Darius, and how it went to great lengths
to prevent deliberate termination of a pregnancy by threatening not only
the woman but also her sexual partner and her father with death, then
perhaps we can appreciate how low-key by comparison this Roman
rescript was. In Persian law consent was irrelevant, for the state was
resolutely determined to prevent abortion under any circumstances. In
Roman law the woman could be punished only if someone felt injured
by the process, and this someone was almost invariably the woman's
sexual partner. If he had consented in the first place, then the entire
process could be kept within the private sphere. Considering these
implications we can reach the conclusion that Tryphoninus and Marcian reflect the philosophy of this law quite accurately when they
understand that the husband's consent was an important factor in this
procedure, even though this term was not included in the actual letter
of the rescript.

In sum, the existing evidence suggests that abortion was not illegal in
the ancient world until the third century AD. Insufficient scientific data
and ambivalence over the status of the unborn, socio-economic and cultural structures that allowed a greater degree of individual freedom, and
political structures that functioned better with small populations, all
contributed to the perception of abortion as an individual or family issue,
not a public one. Thus the laws of the Greek city-states, the hellenistic
kingdoms, the Roman republic, and even the early empire did not think
that it was a matter for the law-courts or the magistrates of the state. A
changing political climate in the Roman empire, perhaps more noticeable
when Rome started feeling the pressure of outside dangers, made the
Romans worry about their ability to keep their identity and control the
vast territories they had conquered, and contributed to increasingly hostile attitudes towards a practice that appeared to be a threat to the
population of Rome, and especially its old, great families, and therefore to

her capacity to rule the world. It is probably not accidental that the prohibition of abortion was introduced by Caracalla, the same emperor who sought to increase the numbers of Roman citizens by enfranchising the entire population of the empire.[42]

iii. Lysias frr. 19-24 Carey: an abortion trial in classical Athens

Among the fragments of Lysias we find a few sentences which are reportedly quotations from a speech delivered in a trial over an induced abortion. These fragments, as well as some testimonia on this speech found in later grammarians and rhetoricians, are tantalisingly revealing and at the same time desperately confusing. Despite efforts by previous scholars, the basics of this intriguing trial remain largely a matter of speculation. But before we attempt a reconstruction it is necessary to consider carefully the relevant fragments and testimonia:

1. Theon *Progymnasmata* 2,69, Spengel (fr. 20b Carey): A number of disputable arguments have already been put forward by the orators ... as in the speech of Lysias 'On the Abortion'. ... In that speech the question is whether what is carried in the womb is a human being, and whether women can have abortions without fear of a penalty. Some people claim that these speeches were not written by Lysias, but it would be beneficial for young people to read these too for the sake of exercise.

2. *Lexicon Rhetoricum Cantabrigiense*, p. 669,20 (fr. 19 Carey): There was a penalty against those who failed to pursue a public lawsuit (*graphê*). Lysias in the speech 'Against Antigenes, On the Abortion' (says): *'Think what Antigenes here has done; although he has prosecuted our mother, he wants to marry our sister and at the same time carry on with the prosecution in order to avoid paying one thousand drachmas, which one is obliged to pay, if he fails to pursue a graphê.'*

3. Sopater *Ek diaphoron tina chrêsima* (ed. H. Rabe *RHM* 64 [1909] 576) (fr. 20d Carey): Lysias is dealing with a medical question, which he paradoxically converts into a rhetorical subject in the speech 'On the Abortion', where Antigenes is accusing his wife of homicide because she had an induced abortion; he maintains that she had an abortion and prevented him from being called the father of a child.

4. Sopater *Commentary on Hermogenes* 5,3 Walz (fr. 20c Carey): There are also medical and philosophical questions; an example of a medical question is the one discussed by Lysias, namely whether a man who made a woman have an abortion has committed murder; for it is necessary to know if it (sc. the foetus) was a living being before it was born. And this is a matter pertinent to medicine and natural philosophy.

5. *Prolegomena on the Staseis* 7,15 Walz (= *Prolegomenon Sylloge* 13,200 Rabe) (fr. 20a Carey): Some of the arguments are political, or philosophical, or medical, while others are mixed, since the main question is political but the material may be medical or philosophical. ... Mixed arguments are like this: someone has hit a pregnant woman on the abdomen and he is on trial for murder. Here the main issue is political, but the material is medical. ... For example Lysias in the speech 'On the Abortion' where the person responsible is on trial for murder goes to great lengths to prove that the

foetus (*brephos*) is a living being, and says everywhere '*as the doctors and the midwives have stated*'.

6. Harpocration s.v. *amphidromia* (fr. 22 Carey): Lysias in the speech 'On the Abortion', if the speech is authentic (cf. Apostolius Paroem. *Centuria* 2,56).

s.v. *themisteuein* (fr. 23 Carey): Lysias in the speech 'On the Abortion', if it is authentic (cf. Lexicon Vindob. s.v.).

s.v. *hupologon* (fr. 24 Carey): Lysias 'On the Abortion', if it is authentic.

7. Pollux 2,7 (cf. Harpocration s.v. *amblôsis*): *amblôsis*: as Lysias.

8a. Hippocrates *Epidemics* 1,2,19: The wife of Antigenes, the one living near Nichomachos' place, produced a foetus which was fleshy, with the major organs already shaped, about four fingers long, but without bones, and then round and thick. Before labour she became asthmatic; then during labour some pus came out, as if from an abscess.

8b. *Galen's comment on this passage* (17A, 371): this birth would have been wondrous if it did not create suspicions that it was the product of an induced abortion.

9. Antiphon Sophist fr. 38: and *amblôsis*, as Lysias, and *amblôma* as A[....

10. Photius *Lexicon* A 1163: *amblôsis* and *amblôthentes* as Lysias mentions.

Theon and Harpocration express doubts over the authorship of the speech, and since so little is preserved there is no way of telling whether it was written by Lysias or not. However, we could date the speech to the early fourth century BC if we could identify the wife of Antigenes mentioned in the Hippocratic passage (no. 8) with the wife of Antigenes around whom the speech revolves. The Hippocratic passage refers to the abnormal foetus of a certain woman called the wife of Antigenes, and Galen explains this abnormality as a probable result of interference with the pregnancy in order to terminate it (most likely by means of drugs). It would be a considerable coincidence if this woman were a different person from the wife of Antigenes who was in the centre of this lawsuit. If the identification is correct then the speech could have been written by Lysias for a lawsuit that went to court early in the fourth century.[43]

This identification would also supply important details concerning the circumstances of the abortion. The wife of Antigenes went to labour under circumstances which the doctor considered extraordinary enough to merit a record. During labour she had an asthma attack, and some pus came out, as if from an abscess. Then an abnormal, obviously dead foetus was extracted. Galen understands that these abnormalities should be explained as a result of drugs taken in order to procure an abortion.

Who should be considered responsible for the abortion – the woman herself or her husband – depends on the interpretation of the remaining evidence, and this is not an easy task. First of all, it is not easy to tell who has prosecuted whom. It is characteristic of the confusion to find Sopater saying in no. 3 that Antigenes was the prosecutor and his wife the defendant, while in no. 4 he seems to imply that Antigenes was the defendant. Among the rest of the sources Theon implies that Antigenes was the prosecutor and his wife the defendant, while the *Lexicon Rheto-*

ricum Cantabrigiense (no. 2) and the *Prolegomena* (no. 5) appear to suggest that he was the defendant. The type of the lawsuit is also uncertain: while Sopater (nos 3 and 4) and the *Prolegomena* (no. 5) unequivocally state that this was a murder trial (a *dikê phonou*) and therefore a private lawsuit (like all homicide trials), one of the few direct quotations allegedly coming from this speech (no. 2) seems to suggest that it was a *graphê*, namely a public prosecution.[44] The differences between the testimonia seem irreconcilable at first sight, and have caused great confusion in scholarly opinion.

Harrison, on the basis of the quotation in the *Lexicon Rhetoricum Cantabrigiense* (no. 2), understood that this particular lawsuit was a *graphê* initiated by Antigenes, a relative of the woman's dead husband, who at the same time was claiming a daughter of the family in marriage.[45] Harrison thinks that Antigenes stepped in on behalf of his dead relative, because when the father was dead, the law permitted anyone to bring a prosecution through a *graphê amblôseôs*. Alternatively he suggests that the law permitted a public prosecution because the actual victim was the embryo itself, and since it could not defend itself, anyone should have the right to do so. Harrison also accepts the evidence of Pseudo-Galen (19,177) that a prohibition on abortion was introduced by Solon (see also the discussion in §ii, and the translation of Pseudo-Galen in Appendix 1). In recent years S. Adam was prepared to follow Harrison's line of argument and agree that abortion was a criminal offence in classical Athens.

There are fundamental flaws in Harrison's interpretation. First of all, as I have already stated in Chapter 5, there is not a single scrap of evidence from the classical period suggesting a perception of the unborn as the victim. It is not until the republican period that we find such views in circulation (in Cicero, Ovid and Chariton). On the basis of the existing evidence, to suggest that Athenian law was based on such perceptions would be a violent anachronism. Moreover, to go so far as to consider a text as rhetorical and chronologically remote as Pseudo-Galen to be a reliable historical source for Athenian law would be beyond the boundaries of common sense. The author of this study simply drops the names of the two famous lawgivers in the ancient world (Solon and Lycurgus) at this point in the discussion because this suits his argument. I would find it hard to believe that we are provided here with any form of serious historical information (see also §ii and my notes in Appendix 1, ad loc.). On the whole, Harrison's interpretation of the case is mere guessing, and shows complete disregard for every other piece of evidence on this speech. This interpretation ignores the explicit references in Sopater (no. 3), and the *Prolegomena* (no. 5) that this was a homicide trial, and also disregards the other two major testimonia, namely the evidence of Theon (no. 1), and the other passage of Sopater (no. 4). For all these reasons I consider this interpretation untenable.

Harrison believed that G. Glotz had completely misinterpreted the passage, when he had stated in no uncertain terms 'Il n'y a pas de *graphê amblôseôs*; on doit recourir à une *dikê phonou* (there is no such thing as a *graphê amblôseôs*; one has to return to a *dikê phonou*)'.[46] Among the arguments put forward by Glotz there is one which I find irresistible: 'if Athenian law defended the life of the foetus, there would be much stronger reason to defend that of the new born'. Athenian law obviously did not recognise an automatic right to life before the ritual acknowledgement of the child and its acceptance into the community through the ritual of *amphidromia* (cf. no. 6) (which normally took place a week or so after birth). So common sense would clearly suggest that Athenian law did not step in to defend foetal life. According to this interpretation of the case Antigenes could not prosecute his wife for the abortion, simply because it was not illegal, and this is why he resorted to a homicide trial (*dikê phonou*), in order to obtain redress for the abortion which as the father he perceived to be a grave personal injury. The view of Glotz that this was a homicide trial, and not a lawsuit based on a law specifically dealing with abortion as a criminal offence, was accepted by Lipsius and Nardi.[47] The latter agrees that this was a *dikê phonou*, even though he cautiously avoids further speculation on the details of it, evidently discouraged by the contradictions that seem to dominate the primary sources.

Before one can accept that this was a homicide trial by Antigenes against his wife there are some serious problems to be resolved. First of all we need to examine the sources and see if they can be fitted into this interpretation of the case, and then we need to answer some difficult questions on Athenian legal procedure. The first passage of Sopater (no. 3) appears to be the clearest and most complete of all the testimonia. According to it Antigenes is the prosecutor and his (probably former) wife the defendant. He is accusing her of homicide through an ordinary *dikê phonou*, because she had an induced abortion evidently without his consent. In order to be able to prove that this was homicide Antigenes would need to prove first that the unborn is a human being in its own right, and this would be a key issue in his line of argumentation. As I have stated in §ii, the human status of the unborn was probably not explicitly recognised by Athenian law. Therefore it would be essential for the prosecutor to prove that the aborted foetus ought to be considered as human in the eyes of the law, because otherwise a homicide charge could not stand. In order to be able to do that he would need to provide legalistic arguments like those which we find in the study *Whether what is carried in the womb is a living being* (see Appendix 1). He could also explore current medical and philosophical theories on the status of the unborn, and substantiate these arguments with testimonies from expert witnesses. The passage from the speech quoted in the *Prolegomena* (no. 5), '*as the doctors and the midwives have stated*' suggests that he did provide testimonies of this kind. Probably a number of male doctors were summoned to give evidence concerning the human status of the unborn. These doctors may have voiced their own professional opinion as well as that of some midwives with whom they had a consultation before appearing as witnesses. Thus Lysias (or whoever wrote this speech) created a fascinating blend of rhetorical argument and medical theory, much admired by later rhetoricians.

Theon (no. 1) is so impressed by this extraordinary line of argumentation that he recommends students of rhetoric to read the speech even though he suspects that it is not authentic Lysias. The passage of Theon supports an interpretation of the case as presented above. The phrase 'whether women can have abortions without the fear of a penalty' implies, I think quite clearly, that it was the wife of Antigenes who was on trial after an induced abortion, not Antigenes himself. Theon's statement that the human status of the unborn is the key issue in this speech also corroborates this understanding of the case. It makes perfect sense to think that the woman is facing homicide charges for having an abortion, while the man is arguing that she had killed his child and therefore she should be treated as a murderess by the law because the foetus was a human being after all.

The passage of the *Prolegomena* (no. 5) is less straightforward, yet I think it holds the key to our understanding of the entire case. At first sight it seems to imply that Antigenes is on trial for having kicked his pregnant wife. However, a more careful consideration of the passage reveals a clear division into two parts. There is first a general part ('Some of the arguments ... medical') where the author explains what he means by medical, philosophical, or political arguments, and uses a very well known example of a mixed argument where a political issue is entangled with a medical matter: 'should someone who hit a pregnant woman on the abdomen and caused an abortion face homicide charges?' This example we can easily identify as a resonance of the famous passage from Exodus (21:22-4), which is very often quoted in debates over the ethics of abortion in later antiquity (on the passage and the intense controversy that it has raised see Chapter 2 §iv). Therefore, this example is a famous *topos* that often figures in such discussions, and totally unrelated to the particular circumstances of this trial. When the author of the *Prolegomena* starts speaking about the present trial he marks the transition from the general part to this specific case by saying 'For example Lysias in the speech "On the abortion" ...'. It is only what follows that is related to the circumstances of the present trial. In this section ('For example ... *stated*') we find nothing that would not completely accord with the version of events as presented by Sopater (no. 3) and Theon (no. 1). In fact this section corroborates this version of events by stating that the key issue is the status of the unborn, and that the orator has gone to great lengths to prove that the unborn is human by presenting, in addition, expert witnesses to testify to this effect. This would fit very well into the context of a homicide trial against the wife of Antigenes.

The observation that the phrase 'should someone who hit a pregnant woman on the abdomen and caused an abortion face homicide charges?' is a *topos* frequently appearing in discussions over the legality of abortion, and not relevant to the circumstances of this particular lawsuit, would help us explain the other passage of Sopater (no. 4) and remove the discrepancy between this author's two passages. We must understand that here Sopater is speaking in general terms. He has explained that some rhetorical questions are related to medical and philosophical topics. As an example he has cited the speech of Lysias 'On the Abortion'. He certainly had read it some time ago (as passage no. 3 clearly suggests), and was probably fascinated by this paradoxical[48] blend of rhetoric, medicine and philosophy. He could even remember that the speech deals with the question of the human status of the unborn, and that it was a homicide trial. But, in addition, he has inserted somewhat carelessly and without clear warning a *topos* often to be found in this kind of context. If we interpret this reference to the 'man who made a woman have an abortion' as a *topos*, and not a reference to this particular trial, then this passage of Sopater is not inconsistent with his other reference to the speech 'On the Abortion', and the other testimonia concerning this text. It accords with the interpretation of this trial as a homicide trial against the wife of Antigenes, with the human status of the unborn being the main point of contention and the key issue in the argumentation line adopted by the prosecution.

The only passage that is really impossible to fit into this pattern is from the *Lexicon Rhetoricum Cantabrigiense* (no. 2). The information provided by this passage is absolutely irreconcilable with the information on the abortion trial provided by the other sources. First of all, this is obviously a defence speech in a public lawsuit, a *graphê*, initiated by a man called Antigenes, whom for the sake of convenience I will call Antigenes II. However, according to the other sources, the speech concerning the abortion is a prosecution speech delivered in a homicide trial, which would always be a private lawsuit, a *dikê phonou*, by a man called Antigenes (whom I will call Antigenes I). I cannot see how these differences could be bridged. However, they do not need to be bridged: the only indication that associates passage 2 with the abortion trial is the assertion of the lexicographer that the fragment comes from the speech 'Against Antigenes, on the Abortion' (*Kata Antigenous, peri tês amblôseôs*).[49] The actual quotation gives no indication whatsoever that the lawsuit involving Antigenes II has anything to do with the abortion. The title of the speech in the abortion trial as given by Theon, Sopater, the *Prolegomena*, and three times by Harpocration, is simply 'On the Abortion' (*Peri tês amblôseôs*). This is not decisive *per se* as these sources might be giving a shorter version of the title. However in the light of the above-mentioned discrepancies it acquires significance. The original title of the speech directed against Antigenes II probably was 'To Antigenes' (*Pros Antigene*). This speech is the defence speech delivered in a trial initiated through a *graphê* by Antigenes II, against a woman who is defended in court by her adult sons. It is an attack against the prosecutor, Antigenes II. The speech written for the abortion trial is entitled 'On the Abortion' (*Peri tês amblôseôs*), and it was a prosecution speech delivered in a homicide trial by Antigenes I against his former wife because she had an abortion without his consent. The attribution of both speeches to Lysias would be far-fetched but not inconceivable.

Here is a summary of the events surrounding the abortion trial, as I understand it: The wife of Antigenes I had an abortion with some complications but undoubtedly she recovered well after labour. The attending doctor recorded the complications of the labour and the abnormalities of the dead foetus, but did not express an opinion over the cause. Probably he was uncertain and could not tell whether the abortion was spontaneous or induced by means of drugs. Galen, however, commenting on this record several centuries later, explicitly declares that the circumstances were suspicious, implying that drugs taken in order to procure the abortion were the cause of these abnormalities. At any rate, Antigenes suspected that his wife's abortion was deliberately procured by means of drugs, and felt hurt and angry. He might even have been in a position to confirm that she had taken drugs, and he was determined to avenge the injury to his emotions, his interests as a father, and the damage to his *oikos*. Nothing would deter him from seeking for revenge, not even the fact that the laws of the city did not consider his wife's action to be an offence. He was convinced that she had killed his child, and saw himself in the role of the avenger of his dead child's life. He believed that his wife deserved the same punishment as the killer of any other human being, and decided to bring homicide charges against her. But here he had a problem. Since Athenian law did not explicitly recognise the unborn as human he had to convince the *basileus*, the magistrate in charge of accepting homicide cases, that the killing of the unborn was nothing less than murder. The *basileus* could refuse to process the lawsuit, if he thought that the procedure was not appropriate. But if the *basileus* refused, Antigenes might turn his wrath against him.[50] This particular *basileus* obviously did not refuse: perhaps he was genuinely persuaded by the arguments of this forceful man, or maybe he simply wanted him off his back. By accepting this lawsuit the *basileus* certainly chose the safest option for himself. Beyond that point the whole procedure would be in the hands of the court. We can assume that this court was no other than the Areopagus Council, the most venerable court in the city. Antigenes was accusing his wife of deliberate homicide, and such cases fell within the jurisdiction of this awesome body. The Areopagus had a tremendous reputation for fairness, and we can understand why.[51] It tried only homicide cases, membership was for life, and each of its members had considerable administrative experience prior to becoming an Areopagite, since it was exclusively composed of persons who had served as senior magistrates (archons). Moreover, the Areopagus had the right to conduct its own investigations before the trial, if it so wished, and be independently prepared for the hearing.[52] These criteria probably made it the most experienced homicide court that has ever existed. Antigenes won the first round and succeeded in his attempt to have this unconventional case sent to court, but to win over this formidable body would be the real challenge. To convince or intimidate a single magistrate into accepting that abortion amounts to murder might have been fairly easy for this determined man. But to convince the Areopagus Council that the homicide law of Dracon should be extended to cover unborn children would not be as easy. Substantial arguments would be needed to prove that a foetus is as human as a born child.

During the trial the burden of proof fell upon the prosecution. Antigenes had to prove to the Council that the law should recognise the foetus as a child, and therefore its deliberate destruction as intentional homicide. The study *Whether what is carried in the womb is a living being* gives us an idea of the sort of legal arguments that he might have used.[53] He could claim that an unborn heir was recognised as such, since, according to Attic law, the final settlement of an inheritance was to be delayed until the birth of the potential heir or heiress. He could also mention that a pregnant woman who had no other children could choose to remain in her dead husband's house until she gave birth. All these arguments might be legally sound, but probably not enough to convince the court to sentence someone to death for intentional homicide. Antigenes knew that he needed something more substantial, and sought to provide this argument in the form of expert opinions by medical practitioners. In the trial he went to great lengths to prove that the foetus was a human being in its own right. He probably quoted some of the medical and philosophical views on the status of the unborn that were in circulation in the early fourth century BC, and sought corroboration from expert witnesses. He invited doctors to convey their own opinions, and those of some midwives too. Now, considering that there was no cross-examination of witnesses in fourth-century Athenian courts, and that each side invited its own supporting witnesses, we can be fairly certain that the doctors whom Antigenes invited testified that the foetus was a human being, at least at this stage of its development. If the doctors whom Antigenes invited held the dominant view in the classical period, that once a foetus is formed it should be considered as a human being (see Chapter 2), then they should be in no doubt over the status of this particular foetus. The medical record (passage 8a) states in no uncertain terms that the major organs were formed, and this fact should lead the doctors to consider that it was already a human being.

Antigenes set up a formidable case, but the Areopagus was not convinced. I think we can safely draw this conclusion from the fact that women in the classical period, and in later years until the prohibition of abortion by Caracalla, could have abortions without fear of the law. If the wife of Antigenes had been convicted this would have created a precedent that might encourage others to use the homicide law for the prosecution of women who had abortions. But there is no evidence that such a possibility was present when Athenian women were considering or even attempting abortions. The drugs might threaten their lives, the law did not. Why the Areopagus was not convinced we cannot tell for certain. It is possible that this experienced body found the argument that abortion amounted to homicide, since the foetus was formed and therefore human, to be contrived and far-fetched. Lengthy philosophical theories on the status of the unborn might fascinate philosophers and rhetoricians, but could prove insufficient to influence seriously the sober judgement of this court. The defence might argue that abortion was not a criminal offence in Athens, and therefore the woman should not be punished for something that was not a crime in the eyes of the law, or alternatively they could play safe and claim that this abortion was not induced, but spontaneous. If they had access to the medical record provided in the *Epidemics* (passage no. 8a), they could present it to court and argue that the attending doctor nowhere states that the abortion was deliberate. This should be sufficient to induce an element of reasonable doubt that could sway the judgement of the Areopagitai. The defence could also plead for the sympathy of the court on the grounds that the woman had suffered enough by losing her child, and that she certainly did not deserve to be killed as a result of this misfortune. Considering that conviction by this court for deliberate homicide could only carry the death penalty, the members of the Council would certainly think seriously before pronouncing a 'guilty' verdict. In the end, no one could know what each Areopagite had in mind when he cast his vote. What finally mattered was the fact that for the majority of the Areopagus this particular abortion did not deserve to be avenged by the death of the woman.

Many of the details of this unconventional lawsuit remain obscure, and we do not have further information concerning the affairs of the family involved. However, the arguments that were exchanged that morning at the foot of the hill of Ares were to remain bitterly controversial and are still exchanged in television studios and discussion platforms all over the world.

iv. The trial of Cicero's Milesian woman

We know little about the actual circumstances under which an unnamed woman from Miletus was sentenced to death after having an abortion. The main source for this case is a reference in the speech of Cicero *Pro Cluentio* (32):

> I remember a Milesian woman, when I was in Asia, who was sentenced to death for having a self-induced abortion by means of drugs, having been bribed to do so by the heirs in reversion, not unjustly, because she deprived her husband of the hope of becoming a father, the memory of his name, the successor to his generation, the heir to his family, and the city of a future citizen.

This trial probably took place in 79 BC, when Cicero was visiting Asia during his temporary retirement from the bar.[54] The orator's wording does not allow us to determine with any degree of certainty what exactly was the charge, and we cannot even tell whether she was convicted under

Roman or local Milesian law. However, we can tell for sure that if she was prosecuted under Roman law then the charge could not have been that she had an abortion. This was not illegal until the third century AD, and even after that date a prosecution for abortion did not carry the death penalty. The wording of Cicero (*rei capitalis esse damnatam*) might provide an indication that she was actually prosecuted for homicide. If so, the similarities with the trial of the wife of Antigenes are remarkable. Three centuries later in another corner of the Greek world a woman who had an abortion also faced homicide charges. Only this time the unlucky woman did not escape. She was sentenced to death because, we are told by Cicero, with her actions she had caused grave injury to her husband's feelings and interests. The woman's motives, namely bribery by the alternative heirs, may have played a strong part in her conviction. If witnesses had been presented confirming this accusation it would have been very difficult for the defence to shake off the bad image of the accused created in court. A woman who had killed her own child for the sake of money could easily be portrayed as a monster by the prosecution. The main character in Albert Camus' *L'Etranger* comes to mind, sentenced to death for homicide because he did not cry at his mother's funeral. The bad image of a heartless brute which the prosecution successfully created in the court-room had a much more lasting effect upon the jury's decision than any legally sound argument.

Conclusions

A closer consideration of the evidence suggests that abortion was not illegal until a rescript of Severus-Caracalla penalised it in the early third century AD. The fact that the law allowed abortion is consistent with the religious, political, ethical and philosophical beliefs of the ancient world. It is also consistent with the ambiguity and uncertainty over the status of the unborn that characterises most of the medical and philosophical literature from the Graeco-Roman antiquity. The change of heart in the imperial era was not a result of greater certainty over the biological facts concerning the status of the foetus, or even a greater ethical conviction concerning the wrongs of induced abortion, since these issues continued to be very contentious in the following centuries. The criminalisation of induced abortion was primarily due to demographic policies intended to address the insecurity of the ruling Roman classes. It was a product of the fear that the traditional Roman family and the values that it represented were in danger from the multitude of alien cultures that surrounded them and the barbaric races pressing against their borders. Those who formed the core of the Roman empire feared that if practices that kept their population down were allowed eventually they might lose control, as they would be reduced into an insignificant minority within the borders of their vast state. With hindsight, perhaps their worries were not totally unjustified.

Attitudes to Abortion:
A Historical Perspective

A historian observing the developments and shifts in attitudes to abortion over a period of 800 years is bound to come to the conclusion that these attitudes were tied to several other factors. Abortion is an issue inextricably linked to personal, emotional, religious, cultural, political, social and economic circumstances. There is usually a strong motive behind a woman's desire to have a pregnancy terminated, and this was even more the case in the ancient world, where poor medical care made the undertaking truly painful and dangerous. One would need a compelling driving force before contemplating such a risky ordeal, a motive that would outweigh the risks and pains of the operation. History presents us with plenty of examples in which the motive was stronger than the drawbacks. As outsiders we might agree that this motive was compelling and we might even empathise with the individual. In other instances we might find the motive superficial, strange, or even incomprehensible. Sometimes we may not be able to appreciate fully the cultural background behind a woman's actions unless we are prepared to step outside our own system of beliefs, and our own culture, and put ourselves into her shoes. By doing so we might still disagree with her decision, and we could even maintain that we would have acted differently in that situation, but at least we can acquire an insight into her motives, and perhaps understand why in her eyes these motives appeared to be stronger than any deterrent that nature, society or even the gods themselves had set up.

It may be curious at first sight to find that the dangers and pains of abortion were not sufficient deterrents. The medical and scientific data, as these are preserved in the writings of the great physicians and natural philosophers of the ancient world, leave many questions unanswered. We cannot be sure how efficient oral drugs were, and we can only vaguely speculate on the safety and success rate of surgical and mechanical procedures. But we can be sure about two things: first, that women and their attendants had sufficient knowledge to enable them to procure abortions, and second that the entire undertaking was perilously dangerous and painful. Surely some of the oral drugs were at times effective, and the percentage of successful terminations probably increased when more violent mechanical or surgical means were used. However, serious physicians realised that the more potent the means, the higher the risk for the woman. Success in the operation often went hand in hand with extreme danger or death. Ordinary men and women might not always appreciate the extent of the danger, and often mixed myth and magic with fact. However, everyone understood at least this simple fact, that abortion could cost a woman her life.

So, why did they still do it? In this book I have tried to explore the motives of various groups of women against the historical and cultural background in which they lived and functioned. I think the orators, historians and dramatists of the ancient world provide us with sufficient evidence to be able to understand the basic parameters of contemporary socio-economic, legal, religious and cultural settings. This allows a good insight into the motives of various groups of women. But in the end I argue that it all came down to one simple fact: if the woman *from her perspective and in her own mind* thought that continuing with the pregnancy under existing circumstances would make her life unbearable, then she would not be deterred either by law, or religion, or even the real threat against her own life.

Such being the realities of abortion, the ceaseless debate over the status of the foetus, namely whether it should be considered to be a human being in its own right before birth, or not, may seem hopelessly academic. The complicated, and often flawed and confusing arguments that we read in medical handbooks, Platonic and Aristotelian studies, philosophical or theological works, and even in two Pseudo-Galenic studies specifically addressing the issue, were irrelevant for the ordinary woman who faced an alarming situation in her hands and had no knowledge or time for refined arguments over the beginnings of human life. However, it is very constructive for us to follow this debate. It reveals that the ancient world did not have any certainty over the status of the unborn. People did not tend to think of the unborn as a human being with an independent right to life, but they were not prepared to discard this possibility either. Poor knowledge of human anatomy and imperfect understanding of the stages of pregnancy may have contributed to this uncertainty. Some might say that the foetus was human from the moment of conception, others maintained that it acquired human status at the more advanced stages of pregnancy, others argued that it did not really become alive before it could breathe air after birth. But there was no consensus, and the ordinary man probably did not understand most of this complex and inconclusive debate. The ordinary person remained undecided, if not unconcerned with such difficult and complex questions.

Now, at least in the case of the Greek city states this is very significant, because the ordinary man was also the lawgiver, the judge and the magistrate. If the ordinary assembly member in Athens had no fixed ideas regarding the human status of the unborn, he would not bother to propose or vote either laws intended to safeguard its life, or laws allowing its destruction. So the fact that there was no consensus, or even any kind of

firm conviction over the human status of the unborn became very significant, because it formed the basis of attitudes towards abortion which could
be considered as tolerant. This is not to say that most Athenian men, and
men in other parts of the ancient world, approved of abortion, or that they
did not care if one of the women under their authority went ahead with it.
The case of Antigenes versus his wife indicates that hurt feelings and
acrimonious disputes could arise, and the generally disapproving tone of
the majority of ancient authors when speaking about abortion suggests
that most people did not feel particularly comfortable with the subject.
However, in addition to what I mentioned above, there was a number of
further reasons why the Greeks, and the Romans until the third century
AD, did not think that the laws of the state ought to be concerned with
abortion.

First of all, the men who made the laws were often ignorant of such
undertakings because their daughters or wives kept them secret. Second,
they did not perceive abortion as a serious threat to the general interest.
Individual men, such as Antigenes, might feel that their family and their
own personal interests as men, fathers, and citizens had been harmed, but
collectively the citizens of the city-state or the Roman republic did not feel
that this was a public matter, something which threatened the structures
and existence of the state. The Greek city-states did not aim at large
populations, and in the Roman republic and early empire clearly the
birth-rate among the leading orders was low too. Repeated measures by
emperors to stimulate a higher birth-rate and strengthen family life
should probably be interpreted as proof that a stimulus was necessary,
because in reality people did not go for big families. Thus the Greeks and
the Romans until the first couple of centuries into the Christian era
generally did not view abortion as a threat to the safety of the state.
However, from the time of Cicero we can see the first signs of a change.
Increasingly the Romans felt threatened in their position as rulers of the
world, and this growing insecurity changed attitudes and led to a perception of abortion as a practice that was bad for Rome, and to its eventual
prohibition.

It seems clear to me that these political and demographic trends had an
influence upon the perception of abortion by religion. The religions of
pagan Graeco-Roman antiquity are probably a unique phenomenon in
human history in the sense that they were human-centred, not god-
centred. There was no supernatural authority outside this world holding
the absolute truth and transmitting it to humans by means of a holy book
or the teachings of some holy man. The gods of the Greek and Roman
pantheon were modelled on humans, looked human, acted human, and
they were by no means examples of good behaviour. So, what was good,
what was bad, what was holy or unholy, what the gods would find
acceptable, depended directly upon the political and cultural set of values
that each group or individual chose to follow. So, if people were not
collectively vocal in their condemnation of abortion, we can understand

why religion was not particularly critical either. Most individuals might feel uneasy in the sense that they did not want such acts taking place in their house, and so religion accommodated this sentiment by equating abortion to impurity, something that would need ritual cleansing, as death, or childbirth, or menstruation did. But since most people had no firm conviction that abortion was murder, Greek and Roman religion did not make this equation either. Christianity did make this equation, but there the parameters of the dogma itself were very different, and by that time abortion was much less tolerated in society as a whole and had already been declared illegal.

Inaccurate knowledge of many facts surrounding the progression of the pregnancy, insufficient data on embryology, and social attitudes that did not necessarily view abortion as a violation of the laws of the gods or those of the state, contributed to an ambivalent perception of abortion by Greek and Roman doctors. Since there was no official state policy on the matter in any part of the ancient world until the third century AD, they had the freedom to perform abortions or refuse them as their own professional, moral and personal considerations suggested. I think that we can safely conclude that no serious physician in the ancient world wanted to be seen as an abortionist. Frequently in the Hippocratic Corpus drugs used for abortions are disguised as emmenagogues (medicines designed to bring on menstruation). Later physicians make more explicit references, but still try to distance themselves from the practice. Let us remember Soranus, for example, who recommends abortion only if the woman's life is at risk. Obviously he did not want to be perceived as an advocate of abortion at will. These doctors probably had first-hand experience of abortion, but they did not want to own to it. Perhaps they understood it as a practice contrary to their main duty to do no harm. So perhaps the Hippocratic Oath and the stern prohibition of abortion in it may not be a marginal product of a closed sect, but a mainstream document reflecting the feelings of many physicians of the time. This stipulation of the oath is certainly consistent with another clause that follows almost immediately afterwards: 'I will abstain from all intentional wrong-doing and harm.' However, even if we conceded the point that most doctors had moral reservations in relation to abortion, it is clear that under certain circumstances they were prepared to perform it, and these circumstances need not always coincide with sound medical reasoning.

So is what we read in the Oath and many other medical texts just lip-service to principles? Or should we go as far as to speak about blatant hypocrisy? Before we rush to call people like Soranus or Galen hypocrites we should pause for a moment and consider the actual circumstances of women seeking abortions and the human response of their medical attendants. Many of these women were probably very distressed, desperate, in serious trouble, in a bad mental and emotional condition. The doctors had to consider these facts too, as they had to think of the well-being of their patients as a whole, especially since most ancient doctors had a clearly psychosomatic perception of health and disease. They might also empathise with the distress of their patients and understand that the reasons behind the request were compelling and serious. After such considerations they might come to the conclusion that high moral standards are desirable, but not always applicable in real life. They might feel that it is one thing to theorise and philosophise about the concepts of movement and sensation, the nature of the foetus, the stages of its development, the moment of its animation, the profound mysteries of the soul, and the phenomenon of life, but certainly it is another thing to have to respond to a real-life crisis. Sometimes this would require them to bend the rules, to set aside high moral principles and philosophical theories, and deal with the crude reality.

Abortion has been debated for thousands of years. Much of this debate has been concerned with high moral standards and principles. However, in practice abortion has been an act that has little to do with high principles, and much to do with compelling circumstances. History clearly suggests that talk of principles has proved ineffective when balanced against the gravity of the circumstances that urge a woman to seek a termination. This does not mean that the debate is over, and that moral issues are irrelevant. It simply means that along with such considerations we need to remember the gravity of the circumstances, because in this instance it might be the most decisive factor.

Appendix 1

Pseudo-Galen
Whether what is carried in the womb is a living being (19,158-181 Kühn)

Introduction

The study *Whether what is carried in the womb is a living being* is preserved among the works of Galen, even though it was not written by him. One hardly needs to resort to detailed linguistic or philological arguments in order to disprove Galenic authorship. Galen mentions in one of his authentic works that he once encountered a Platonic philosopher who explained to him the theory that the foetus is animated and a living being from the moment of conception, and made references to the universal soul that animates everything.[1] However, Galen was not convinced and flatly rejected the theory of animation at conception. The present study appears to be a typical product of that Platonic school of thought which Galen has rejected. It promotes the theory that the foetus is animated at the moment of conception, makes extensive reference to the immortal soul that animates the universe, and betrays a substantial number of Platonic influences, some totally superficial, others more profound. In addition to this irrefutable evidence, this is not a medical study, and it certainly does not bear the marks of Galen's pen, such as his detailed knowledge and spirited discussion of previous medicine, his philosophy, or his teleological cosmology. The author of this study does not seem to know any of the works of Soranus and Galen, which might provide a clue for the date at which it was composed. Since the author is aware of Stoic views on the foetus, and probably hellenistic medicine, and advances a thesis which, according to the aforementioned passage of Galen, was fashionable around the middle of the second century, it would be a fair guess to say that this treatise was written in the first half of the second century AD.

It is an essay in the form of a rhetorical exercise, a literary form familiar to us especially from the period of the second sophistic. It betrays influences from a whole range of different theories on the soul, the body, the universe and human nature, and stands as a unique specimen, a blend of ideas and cosmologies brought together in a manner that suits the specific argument that the author is trying to win at any particular moment. What matters to the author is not the consistency of the argument, but demonstrative prowess, scoring points, even if one has to bring together perceptions and views from very different, if not directly opposing, theories. In this respect the study has a much closer affinity to rhetoric than to philosophy. The author moves between medicine and cosmology, expands on the functions of the soul, and concludes with references to contemporary inheritance law and Greek mythology. Thus his line of argumentation is certainly remarkable and deserves closer study, and moreover it betrays an underlying existentialism which I find inviting and captivating.[2]

The format of the study is in many ways typical of a rhetorical exercise. In section 159 the author refers to the present argument in terms that would be suitable for a law-court trial. He presents himself as the speaker for one side, while those who reject the view that the foetus is fully human are presented as the opposing litigants. The readers must act as the jury, and his task is to convince them that he is right in the same way as a litigant would try to persuade a jury to embrace his cause in an ordinary trial. Moreover, there is a number of striking rhetorical elements scattered throughout the entire study. For example, at one point (174) he clearly echoes arguments similar to those in Lysias 10 *Against Theomnestos*, and in the closing section he uses direct discourse and addresses the embryos as if they were present in the court-room and he could make a direct emotional appeal to them.

The author has taken over a number of arguments and ideas from previous literature. He quotes Hippocrates several times, and is quick to acknowledge his debt to him. Presumably he expected these references to the great master to increase the authority and power of his arguments. He also acknowledges his debt to Plato and Democritus. However, in most instances he does not identify his sources nor acknowledge his debt to other classical authors. I intend to present the results of my research into the sources and origins of his arguments more thoroughly elsewhere; here it suffices to say that I was able to detect plentiful Platonic and Aristotelian influences, knowledge of Empedocles, Anaxagoras, and probably other Presocratic authors, awareness of Stoic theories on the nature of the universe and the process of animation of the unborn, probably some knowledge of hellenistic medicine, and certainly good knowledge of Herodotus and Greek mythology. The author seems to borrow a number of arguments and data from previous authors, which he has rearranged to suit his purposes, without particular concern over their impact on the cohesion and consistency of his overall thesis. For example, while he is arguing passionately that the foetus ought to be considered fully and completely human from the moment of conception, he adopts the Stoic view that the foetus is only potentially human at two different points, and then continues with his own line of argumentation, almost unaware of the seriousness of these contradictions. The most likely explanation is that the author sometimes uncritically adopts views of others which in essence would contradict his own argument. However, even though his account may at times be inconsistent and perhaps unoriginal, it is clearly focused; it is a passionate defence of his belief in the full human status of the unborn from the moment of conception.[3]

From the outset the author exhibits awareness of the complexity and difficulty of the issues involved. He seems to understand well that a human being is more than a biological unit, and this is why he is prepared to place the question of the status of the embryo in a cosmological, religious, legal, social and historical context. He begins his argument by saying that man is a 'loan and particle' of the greater world, the universe, and therefore any enquiry into the identity of man should begin from an exploration of the nature of the universe, the *kosmos*. The universe itself, as the author understands it, is a living being and was so from the moment of its creation, from 'its foetal stages' (162). The author has accepted the Platonic and Stoic beliefs in a living universe, and adapts them to suit his argument. Then in a passage with seemingly Anaxagorean influences he presents the 'soul, or primordial spirit' as the creator of the universe, the element that puts order into chaos by separating the four Empedoclean elements of fire, air, earth and water. The point he is trying to make is that since the universe is a living being and has always been so from the moment of its creation, man, who is a particle of the universe, is also a living being and has always been so from the moment of conception. The soul, or primordial spirit, or air, or whatever one might call this universal force that brought everything to life (and the author does not want to call it by any specific name at this point), is what animates the foetus, and does so from the very beginning.

Consequently the author feels the need to explain exactly how the process of animation works and how the soul enters the foetus. Here he calls upon the assistance of previous medical literature, and in particular the great Hippocrates. He accepts the view that the seed comes from the whole body and this is why, along with the other components, a segment of the soul is contained in the seed and grows along with the foetus. While still in the uterus the foetus performs all the basic functions of a human being. It breathes air that enters the uterus either through the mouth or through the rear end, it feeds from suckers that grow on the walls of the uterus, and is even in the position to separate useful nutrients from harmful or useless substances and reject the latter. According to the author, the foetus behaves like a human being in the uterus, and it is only a matter of time before it can reach its full potential. This is why, he argues, one should not fuss about words and terminology, but simply call the embryo a living human being from the start. The soul is necessary from the beginning as the governing power of the body, and this is why nature has placed it there. The author quotes Hippocrates by saying that nature cannot be taught, and that it does things for its own reasons. It equips all living beings with the necessary tools to survive and reach their potential. So how is it possible that nature could fail to equip man with a soul? In a passage with Platonic resonances it is argued that, since man is the most divine of all living beings and the only one with the potential to be similar to god, the self-taught and wise nature surely gave him the equipment for this purpose, namely the soul, which is only a fragment of the soul of the universe, from the moment that he was created.

In the final section of the study the author presents arguments derived from law, social practice, history and mythology. He starts by arguing that if the foetus were not a living being, its destruction by means of an abortion would not have been deemed as illegal by the great legislators of the past. In one sentence he presents the two great lawgivers of the past, Solon and Lycurgus, as joining forces and declaring abortion illegal. He then continues by saying that these men were simply emulating the works of their predecessors, the gods themselves, who had been the first lawgivers. The historical accuracy of this piece of information, namely that abortion was illegal in the past, ultimately because it was an act that would appear as abominable in the eyes of the gods, is highly questionable, since neither Greek law nor Greek religion condemned abortion (see Chapter 6). On the other hand, the reference to the inheritance laws and family practices in relation to the human status of the embryo contains more historical truth, for the laws of the Greek cities did indeed make specific allowances for unborn heirs (see Chapter 5). Further corroboration of the view that the unborn child is no less of a person than the grown man is sought in Greek mythology and historical memory. Several examples of illustrious men are mentioned whose arrival and future accomplishments had been announced by dreams or omens well before they were born. The argument is that these persons were the men that they were even before they were born. The rhetorical plea to the unborn embryos to emerge into this world without fear concludes the study in a manner that perhaps would be more suitable to a court-room.

The author understands that human identity encapsulates several different dimensions, and seeks to prove that the foetus is a living being and fully human from the moment of conception in relation to all these. He invokes medical science, the law, religion, history and mythology. Moreover, he seeks an answer beyond the limits of this earth. He tries to see the foetus as a particle of a living universe. In this universe all elements of the creation have an inherent purpose of existence. This purpose was assigned to them by the force that created the *kosmos*, and the necessary tools for the fulfilment of this purpose were offered to each element by the creator. A human being as part of this living universe is equally subject to this teleology as any other being. As such it has been offered all the tools that would allow it to fulfil its purpose from the moment of its creation. And since it is the only being that can rise above this world, take a glimpse at its creator, and come to resemble god, at the moment of its creation it was equipped with a soul, a segment of the universal soul that pervades the *kosmos*, in order to guide it towards the fulfilment of its destiny.

Translation [4]

[158] **Chapter 1:** The same issue which has been a subject of investigation among students of nature and philosophers up to the present day, namely the search for the nature of all things, has also been a matter of concern for the Asclepiads and their descendants when they investigate the ambivalent perception of the embryo growing in the womb. As those who investigate the whole have not clearly stated whether it is a living being or not, in the same manner the leading figures in the art of medicine have left the issue concerning the nature the growing child still unspecified. [159] Thus, since the issue is difficult and challenging and still unresolved, we must listen together to what has been said on it; for I, the speaker, and you, the judges, have a common share in human nature in the way of Socrates, and this is why we should be rather content with what has been said, instead of seeking things beyond what is appropriate. According to Plato, god first knows what lies above ordinary comprehension, and then his follower, and his favourite among men. So let love be present, while envy or insolence should be absent from those who attempt such endeavours, because then we can proceed into these fields further motivated by love, while you will forever enjoy favour among your fellow humans and unenvied virtue. However, since we shall speak about a small world, namely man, we will start from the big one, of which we are a loan and particles. If the nature of the latter becomes more comprehensible to us, we will be in a position to see human composition more clearly too. So before we attempt the second we need to define first what is the world. [160] The essence of what is human will be easily specified if the general terminology offers a wholesome explanation. Let us explain what is a living being before it comes to existence, in order to reveal the nature of all seed by defining this particular term. A living being is an essence with soul and sense, as far as the generic characteristics of all its categories are concerned. Now, up to the point that it is simply defined as such it can be inclusive and all-encompassing. However, once differentiating characteristics are added then the general kind presents variations as it is divided into species. So, let us see if the world is a living being, and if it was so at the beginning, and then if it had a complete nature.

The world is a system consisting of the sky and the earth and the natures in between and water and air; and the leader and primal spirit, which some philosophers call soul, or unit, or atom, or fire, or, in accordance with its own character, the primal spirit, pervades all of them. These existed from the beginning even before they were given this name, but then they were mixed together without differentiation, and as some people say, [161] they were called 'material', but now they are called 'world' because they are arranged neatly and in an orderly manner, and they move with rhythm and pattern. For I would consider those who claim that the whole of this is immovable to be immovable themselves and similar to stone. The world has been constructed complete from complete units, perfect from perfect ones, and self-sufficient from self-defined systems. It was and it will be a living being in motion. At an early stage it possessed in seminal form the potential of reason, which brings everything together, but when it was separated and came forward from the darkness it demonstrated the prowess of its inbuilt potential by presenting here earth and there water. And wherever it directed fire and air, with constant expansion it succeeded in illuminating the whole by virtue of the nature of the elements, and by using the sun and the moon as eyes with their clarity and bright shine it became the guide to all motion. Thus it was mixed with the world from the moment that the latter was created and first consolidated into its present nature. So, the universe then was, and apparently still remains, the first living being, and animated, and intelligent. Therefore no one would dare to suggest that it was not a living being [162] from its foetal stages. For how could the universe produce wholesome beings if it were not wholesome itself? In the same manner one would not call what is carried in the womb a living being if something were missing, as a coppersmith or a blacksmith or a sculptor or a ship-builder, or some such, would not be able to claim that he had delivered a completed product if a hand or a foot were missing from the statue, or the sharp edge from a knife, or the helm from a ship. A product is perfect only when it is complete and wholly assembled and nothing is missing. Thus, the world as well as what is carried in the womb could never be considered as perfect unless from the very first moment of their existence they had received the essence of everything.

Chapter 2: After explaining that the universe was a living being, and for this reason it remains one in the present, now we will come to talk about man who is second after the universe. That man is a living being, and why, (namely because, [163] when the child was in the womb, it had the same needs as any other living being) has been said and preordained and declared, as if from the Delphic tripod, on behalf of the Asclepiads by Hippocrates. He attributes its first constitution and apparent living status to the whole, because he is aware that it could not possibly exist as a self-defined being, unless it drew its living status from the whole. He says: 'the seed comes from the whole body, and from healthy parts it is healthy, but from sick parts it is sick.' He said that it is part from the entire body, and a complete total from a complete total. And, far from maintaining that it is not a living being, he even answered in advance a possible objection on the grounds that disabled children are not complete. Seed that lacks nothing in terms of complete-ness produces healthy persons that have everything, while seed that is incomplete produces handicapped people. There is nothing wondrous about this: how could it become healthy if it was not healthy at the moment of creation? Health is a possible state only for something that has the inbuilt potential even before it has been created, and only because it has the inbuilt potential to be healthy can it realise this potential after it is created. For among those things that do not exist, [164] some have not yet been created at all, while others have the potential, like the neuter seed. This has the potential to become a living being, this time for real, when it is used to create a human being. Some others, however, neither exist, nor have the potential to exist, nor have reason, since it is not part of their nature, because they do not possess either the reason of something that has been born, or that of something which will be born. So, following Hippocrates, what is carried in the womb would rightly be considered to be a living being, because it was created by seed from the whole human being and was thus given the potential of the whole human being. Moreover, he did not only declare that it comes from the whole and that it is a living being, but also demonstrated that even in terms of quantity it possesses the principles of the whole, and the same potential as those from which it has sprang. 'For twins are born from the same womb, and the uterus has recesses and curves.' There it is possible to understand clearly that the seed deposited into the womb has the same potential, as the nature of the living being. For, even though it is small in terms of quantity it becomes large because of its potential, and shows that the initial cause of this was its essence as a living being. No one would argue that the fire dispersed in [165] firestones or limestones is not a fire, because it is not burning. It certainly becomes an actual fire when it comes in contact with the wood and the wind from everywhere outside. In the same manner, one would truthfully call 'living being' the seed deposited into a woman, because it already has the potential to be a living being. Then, it actually becomes a living being as soon as it comes out of the womb, and comes in contact with the one who gave it the initial existence. Since it is a particle and a fragment of the great living being, namely the universe, while it stays in the recesses, and nests there, it remains in a mixed state. However, once it is separated and emerges out of this depth, as if from chaos, it embraces its own nature with actions which indicate that it actually exists. It starts moving by itself, and directs its shining eyes everywhere imitating the nature of the sun and the moon, and turns the mind following the trajectory of its own creator.

Chapter 3. It would be possible to prove wrong those who said that what is carried in the womb is not a living being if we were to examine what has been said. [166] I will now explain how many and what kind of things a living being does. As a living being consists of a soul and a nature, it needs food and air, because the soul is fed with air, while the nature is fed with liquid and solid food. Now, we will find that what is carried in the womb is making use of all the resources, the ones needed for the motion of the soul, and those needed for the development of the nature. Hippocrates thinks that it swallows, and says that it breathes through the mouth and the nose. Some of the Asclepiads think that it also sucks milk from the suckers in the womb and digests, since it is necessary to digest what has been consumed, even though it receives the nutriment already highly processed by the mother. But it would not be possible to assimilate the received nutriment unless the nature suitable to receive it is already present. It would be necessary for the one who feeds the nature of the child to resemble the one who is fed. Then it would be ready to give and take the works of nature, and be prepared to make distinctions and single out what is alien. Thus the biles, [167] and all the humours are made once the food is separated. Moreover, one should not think that the only nutrient material for the embryo is the one that comes through the umbilical cord to the liver, because it is also fed through these avenues, and especially the most perfected ones, and when the nutrient goes down that route, it enjoys food. Do not think that because Hippocrates said 'the first nutrient is supplied through the umbilical cord' he was not aware that it is also fed through the mouth, for he mentioned that route too, as it has been explained above. The fact that once it is born it is instinctively drawn to the breast provides additional proof that it is fed through the mouth while still in the womb, otherwise it would not rush so quickly in this direction if it had not already been accustomed to it. And it has the ability to break the ingested nutriment into vapour and spirit, and easily adds it to each one of its own particles. It can also turn the nutriment from the seed into humours and the one from the humours into flesh, veins, nerves, arteries, bones, guts and limbs. It becomes much from little, and big from small, while its capacity to grow allows it to expand and become complete until it has reached the limits of its inbuilt potential.

[168] **Chapter 4:** We have sufficiently illustrated in our speech the works of nature in the womb. In the following lines I will try to demonstrate that it also possesses soul and intellect. Since the sensory organs are constructed in such a

manner that the powers of the soul can be transported through them, the sight through the eyes, the hearing through the ears, the taste and smell through the tongue and the nose, and the touch through the hands and body contact, it is obvious that no part of the body has been left idle. However, the embryo in the womb is predetermined to have the aforementioned places, and it already has from the beginning the essence of the soul and the brain, which is its place of residence, implanted in the recess of the head. It is clear that, along with the ejaculation of the seed into the uterus, the creator of the world sowed the soul too, in order to provide, along with the body, its governing power. We know that those who create instruments construct them in such a way as to be able to fulfil certain functions. [169] The ship-builder constructs the keel underneath the ship so as to be able to cut through the waves and serve as a wall and safe barrier against underwater rocks. The flute-maker shapes the copper into long tubes suitable for receiving the wind blown into them. The musician stretches the strings so that they can produce a harmonious tune. The person who prepares healing medicines does so for the purpose of curing disease. The general gives tactical orders to those in battle-formation so that they can sustain an attack by the enemy. As those who perform any of those functions do so in preparation for a certain task, in the same manner nature creates each organ inside us for the purpose of performing a certain task. So, the nature of the nerves, which is the residence of the soul as it grows together with the spirit, indicates that the soul is created simultaneously with the body. And if the eye cannot see yet, and the tongue cannot taste, and the ear cannot hear, and the touch cannot actually feel the hot, or cold, or moist, or dry, still this potential exists latent, and soon after the baby is born [170] it can do all these. But, I would dare say that inactivity is action, because keeping the eyes shut, and the nose contracted, and the ears inactive, while still in the uterus, is the work of a commanding soul. On the other hand, one could not argue that the tongue of the foetus does not experience taste, or that it does not sense the quality of substances, and this can be proven through the investigation of accidents. We know that often children died in the womb because of the bad quality of orally consumed substances, as they turned away and rejected the food. Nature conveyed this information through the capacity of the tongue to taste, in the interests of the self-preservation of the foetus. Breathing is also the work of the soul in embryos, since they breathe through the mouth, as we have already mentioned. This also indicates that the soul and the seed are both present in the creation of the nature, because most doctors have defined breathing as an activity of the soul, not one of the body. It would be childish to argue that breathing is not an activity of the soul on the grounds that those who are asleep are still breathing [171] spontaneously, even though breathing can be intentional too. While the living being is awake, the soul is in charge of all actions; it sees, hears and functions through the rest of the sensory organs, it moves, and becomes aware of things through the senses, and is in charge of everything. By spreading itself in all directions and diffusing itself through the organs if performs all necessary functions. In the same manner, at night-time, it contracts and brings itself together, and it is not disturbed by what can be seen, or alerted by what can be heard, or distracted by what can be felt through smell, or altered by what is encountered through touch, or getting tired by running or walking or other physical exercise, or getting involved in such things, and so it can perform the function of breathing. Alternatively, we may suppose that nature willingly does what it should do, and not because someone else is doing it on its behalf, while the soul, since it participates in a more divine share, does not follow the same course of action. The nature is mortal and earthly and outside the boundaries of the intellect, and it does not possess the ability to reason. It knows only the mortal world, and is corruptible. However, the soul [172] is a segment of the universal soul, and possesses the knowledge of the celestial chorus, and on its way towards its own kind it surpasses the earth, it turns away from the fallacy of the water, it rises into the air, becomes superior to fire, and encounters the celestial divinity. It often sees the place above the sky, mixes with the supreme master, becomes a traveller of those places above, encounters its own kind, and is aware of its origins, even though it may be living in a body. The universal father knows everything through the eyes of the soul. So, no one should argue that breathing while the body is idle in sleep takes place without the knowledge of the soul. The soul is more capable and stronger than the body in everything. The body has the same capacity whether one is asleep or not. It digests, distributes, separates, adds and develops in both instances. However, only the soul of those who are awake does what is appropriate for the body, while the soul of those who are asleep cannot.

[173] It would be inappropriate, since we have sufficiently demonstrated that what is carried in the womb is a living being, not to present additional external proof in support of what has been said so far. When we see flies and worms crawling from the wood after they are born, as if it were a uterus, we call them living beings. Then, do we still doubt that what becomes alive in the womb ought to be considered a living being? Hippocrates has specifically declared the following: 'Non-living things come to life, living beings come to life, parts of living beings come to life. Nature is not to be taught.' Perhaps he shouldn't have said 'non-living things', or he should have said 'parts come to life'. But he omitted this, and used, instead, the name for the perfected product, so as to make us consider it as a living being from the very beginning of its existence. In a more gallant and less controversial mood he declared: 'Nature is not to be taught.' So, if anyone by any means or reason sought to create life, he could refer the matter to the unteachable nature that gives birth to everything. This reference to nature alone would be sufficient to reject the opinions of the non-believers who claim that the foetus is not a living being. She gives every being [174] the means to life, and to the foetus completion, so that it can be a living being. So, how is it possible to call a combination of body and soul a 'living being', but deny the name from this particular being? It would be as if someone invited to categorise fire would acknowledge that something had the burning quality of fire, but still refused to call it by that name. Or again, if the sun was throwing light upon the darkness, he would acknowledge that it was happening but refused to call it 'day'. Or, if someone who agreed that a combination of liquid and solid substances is nutritious, still refused to call it 'nutriment', or, someone who would agree that copper or steel can cut refused to call the cutting edge a 'knife'. However, no one who would see the dark air being lit by the sun would refuse to call this phenomenon 'day', nor would anyone refuse to call the action of burning a 'fire'. No one would refuse to call something that could perform the act of cutting 'a knife', nor would any one refuse to call the seed that is becoming alive and acquires life by its appropriate name.

[175] We have successfully demonstrated that the embryo possesses nature and soul and the energies of each one of them, and that it is a living being. It remains to demonstrate that what is still inside the womb is a living being. If one enquired about the logic of nature, they should know that she does everything self-taught and self-learned. It is easy for us to state that worms are not born from plants, and wasps and bees are not born from horses and oxen, but they are simply born by nature. No one teaches the birds how to fly, or us how to understand, see and hear. But we see the birds flying and ourselves being able to understand and see without learning. The self-efficiency of nature is somehow secret and hidden and much deeper than our own perception. Therefore we should not doubt that giving life to the embryos amounts to animation. They do not learn the tasks

pertinent to human beings by someone else after they are born, but while still in the womb they swallow and digest and can distinguish the given nourishment, and consume the purified one, **[176]** while they reject the surplus. For when the embryo is born there is a secretion of the surplus. And the discharge from the bowels called 'meconion' contains parts from all the food of the embryo, and so is the liquid contained in the urachus. The wise old man says 'the belly is receiving air from breathing through the mouth, and so do the bowels, and even the *kusaros* offers a way too', for excrement dropping little by little finally arrives to the rectum. Evidently he (sc. Hippocrates) calls the rectum *kusaros*. And no one should mislead us to think that it is impossible for the embryo to receive food through the mouth because the amniotic membrane is deposed around it. Nature is capable of providing a passage through the pores, and a sufficient way to what is appropriate. Democritus says that a human comes from a human, a dog from a dog, and an ox from an ox. Man who has had a glimpse of the heavenly, and can see the nature inside us, must not be ungrateful and claim that what is carried in the womb is not a living being, made complete from complete by its creator. Otherwise the newborn would not possess human reasoning, if it were not born with the perfect potential to reason, nor the ability to perform all the tasks that those from whose seed it was sown can perform, even though it did not possess the full range of abilities to perfection. **[177]** As the marks of imperfect seed, either in terms of quantity or in terms of quality, are inherited, whether they result in more or less limbs, or in the forms of other animals, in the same manner perfect and clearly formed seed possesses the perfect pattern of a living being. What is missing hinders the whole nature, and is responsible for missing limbs and imperfections in the foetuses, and for that reason they cannot be considered living beings at this stage. However, this same element, if it is not hindered it becomes alive from the seed. So, let no philosopher, who may be uninitiated to all this, or a physician follower of Asclepius, who may be ignorant of the nature of man, denounce and alienate the embryos. Instead, he should review his opinions, and learn from his seniors, or be reminded by his parents that he too once was an embryo. Then he was formed perfectly by his mother in the womb, and his stock came to existence by someone's sperm, and therefore he need not misinterpret nature. **[178]** It is easy to slander nature's laws, and for those created by earth to say that all her other creations, born under the same principles and incubated in her bosom, are living beings, but what was incubated in the womb is not. Or should we say that wheat will be born from wheat, and members of the same species from other seeds, and from plants other plants of the same nature as their parents, but a human being, the most divine and superior of all beings, the one potentially similar to god, does not possess the same degree of divine nature as his parents?

But we shall also demonstrate that the embryo is a living being by examining law and practice. We shall ascribe the cause of living to nature, but the cause of living well to the legislators in charge of the well-being of the soul. For these are the tasks that the laws perform: they prevent bad things from happening, and safeguard the good things of the present or those that are to be acquired in the future. So, those men who established the laws demonstrated that what is carried in the womb is a living being with two unshakeable kinds of proof. First they ordered the punishment of the person responsible for the abortion. **[179]** Then they allowed even those who have not yet been born to inherit. They did so because they knew better than most people, and because they imitated the works of the gods. The task of introducing laws is first and foremost a divine one. The father of all among the gods put everything in order with laws. The world is moving in accordance with his ordinances, and each one of the planets moves within its own sphere at the ordained time, and the sun and the moon move along their preordained routes. The earth was fixed by order of the creator, and water was poured, and air was spread, and fire was thrown, and each element retains its own function afraid to exceed the specifications of its own laws. Zeus gave laws to the Cretans, the Pythian to the Spartans, and Athena to the Athenians. Their students, the lawgivers, Solon and Lycurgus, unambiguously clarified the status of embryo in the aforementioned provisions. If it was not a living being they would not order the punishment of those responsible for the abortion. But, because they considered it to be a living being, they introduced sanctions. Who would exact revenge upon an obviously perfected human being on behalf of something that never was human in the womb, and had not come to life in the first place? [180] And who would abandon an inheritance on the grounds that he does not know whether the embryo is a living being? How will you try to prove that what is in the womb is not a living being? Who appoints as his heir someone who is not believed to exist? Who will declare that one who is the object of doubt ought to be put in charge? Even before he was born, Pericles was already formidable among the Greeks because of a dream, and likewise Peisistratus was already a tyrant. As soon as Olympias was pregnant with Alexander, everyone was saying that he was the son of Ammon and king of the entire world. Cypselus was still in the process of animation when he was understood to be the leader by the Bacchiads, who were intimidated by an apparition. It is also said that Hecuba was afraid of Alexander even before he was born, because she was intimidated by a very strange vision, and that all the Phrygians were already suffering from the fire that was not yet born. Alcmene, when she was going to give birth to Hercules, seemed formidable to the enemy soldiers, and destroyed the courage of the enemies simply by having the child in her womb. [181] Far from suggesting that the embryos are not living beings, they confirmed not only that they are living beings, but also that they are braver than human nature, even while they still remain rooted in the womb.

But let me address the embryos themselves, since they have acquired full human form. Come out of the recesses without the fear that you might be deprived of your generation, or lose your family and your fortune. The slander of many, and the wickedness of those who commit crimes against nature will not erase you. You yourselves will become the avengers, like Pericles, Peisistratus, Paris, like Alexander the Macedonian and Hercules.

Commentary

158. Asclepiads] Namely, medical practitioners.

As those ... unspecified] On the term 'living being' (Greek: *zôon*), and in general the significance of the terminology related to the stages of the development of the foetus, see Chapter 2. From the outset the author draws a distinction between the investigation of an issue in general terms, that is, as part of the big picture, the nature of all things, and the investigation in specific terms. The philosopher would carry out the first type of investigation, while the specialist in a certain art, the doctor in this case, would carry out the second. This distinction is important for the evolution of the author's arguments, because he is going to approach the issue first in general terms as part of the nature of all things, and then in specific terms.

159. I the speaker and you the judges] The author speaks as if he were delivering a speech in court and his readers were the jury. But, while he describes himself by using the standard forensic term for a litigant in court (*ho legôn*), he does not go so far as to use the standard term for a jury to describe his readers (*hoi dikastai*); instead he calls them 'judges' (*kritai*).

God first ... among men] Probably a reference to Pl. *Phd.* 108e-115a, where the souls of those who have led an exceptionally holy life are liberated from the earth and reach the higher place above it, the 'pure residence' (*katharan oikêsin*). There they can see much more clearly.

A small world ... particles] The perception of the universe as a living, ensouled being is commonly associated with the Stoics (the relevant sources and previous bibliography are provided in the excellent article of H. von Staden 'Hellenistic theories of body and soul' in J.P. Wright & P. Potter [ed.] *Psyche and soma*, pp. 96-105). However, it undoubtedly has its origins in Presocratic philosophy (Anaxagoras, Anaximenes et al.) and is first presented in a clear and articulate manner in Pl. *Ti.* 29d ff. and *Lg.* 896e ff. See also T.M. Robinson *Plato's psychology* (Toronto 1995); M. Lapidge, 'Stoic cosmology' in J. Rist (ed.) *The Stoics* (Berkeley & Los Angeles 1978) 161-85; A.A. Long, 'Soul and body in Stoicism' *Phronesis* 27 (1982) 34-57. On topics relevant to embryology see D. Nickel 'Stoa und Stoiker in Galens Schrift De foetuum formatione' in J. Kollesch & D. Nickel (ed.) *Galen und das hellenistische Erbe: Verhandlungen des IV. internationalen Galens-Symposium, veranstaltet vom Institut für Geschichte der Medizin am Bereich Medizin (Charite) der Humboldt Universität zu Berlin, 18-20 September 1989*, Sudhoffs Archiv Beihefte 32 (Stuttgart 1993) 79-86.

160. The world ... pervades them] The author's indecision as to what he should call this entity is consistent with the fact that he borrows elements from very diverse philosophical systems as this suits his argument at any particular moment.

161. World] Greek *kosmos*, from the verb *kosmein*, 'to arrange in order'. I was obliged to use two different English words, namely 'world' and 'order', to translate *kosmos*. The Greek word has both meanings, and in this passage it appears first meaning 'world', and one line below it appears meaning 'order'.

At an early stage ... water] The author seems to follow Anaxagoras' theory that 'the mind' arranged the world in order, however, while Anaxagoras believed that 'the mind' was not mixed with anything and that it existed as self-defined, the author of this study maintains that 'the mind' (or 'primal spirit') was inseparably mixed with the universe from the beginning, and this point is crucial for his argument. It serves the purposes of the author to present the 'mind' or 'soul' as mixed with the universe (the *kosmos*). His argument is that, as the universe has been animated by the primal spirit from the moment of its creation, so the human body is animated by the soul from the moment of its creation, since the latter is a particle of the universe. See also J. Annas *Hellenistic philosophy of mind* (Berkeley & Los Angeles 1992).

162. foetal stages] The original *ekuisketo* would be literally translated as 'from the time that it was carried to term', and this is obviously a metaphor. The universe once was in a foetal stage, like a living being, before it was born.

163. Delphic tripod] The reference to the Delphic tripod is meant to underline the authority status of the great Hippocrates. His statements carried similar weight for students of medicine as Apollo's words in the Delphic oracle. It may be noteworthy at this point that Hippocrates is the only medical authority explicitly mentioned by the author of this study, even though he has probably consulted other medical authors too. The reason would be that he tries to strengthen the authority of his statements by invoking the authority of Hippocrates, while he might consider that other medical authors did not carry the same weight as witnesses.

Living status] The original word *zôotêta* is a difficult term to translate: it implies the energy of life, the status of a living being.

The seed ... sick] Hip. *Sem.* 7,484 (10).

164. Potential] *dunamei* would mean to have the potential to become something, while *energeia* would mean actually to be something, to have realised that potential. The contrast between 'actual' and 'potential' is exploited much more extensively in another study with a similar subject, also wrongly attributed to Galen, the treatise *To Gauros, on how embryos are animated*.

For twins ... curves] Hip. *Nat. puer.* 7,540 (31).

165. In the same manner ... existence] The author contradicts himself at this point. Throughout the study he is striving to prove that the foetus is a living being from the moment of conception, but here he adopts the Stoic view, that the embryo is only a potential living being in the womb, and actually becomes a living being after birth. I think the contradiction is due to the fact that the author uncritically adopts Stoic views at this point.

166. Nature] The use of the word 'nature' instead of 'body' also has Stoic resonance (see H. von Staden in J.P. Wright & P. Potter [ed.] *Psyche and soma* 96-105 for the sources and relevant bibliography), and was adopted by Galen too (4,372; 7,55; 9,612-13; R.J. Hankinson 'Galen's anatomy of the soul' *Phronesis* 36 [1991] 197-233). Nature and soul together constitute the whole person.

air] The Greek word *pneuma* means 'spirit' and 'air'. Here the concept of the soul is clearly biological. It is presented as an integral part of the being, and not as an external force that needs nutrition, which is provided by breathing. So, perhaps 'air' fits better in this material context. The association of the soul with air originates from the Presocratics, in particular Anaximenes (Aet. 4,3. 387; Simp. *Phys.* 6r 24. 26; *Dox.* 476; Hipp. *Philos.* 7; *Dox.* 560) and Diogenes of Apollonia (frr. 4 and 5 D-K = Simp. *In Ph.* 151,28). On Presocratic beliefs about the soul see W.K.C. Guthrie *A history of Greek philosophy* I & II (Cambridge 1967 & 1969). This association was adopted by Hippocratic medicine (*Nat. Puer.* 7,496-8 [17], *Vict.* 6,428-484 [1,9] and 6,500 [27]), and became widespread in subsequent centuries. See also J.P. Wright & P. Potter (ed.) *Psyche and soma* passim for relevant bibliography and references.

Hippocrates ... nose] Hip. *Nat. puer.* 7,498 (17).

Now ... alien] This is a clumsy and almost incomprehensible passage, and the constantly shifting concept of the word '*phusis*', sometimes meaning 'body' and sometimes 'nature' is partly responsible for the difficulty. What the author is trying to say is that unless the foetus and the mother had the same nature, then nutriments processed by the mother would not be suitable for the foetus. The point, of course, is that the foetus is as much a human being as the mother is.

167. The biles and all the humours] This is an unorthodox theory. In the standard version of the humoral theory, the two biles, the yellow and the black, are two of the four humours of the body, not separate substances. A textual corruption cannot be ruled out, however, it is possible that this author has adopted his own version of the humoral theory, perhaps with the hellenistic influence that there are more than four humours.

The first ... cord] Hip. *Vict.* 9,108 (30).

168. It is clear ... power] This argument is crucial for the author's thesis. The same view was held by the Pythagoreans: see Chapter 2 §i.

170. I would dare ... soul] The author realises that he has contradicted himself by saying here that the embryo is only a potential human being and elsewhere that it is completely and perfectly human from the moment of conception, and tries rather desperately in this sentence to salvage the argument and give some coherence to his reasoning.

171. While the living being ... everything] The author here follows the Hippocratic study *Regimen*. See also G. Cambriano 'Une interprétation "material-iste" des rêves, du Régime IV' in M.D. Grmek (ed.) *Hippocratica* (Paris 1980), and B. Gundert in J.P. Wright & P. Potter (ed.) *Psyche and soma* 24.

172. A segment ... fire] Apparently a rhetorical and contrived reference to the four Empedoclean elements, upon which creation was based, namely earth, water, air, fire. This perception of the soul as an 'amphibian' entity (in the words of T.M. Robinson 'Mind-body dualism in Plato' in J.P. Wright & P. Potter [ed.] *Psyche and soma* 48) having a share in both celestial and worldly things, is also found in Plato's *Phaedo*. See also R.T. Hankinson 'Galen's anatomy of the soul' *Phronesis* 36 (1991) 197-233.

173. Non-living ... taught] Hip. *Alim.* 9,112 (38).

174. So, how is it possible ... day] The argumentation is clearly rhetorical at this point. See the interesting parallels in Lys. 10.

176. The wise ... too] Namely, Hippocrates (*Nat. puer.* 7,498 [17]); this passage is an almost word-for-word quotation. However, obviously the author here does not understand the meaning of the word *kusaros* (etymologically connected to *kusthos*, a better-known word for vulva). He thinks that *kusaros* is the rectum, and on this basis, he misinterprets the Hippocratic passage, and adapts its meaning to suit his purposes.

Democritus] See Wagner ad loc. for the sources on Democritus.

177. Then he was ... womb] According to the author, a human being comes into existence by his father's seed, while the mother's contribution is to form this seed. This is the only indication of the author's views on the process of conception, and the contribution of each parent in the entire study. Considering how vague and marginal this reference is, we can safely conclude that the role of the sexes in the reproductive process was not one of the primary concerns of this author. This is not surprising, since such theories would be rather irrelevant for the bulk of his argument that concerns the embryo.

179. Their students ... provisions] For further discussion of this passage see Chapter 6 §ii.

Peroration: A rhetorical ending, where the author addresses the embryos, as if in a courtroom with the embryos present. The value of this passage as a historical source is significant. The author states that the majority of people in his time found nothing wrong with induced abortion. Even though the mere existence of this study probably suggests growing opposition, this passage clearly states that most people in his time did not consider the destruction of the foetus as morally wrong. In his rhetorical address to the foetus the author implies that the dangers are loss of one's family, family name and property. These would mean nothing to a dead foetus, but certainly they would mean a lot to the father who had been deprived of his son and heir. So, although the foetus is presented as the potential victim (and this is significant *per se*), the author actually refers to the interests of the father (see the discussion in Chapter 5 §i.). The Ciceronian passage quoted in Chapter 5 comes to mind.

Appendix 2

Abortion, the Hippocratic Oath, and the sacred ordinances of the Philadelphia inscription (*LSA* 20)

This inscription from Philadelphia in Lydia contains ordinances regulating entry into the private sanctuary owned by a certain Dionysios. This is a striking and significant document that has attracted a lot of attention.[1] The document is dated to the second/first century BC by the overwhelming majority of scholars. Its peculiarities are many and astonishing. As far as the composition is concerned, it seems to me to betray a dependency upon classical authors which would be totally uncharacteristic of such documents. Its content is even more startling: it promotes an ethical system which would be much more in place in an early Christian context than in a pagan Graeco-Roman religious setting. It is outside my purposes here to deal in detail with all the intriguing issues that this document raises, but it is necessary to discuss briefly the permanent ban from the temple of all persons who have attempted abortions, contributed to their procurement, or disseminated information concerning abortifacient techniques and substances. I maintain that this document is out of line with the sacred laws of the Greeks on the issue of abortion, and this should be explained as a result of direct dependency upon the stipulations of the Hippocratic Oath concerning this matter. Another important issue which will need to be briefly discussed concerns the ordinances of the inscription which provide corroborating evidence for one of my main arguments in this book. I have argued that while in the classical, hellenistic and early republican period the father of the unborn is seen as the chief victim of abortion, from the first century BC onwards the foetus becomes the focus of the debate and is seen as the innocent victim of maternal cruelty. I maintain that this text offers further support for this argument. Here I provide a translation of the inscription in its entirety and attach a brief commentary on the relevant sections:

Translation

Good Fortune

   The ordinances given to Dionysios in a dream concerning entry into his sanctuary for men and women, free and slaves, have been written down for health and common salvation and the highest glory. In this sanctuary altars of Zeus and Hestia, his assessor, and the other gods Saviours and Prosperity, Wealth, Virtue, Health, Good Fortune, Good Spirit, Memory, Graces and Victory are established. Zeus gave Dionysios the ordinances in order to perform the purification, cleansing, and mysteries according to the traditional custom and as ordained here.

   Men and women, free and slaves, upon entering this sanctuary must swear by all gods that they have not known anything insidious against a man or a woman, or an evil drug that could be used against people, and that they neither know nor employ evil incantations, or philtres, or abortifacient drugs, or contraceptives, or anything else which could result in the killing of a child, and that they do not employ such items, or give advice, or relate information about them to anyone, and that they will be benevolent towards this sanctuary depriving it of nothing. And if anyone either practises or contemplates to practise any of the above, (they must swear) that they will not allow or hide it, but that they will reveal and resist it. A man (is to swear) that he will not corrupt or advise anyone else to corrupt a boy or a virgin, or besides his wife another woman who is with another man, either free or slave. And if he tells someone (that he has done any of those things), this person (is to swear) that he will expose such a man or woman, and that he will not hide it or cover up for them. A man or woman who commits any of these acts is not to enter this sanctuary. For great gods have been established in it and they watch for such actions and will not tolerate those who have breached the ordinances.

A free woman must be chaste and must not know the bed of another man except her husband. And if she does have intercourse with another man, such a woman is to be considered as not chaste, but polluted and full of filth inside, and unworthy to pay her respects to the god in whose honour this sanctuary has been built, or be present at sacrifices, or take part in purification and cleansing, or view the mysteries being acted. And if she does anything prohibited by the ordinances of this inscription, a great curse will befall upon her from the gods for having ignored these ordinances. The god does not wish or want any of this to take place, but wishes to see these ordinances obeyed. The gods will be propitious to those who follow them, and will always give them everything good that gods bestow upon the people they love. If anyone disobeys, they will hate this person and impose upon them the greatest punishments.

These ordinances have been deposited with Aggdistis the most pious guardian and mistress of this sanctuary. May she inspire good thoughts in men and women, free and slaves, to follow the ordinances recorded here, and during the monthly and annual sacrifices let those men and women who have faith in themselves touch this inscription, where the ordinances of the god are recorded, so as to become clear who is following these ordinances and who is not.

Zeus Saviour, accept the touch of Dionysios propitiously and favourably and kindly offer good rewards to him and his family, health, salvation, peace, safety on land and sea, ... and equally ...

Commentary

The richness and peculiar character of this text never cease to amaze me. The ethical principles upon which the sacred ordinances of the Philadelphia document are based certainly remind the reader of early Christian organisation. Nardi calls it 'an authentic catechism, which prepares and anticipates that of protochristianity', while Sokolowski believes that 'The universalist and moral character of these ordinances are derived from oriental rather than Greek spirit'. I mention briefly a few of these unusual principles: The dividing lines between men and women, free persons and slaves, although present are softer than they would normally be in pagan antiquity. Slaves are treated as human and violation of their person, sexual abuse, or evil plans against them should be considered by the entire community as offensive as those against free persons. Slave women who are in a relationship with a man (any man at all, even another slave) cannot be sexually harassed or violated. It is a serious crime even to contemplate corrupting a boy or a virgin, never mind actually doing it. Adultery for both sexes (as this would be defined in a pagan Graeco-Roman context) is utterly unacceptable. More important, even the thought of unholy or improper acts such as those mentioned above, or encouragement to engage in any of them, are offences. To know that someone else has such thoughts and not reveal it makes one an accessory to the crime, and therefore an unsuitable person to enter the temple. Thus this fascinating text inserts a dimension of mind control and collective guilt that are totally uncharacteristic of Graeco-Roman antiquity.

Pythagorean, Stoic and oriental influences have been invoked to explain these cultural peculiarities. However, the answer may be simpler. A reader who is familiar with classical literature will not fail to notice two passages. The first is the section which prohibits use, knowledge and dissemination of knowledge on abortifacient drugs and techniques. Nardi has noted the closeness between this document and the stipulations of the Hippocratic Oath banning abortion.[2] He does not go so far as to assume direct dependency of the Philadelphia document upon the Oath, but I would. I am convinced that the author of the inscription had read the Oath, accepted its principles, and translated them into sacred law. This conclusion is not based exclusively upon the sections concerning abortion. It seems to me that several other points in the inscription echo phrases and principles of the Oath. I quote those sections and put in italics phrases which seemingly have influenced the composition of the Philadelphia inscription:

> *I will give no deadly medicine to any one* if asked, *nor disseminate any such information*; and in like manner *I will not give to a woman a pessary to procure an abortion*. With *purity and with holiness I will pass my life* and practise my Art. ... *Into whatever houses I enter*, I will go into them for the benefit of the sick, *and will abstain from every voluntary act of mischief and corruption; and, further from the seduction of women or men, free persons or slaves*.

The parallels between the two documents are unmistakable and probably not accidental. The composer of the Philadelphia document (perhaps Dionysios himself) adopts the strict and unparalleled stance towards abortion taken by the composer of the Oath that has caused so much controversy. Moreover, like the author of the Oath, he does not prohibit only abortion but also knowledge and dissemination of information about any form of harmful or deadly drug or technique. The composer of the Philadelphia document, like the author of the Oath, aspires to a life of wholesome 'purity and holiness', what Sokolowski calls 'une tendence vers la religion universelle et personelle'. Like the ideal doctor of the Oath, the believer who enters the sanctuary of Dionysios pledges to abstain from voluntary acts of mischief and corruption, and especially sexual corruption of boys and virgins. Finally the astonishingly inclusive phrase that appears several times in the Philadelphia document – 'men and women, free and slaves' – is an almost exact quotation from the Oath. In my understanding these parallels suggest beyond reasonable doubt that the person who drafted this document has assimilated several sections and principles of the Oath.

The precise religious and cultural background of the Oath, as well as several conceptual points of this very well known and yet so little understood document, remain the subject of intense controversy. It could be argued that the Philadelphia inscription and the Oath are basically products of the same religious sect, and no rigorous internal objection could be brought against this argument, but there would be no external corroboration for such a view either. Since in Chapter 3, following C. Lichtenthaeler in his objections to Edelstein's Pythagorisation of the Oath, I have argued that the Oath is not necessarily a text associated with a marginal religious sect, but could be considered as perfectly aligned with mainstream medical ethics, I will not pursue further this line of investigation at this point, because it would probably prove infertile. We cannot be sure whether the Oath is associated with a marginal religious sect, and therefore we would not be sure that the Philadelphia document too is associated with a similar cult. The only conclusion which could be considered as provable is that the inscription depends directly upon the Oath in a number of places.

If the interpretation of the Philadelphia document as an echo of the Oath is correct, this makes it a startling discovery, because it would move our earliest reference to the Oath back by two, or possibly three, centuries. So far the orthodox view has been that the Oath is first mentioned in Scribonius Largus, a first-century AD author.[3] Now this text seems to backdate our earliest reference to the Oath to the second/first century BC. Moreover, this kind of dependency of sacred law upon previous literature would be a highly unusual instance per se, like so many things in this exceptional document.

Even more unusual and fascinating in this respect would be the possible dependency of the passage of the inscription which describes why the adulteress should be barred from the temple and the rituals performed in it upon a literary source. Here everything reminds me of a well-known classical text, the speech of Apollodorus 'Against Neaira'.[4] Apollodorus explains that a woman caught committing adultery ought to refrain from the temples and quotes the Athenian law which prohibits her to enter. The orator gives in his narrative an explanation for this prohibition: he states that this is done in order to avoid pollution and impieties being brought into the temples. At another point in his speech, when he refers to a woman who allegedly had taken part in some sacred rituals in honour of Dionysus, he mentions that she ought to have refrained from viewing and performing these mysteries since she was an adulteress. I wonder whether the author of the sacred law of Philadelphia had in mind these passages from the speech. If he did, this, to my knowledge, would be an amazing case of dependency of sacred law upon a literary source.

Such dependencies would make the serious deviation of the Philadelphia ordinances concerning abortion from the sacred laws of the Greeks appear less mysterious and extraordinary. While in Greek sacred law, with minor local variations, abortion is treated as a carrier of miasma similar to that from a birth or death, namely as something not particularly serious,[5] in the Philadelphia inscription it is treated as a much more serious issue resulting in a permanent ban for anyone who is in the business of using or producing abortifacient drugs and techniques, or compiling and disseminating information about them. Here is where I think the author of the sacred law relies upon the Hippocratic Oath.

In addition to this, the Philadelphia document for the first time introduces the idea that abortion is a grave offence against the gods because it deprives the foetus of life. A sharp condemnation of abortion as an act of infanticide is something we often see in later centuries in the writings of Christian theologians, synod rulings and canonical texts, but it is certainly out of line with pagan sacred laws. The explanation I can provide for this striking peculiarity is related to the fact that the Philadelphia inscription probably dates to the first century BC, which would make it roughly contemporary with the works of Chariton, Ovid and Cicero. I have argued in Chpater 5 §iv that, on the basis of the evidence provided by these authors, abortion was first seen as a serious crime which deprived the foetus of its life in the first century BC. Until then it was seen primarily as a threat to the interests and concerns of the father. This text would provide strong corroboration for my view that in this period there was a change in attitudes to abortion which brought the life and rights of the foetus to the centre, and this change of heart eventually led to its prohibition under Roman law.

The Philadelphia inscription anticipates Christian views on abortion, purity of life, communal conscience and spiritual cohesion, but the link between this text and Christianity is not direct. This text is based upon pagan documents such as the Hippocratic Oath and possibly other literary sources which happen to reflect views that became popular in the Christian era. The reason may lie in the fact that Christian authors were searching for their principles in the same direction as the author of the Oath, and the certainty they were looking for was not to be found in pagan relativism, ambivalence and freedom of choice.

Abbreviations

Abbreviations of ancient authors are as in Liddell & Scott *Greek-English Diction-ary*, 9th edition, or the *Oxford Latin Dictionary*, with the following exceptions:

Titles from the Hippocratic Corpus are abbreviated as in Liddell & Scott, but I prefer the citation of passages by volume and page of Littré's edition, because I feel that there is a need to find a consistent and easily understood system of refer-encing for the more voluminous collections of Greek medical works. This is why I prefer a system similar to that used for Plato and Aristotle, this time based on Littré's edition for the Hippocratic Corpus and Kühn's edition for Galen. However, since alternative systems are widely used for the Hippocratic works, I tend to give the alternative references in parentheses. In the case of Galen it seems to me that there is no satisfactory alternative to the citation of passages by volume and page of Kühn's edition, and this is the system that I have adopted consistently.

Ant. = Antiphon orator
PCG = Kassel & Austin, *Poetae Comici Graeci*

The fragments of Lysias follow the numbers of Carey's forthcoming edition; those of Hyperides the edition of Blass. I am grateful to Professor Carey for allowing me to consult an advanced draft of his forthcoming edition.

Works cited in full in the Select Bibliography appear in the Notes with a shortened title; titles that do not appear in the Select Bibliography are cited in full in the Notes. Journals are usually abbreviated as in *L'Année philologique*.

Notes

Preface

1. I frequently use the terms 'classical period' (fifth – fourth century BC), 'hellenistic period' (third – second century BC), 'republican period' (first century BC – first century AD), and 'imperial era' (first century AD – fifth century AD). Sometimes I differentiate between 'early empire' (first – second century AD) and 'late empire' or 'late antiquity' (third – fifth century AD). For the benefit of the non-specialist reader it is necessary to mention that these are not strictly defined periods, but convenient terminology which historians use with a degree of approximation.

Introduction

1. Aleck Bourne in *The Abortion Act 1967* (London 1969) 82.

2. See the discussion in Chapter 3 and Appendix 2.

3. R. Flemming *Medicine* 253. Flemming's account is the most recent, and perhaps the richest one on women in Galen's medical writings.

4. These verses certainly provide sufficient explanation as to why Sappho was so greatly admired and loved in the ancient world, but they do not substantially enrich our understanding of contemporary Greek society. This is personal, emotionally charged, homoerotic poetry.

5. See Mary-Kay Gamel in *Helios* 16 (1989) 183-206; R. Flemming *Medicine* 1-28.

6. E. *Andr.* 355-60.

7. Chariton *Chaireas and Callirhoe* 2.8.6-2.9.6.

8. S.K. Dickison in *Arethusa* 6 (1973) 159-66.

1. Methods of Abortion

1. E. *Andr.* 355-60.

2. Soph. fr. 132 Radt.

3. L. Dean-Jones *Women's bodies* 30; A. Rousselle *Porneia* 24-6; N. Demand *Birth* 65; J. Riddle *Contraception* passim; *Eve's herbs* passim.

4. H. King *Hippocrates' woman* 132 ff.

5. A. Preus in *Arethusa* 8 (1975) 237-63, esp. 251-6.

6. See Phryn. *Ecl.* 179; Eustathius *Com. Il.* T 118; Galen 17A 799; Etym. Gen. A 611; Etym. Gud. A 110; Etym. Magnum s.v. *amblôsis*; Ar. *Nub.* 137 for a metaphorical usage, and Schol. Aristoph. ad loc.

7. D.R. Langslow *Medical Latin* 164.

8. Sor. I 46.

9. This work is thought to be a genuine Hippocratic study, but the authorship of it, as of the other works of the Hippocratic Corpus, remains a highly controversial and complex issue, outside the purposes of this study. See É. Littré *Oeuvres* *complètes d'Hippocrate* vol. 1 (Paris & London 1839) passim; the brief but informative introduction to the first volume of the Loeb series by W.H.S. Jones: *Hippocrates* vol. 1, pp. ix-lxix; R. Joly *Le Niveau de la science hippocratique* (Paris 1966) passim; L. Edelstein *Ancient medicine* (Baltimore 1967) passim; W.D. Smith *Hippocratic tradition*; E. Craik *Hippocrates* 1-13.

10. Celsus *De medicina*, Proemium 8. See also P.J. van der Eijk (ed.) *Ancient histories* 10 and n. 31, and H. von Staden 'Celsus as historian' in *Ancient histories* 251-94. For further studies on Celsus see the collection in G. Sabbah & P. Mudry (ed.) *La Médecine de Celse*; R. Flemming *Medicine* 129 ff.; P. Mudry (ed.), *La Preface du De medicina de Celse*.

11. For further discussion see A.E. Hanson 'The logic of the gynaecological prescriptions' in J.A.L. Férez (ed.) *Tratados Hipocráticos* 235-50.

12. L. Dean-Jones *Women's bodies*; H. King *Hippocrates' woman*; R. Flemming *Medicine*.

13. On medical education in the ancient world see I.E. Drabkin in *BHM* 15 (1944) 333-51; F. Kudlien 'Medical education in Classical antiquity' in C.D. O'Malley (ed.) *The history of medical education*.

14. On Soranus see Ann Ellis Hanson and Monica Green 'Soranus of Ephesus: methodicorum princeps' *ANRW* 37.2 (1994) 984-1075; R. Flemming *Medicine* 228-46; P. Burguière, D. Gourevitch & Y. Malinas *Maladies des femmes*, tome 1, livre 1. *Soranos d'Éphèse* (Paris: Les belles lettres 1988) (the latest edition with substantial introduction and some commentary); P.J. van der Eijk 'Antiquarianism and criticism' in id. (ed.) *Ancient histories* 388-452; P. Minuli in *Memoria* 3 (1982) 39-49, and 'Donne mascoline' in S. Campese, P. Manuli & G. Sissa *Madre materia* 147-92.

15. On the supply and trade of drugs in the ancient world see A. Schmidt *Drogen und Drogenhandel im Altertum*; V. Nutton in *Journal of the Royal Society of Medicine* 78 (1985) 138-45; Jukka Korpela 'Aromatarii, pharmacopolae, thurarii et ceteri: zur Sozialgeschichte Roms' in P.J. van der Eijk et al. *Ancient medicine in its sociocultural context* vol. 1, 101-8.

16. For further information see E. Nardi *Aborto* 590-8.

17. Hip. *Mul.* 8,140 (67). See also *Carn.* 8,610 (19).

18. See for example the potions known as antidotes (*antidota*) cited by Galen in his work *On the antidotes* (14,109 ff. Kühn; cf. Chapter 1 §§ i & ii; E. Nardi *Aborto* 381 ff.).

19. On Celsus see the collection in G. Sabbah & P. Mudry (ed.) *La Médecine de Celse*; R. Flemming *Medicine* 129 ff.; H. von Staden 'Celsus as historian' in P.J. van der Eijk (ed.) *Ancient histories* 251-94.

20. I normally use terms such as 'Hippocratic medicine' or 'Hippocratic doctor' with a purely chronological significance to refer to the medical science of the classical period (fifth and fourth centuries BC). I do not imply a certain school or branch of medicine.

21. Even RU 486, an oral abortifacient licensed in some countries (and recently in the USA), has attracted a lot of criticism as unsafe: see J.G. Raymond, in J.C. Callahan (ed.) *Reproduction, ethics and the law* (Bloomington 1995) 284-99.

22. On methods and medical aspects of abortion today: H. Bequaert Holmes, *Reproductive technology,* 113-92; I. MacGillivray and K.J. Dennis 'Gynaecological aspects' in G. Horobin (ed.) *Experience with abortion* 67-76; M. Potts, P. Diggory & J. Peel *Abortion* (Cambridge 1977) 178-252; G.I. Zatuchni, J.J. Sciarra & J.J. Speidel (ed.) *Pregnancy termination* (Chicago 1979) passim. Chemicals used to induce an abortion at the very early stages of pregnancy, that is before the implantation of the fertilised egg, are conventionally classed as contraceptives, not as abortifacient drugs: see D.T. Baird, I. Cameron & E.E. Baulieu in R. Porter &

M. O'Connor (ed.) *Abortion: medical progress and social implications* (London 1985) 178-210.

23. Sor. I 60.

24. Hip. *Mul.* 8,218. On the term *elatêrion* see C. Lienau *Hippocrates Über Nachempfängnis, Geburtshilfe und Schwangerschaftsleiden* (Berlin: Akademie-Verlag, 1973) 103-4.

25. Hip. *Mul.* 8,170.

26. Hip. *Mul.* 8,172 ff.

27. Hip. *Mul.* 8,152 (72).

28. Since my knowledge of names of plants is rather limited in both languages, I normally adhere to the translations provided by the *LSJ*. However, I have provided the Greek words transliterated for the benefit of those with a special interest in plants and their identification.

29. Hip. *Mul.* 8,176 (78).

30. Dsc. 2,166,2.

31. Dsc. 3,45,1, Pliny *NH* 20,143, J. Riddle *Contraception* 28-9. In *Eve's herbs* (48-50) Riddle mentions that rue contains chalepensin, which is toxic in high dosages.

32. Dsc. 3,4,4. J. Riddle (*Eve's herbs*, 58-9) mentions that birthwort contains aristolochic acid, which can block implantation and interrupt even midterm pregnancies.

33. Hip. *Mul.* 8,154 ff.; Thphr. *HP* 9,18,8; Dsc. 1,10,2; 4,182,3; 4,185,1; 2,156,2; 3,35,3; Pliny *NH* 20,9.143.226.248; 21,116.146; 24,18.29; 26,153; Gal. 11,853 ff.; Sor. I 63. On hellebore see J. Riddle *Contraception* 55. On bracken (*thelypteris*) see J. Riddle *Eve's herbs* 59-60. On poplar see J. Riddle *Contraception* 33-4.

34. *NH* 32,18.

35. The abortifacient qualities of the chaste-tree were probably widely known, considering that it played some part during the fertility ritual of the Thesmophoria: see J. Riddle *Contraception* 35-6 and 59.

36. On the qualities of coriander see M.S. Al-Said, K.I. Al-Khamis et al. 'Post-coital anti-fertility activity of the seeds of *coriandrum sativum* in rats' *Journal of Ethnopharmacology* 21 (1987) 165-73. On parsley, sage, rosemary, thyme and coriander see also J. Riddle *Eve's herbs* 61-3.

37. On the qualities of myrrh see J. Riddle *Eve's herbs* 51-3.

38. Galen 14,109-11.

39. Galen 14,152 ff.

40. E. Nardi *Aborto* 262.

41. G. Negri *Erbatio figurato: descrizione e proprietà delle piante medicinali e velenose della flora italiana* (Milan 1960).

42. On the qualities of squirting cucumber see J. Riddle *Eve's herbs* 53-4; the author mentions that its contraceptive qualities have been confirmed by modern experiments, but its possible abortifacient qualities have not been confirmed so far.

43. See Bibliography for the titles. Other useful studies on the subject are N.P. Farnswort et al. 'Potential value of plants as sources of new anti-fertility agents' *Journal of Pharmaceutical Sciences* 64 (April 1975) 535-98 and (May 1975) 717-54. and also the study by the same author entitled 'Prospects for higher plants as sources of useful fertility agents for human use' in Chang Chai Fen, D. Griffin & A Woolman (ed.) *Recent advances in fertility regulation* (Geneva 1981) 330-64.

44. See for example the thorough and learned discussion by H. King *Hippocrates' woman* 132-56, and B.W. Frier 'Natural fertility and family limitation in the Roman marriage' *CPh* 89 (1994) 323 ff.

45. Galen 14,114 ff.

46. Galen 12,252.

47. Hip. *Epid.* 5,1,53.

48. Hip. *Mul.* 8,706; cf. 8,140.

49. Sor. I 60.

50. Hip. *Mul* 8,154 ff.; 170 ff.; 706, Sor. I 59.

51. Plu. *Lyc.* 3,3

52. Ovid *Amores* 2,13. Ilithyia was the goddess assisting childbirth; considering, however, that an abortion induced with the methods practised in the ancient world would be an experience similar to that of normal childbirth with mild labour symptoms, it is not surprising to see the poet begging Ilithyia to assist his loved one with her abortion troubles.

53. Ovid *Amores* 2,14. Medea killed her children to avenge the infidelity of her partner Jason (E. *Med.* 792-1414) and Procne killed her son Itys to avenge her husband Tereus (see S. fr. 580-95 Radt [*Tereus*], Ovid *Met.* 6,424 ff.). The translation quoted here is that of A.D. Melville *Ovid: the love poems* with introduction and notes by E.J. Kenney (Oxford 1990). I do not agree with the interpretation of Kenney (p. 195) that the poems are satirical or that they 'point to an ironical presentation of a typically masculine attitude'. I find this interpretation insensitive, one of those cases where modern literary criticism has lost touch with the primary emotive function of poetry. One can sense the quiet frustration and angry sympathy running through the first poem in particular. In my understanding, these works are perfectly serious in the expression of raw, true emotion. A more detailed discussion of the historical and sociological content and context is provided in Chapter 5.

54. Y. Courtone *St Basile: Lettres* vol. 2 (Paris: Les belles lettres, 1961) Letter to Amphilochios 188, 2.

55. See for example: E. *Andr.* 355-60; Pl. *Tht.* 149c-d; Plu. *Rom.* 22,3; *Lyc.* 3,3-4; *Mor.* 134 f., Ael. *VH* 13,6; Clem. Al. *Paed.* 184; Ovid *Amores* 2,13-14; Juv. *Sat.* 6,595.

56. A portrait of the word *pharmakon* is given by E. Nardi *Aborto* 16-29 and 355-6 n. 119.

57. Pliny *NH* 25,3,25; Galen 12,251.

58. *pessos*: from the verb *pettein* 'to bake'. *pessos* primarily indicates an oval object, anything resembling a loaf of bread. A vaginal suppository was probably thus called on account of its shape ('en raison de sa forme' in the words of P. Chantraine *Dictionnaire Etymologique de la langue grecque* vol. 3, p. 890, s.v.). E. Nardi (*Aborto* 60) thinks that the word *pessos* meaning 'suppository' is not related to this verb, and that the word is of uncertain etymology, but he is probably wrong.

59. Dsc. 1,128,3-4.

60. Hip. *Mul.* 8,154 ff.; Dsc. 2,163,1; 3,4,4; 1,30,1; 1,14,4; 4,150,7; 2,164,1; 3,35,3; 1,76,1; 1,77,2; 3,6,2-3 (in order of reference in the text); Galen 11,853 ff.; Sor. A.14 and 20. Pliny normally does not make the distinction between oral drugs or pessaries, he mentions however the abortifacient qualities of many herbs and plants, some of which surely were used in pessaries.

61. See the studies mentioned in n. 10.

62. Hip. *Mul.* 8,188 (78).

63. To give one example, oral drugs and pessaries are the two methods employed by Canace in Ovid's *Heroides* (11,39-46). Canace says that her trusted nurse applied some potent pessaries with her own hand, while stressing how important secrecy was in her attempt to induce an abortion, and how the whole undertaking was kept strictly between the two women.

64. Hip. *Mul.* 8,140; Galen 16,180; 19,456; Sor. I 64.

65. Galen 12,50-1.

66. Ps.-Galen 14,480-1.
67. Ps.-Galen 14,481.
68. Sor. I 65.
69. Hip. *Genit.* 7,484 (10,1)
70. Hip. *Nat. puer.* 7,490 (13,2)
71. Sor. I 60.
72. Sor. I 64.
73. Galen 17,653 (cf. 17,635).
74. Theon *Proleg.* 7,15 Walz.
75. Exodus 21:22-5.
76. T.N. Cingomklao in *Abortion: medical progress* 56-60.
77. Sor. I 64.
78. Hip. *Mul.* 8,142 ff.
79. On mechanically induced abortions see also the comparative evidence presented by H.L. Shapiro in Hall (ed.) *Abortion* vol. 1, 183-7.
80. See n. 10.
81. Celsus *De medicina* 7,29,1-10.
82. Hip. *Nat. mul.* 7,380; *Mul.* 8,452.
83. Hip. *Mul.* 8,142ff.480.512.
84. Hip. *Superf.* 8,480 (*CMG* I 2,2,7-8).
85. *embruosphaktês*: Tertullian *De anima* 25,5, and Herophilus T247. Von Staden states that an infanticidal instrument had been used for surgical abortions since the time of Hippocrates (*On the excision of the foetus*: 8,512 Littré). No doubt ancient surgeons would have to be prepared for the eventuality of having to remove a dead foetus, and it is perfectly believable that they had developed some form of knife of hook for such purposes from the early years of rational medicine. As anatomical knowledge improved the instrument might also evolve and become handier and more accurate. Here again it seems to me that we are dealing with knowledge initially pursued for therapeutic purposes, but eventually used for induced abortions too. See also E. Nardi *Aborto* 236 n.75.
86. Sor. I 65. See also Hip. *Mul.* 8,140 and the passage of Celsus quoted above, especially section 5.
87. Galen 17,635; Sor. I 65; Hip. *Aph.* 4,542 (5,31). Cf. also Burguière, Gourevitch & Malinas *Soranos* vol. 1, p. 103 n. 316.
88. Sor. I 64-5; cf. also I 46, I 58.
89. Sor. I 65; cf. Plu. *Mor.* 134 f.
90. Hip. *Aph.* 4,542 (5,31); Galen 17,635 ff., 653.
91. Galen 17,635 ff.; Pollux 4,10.
92. See Flemming *Medicine* 131.
93. On Pliny see M. Beagon *Roman nature* passim; V. Nutton 'The perils of patriotism' in R. French & F. Greenaway (ed.) *Science in the early Roman empire.* J. Hahn in *Sudhoffs Archiv* 75 (1991) 209-39; R. Flemming *Medicine* 131-6. In particular on superstition in Pliny see P.M. Green *Prolegomena to the study of magic and superstition in the Natural History of Pliny the Elder* (PhD thesis, University of Cambridge 1954); 'Pharmacy in Pliny's *Natural History*: some observations on substances and sources' in R. French and F. Greenaway (ed.), *Science in the early Roman empire: Pliny the Elder, his sources and influence* (London 1986) 59-85.
94. Pliny *NH* 28,251; 30,129. On the supernatural in Pliny's history see P.M. Green *Prolegomena.*
95. The standard book on Dioscorides is J. Riddle *Dioscorides on pharmacy and medicine.*
96. Dsc. 2,164,1; 3,131,1; Pliny *NH* 25,115; 27,110.
97. Galen 14,243; Pliny *NH* 30,128.

98. Pliny *NH* 30,130: The woman would have an abortion through her mouth because, according to popular belief, the crow copulated and gave birth through its mouth (Pliny *NH* 10,32).

99. Ps.-Galen 14,480.

100. Dsc. 1,93,1; Galen 12,50.

101. Thphr. *HP* 9,18,11.

102. Dsc. 5,67,1; cf. Ael. *VH* 13,6; Pliny *NH* 14,116; Eustathius *Com. Il.* B 561.

103. Maximus 6,141-275; see also R. Gordon '*Quaedam veritatis umbrae*: hellenistic magic and astrology' in P. Bilde et al. (ed.) *Conventional values of the hellenistic Greeks* (Aarhus 1997) 128-58.

104. Pliny *NH* 28,81.

105. Galen 12,151-2.

106. W.A. Krenkel in *Wissenschaftliche Zeitschrift der Universität Rostock: Reihe Gesellschaft und Sprachwissenschaften* 20 (1971) 443-52.

2. When Does Human Life Begin?

1. B.A. Brody's study *Abortion and the sanctity of human life,* though somewhat dated (published 1975), still constitutes a thorough introduction to the arguments surrounding this important aspect of the abortion debate. See also J. Reiman *Abortion and the ways we value human life*; P. Cozic & J. Petrikin *The abortion controversy*; J. Woods *Engineered death*; H.J. Morowitz & J.S. Trefil *The facts of life*; P. Ramsey *Ethics at the edges of life*; H. Watt *Life and death in healthcare ethics*; R. Dworkin *Life's dominion*.

2. See J. Needham *History of embryology* 2nd ed. (Cambridge 1959) passim; J.M. Oppenheimer in *Arethusa* 8 (1975) 331-43; P. Singer et al. (ed.) *Embryo experimentation* passim; R.W. Beard and P.W. Nathanielsz (ed.) *Foetal physiology and medicine* 2nd ed. (New York 1984) passim.

3. A. Knutson, in a contribution to the debate entitled 'Abortion and Animation' included in *Abortion* (ed. R.E. Hall) vol. 2, 3-18.

4. See R.J. Cook 'Reducing maternal mortality: a priority for human rights law' in *Abortion: medical progress* 211-27; G.W. Corner in *Abortion* (ed. R.E. Hall) vol.1, 3-15; I.H. Porter & E.B. Hook (ed.) *Human embryonic and fetal death*; J. Van der Tak *Abortion, fertility, and changing legislation*; H.J. Morowitz & J.S. Trefil *The facts of life*; P. Ramsey *Ethics at the edges of life*; D. Cornell *The imaginary domain*; H. Watt, *Life and death in healthcare ethics*; R. Dworkin, *Life's dominion* passim.

5. See R.W. Beard & P.W. Nathanielsz (ed.) *Foetal physiology* passim.

6. See A.V. Campbell in *Abortion: medical progress* 228-43; K. Mason 'Abortion and the law' in S.A.M. McLean (ed.) *Legal issues in human reproduction* (Dartmouth 1989) 66 ff.

7. The extent of this ever-increasing problem is reflected in the use of a controversial treatment in the course of a late abortion, which involves the administration of direct foetal intracardiac potassium chloride injection causing immediate foetal cardiac arrest: see J.C. Callahan 'Ensuring a stillborn: the ethics of lethal injection in late abortion' in id. (ed.) *Reproduction, ethics and the law: feminist perspectives* (Bloomington 1995); see also K. Mason in *Legal issues* 66 ff.

8. *embruon* Arist. *HA* 583b11-23; Gal. 17,440 ff.; Sor. I 59; *kuêma* Arist. *HA* 583b11-23; Gal. 17,445; *to kuoumenon* Gal. 17,440 ff.; *to kata gastros* Ps.-Gal. 19,178 ff.; *quod in utero geritur* Augustine *Quaestionum in heptateuchum libri VII, Exodi LXXX*.

9. Juv. *Sat.* 6,596 *homines in ventre*. Cf. Philo *De Vita Mosis* 2,84 (IV p. 220 Cohn).

10. Hip. *Carn.* 8,608-10 (19 ff.).

11. D.S. 1,77,9-10; 5,2. Virgil *Aen.* 6,427-9 (I agree with E. Nardi *Aborto* 228-9 that this passage of Virgil does not necessarily speak about abortions, but it certainly refers to the unborn). Ovid *Heroides* 11,45.

12. Hip. *Nat. puer.* 7,498/500 (18).

13. Galen 4,542-4 (*CMG* I,9,1-12): *gonê, kuêma, embruon, paidion*.

14. Exodus 21:22-5.

15. Philo *De specialibus legibus* 3,108-9 (V pp. 180-1 Cohn), 118 (V p. 183 Cohn)

16. Ps.-Gal. 19,160; see also Appendix 1 and also the extensive discussion of the term in the Pseudo-Galenic study *To Gauros, on how embryos are animated*.

17. Further on this debate see Arist. *GA* 736a24-b8; J.M. Oppenheimer, *Arethusa* 8 (1975) 331-43; A. Preus 'Science and philosophy in Aristotle's *Generation of Animals*' *J. Hist. Biol.* 3 (1970) 1-52.

18. Clem. Al. *Strom.* 8,4.

19. Ps.-Gal. 19,451.

20. Hip. *Nat. puer.* 7,514-28 (22-5), Arist. *GA* 731a1-4; Galen 4,542-3 (*CMG* 1,9); see also the Pseudo-Galenic study *To Gauros, on how embryos are animated*, where the comparison between the foetus and a plant is the subject of extensive discussion.

21. Plato is presented as the main representative of this view in the Pseudo-Galenic study *To Gauros, on how embryos are animated*; see also the aforementioned passage of Clement.

22. Plu. *Mor.* 907d; cf. also Chapter 2 §iv. I translate *phusikê* as mechanical and *pneumatikê* as conscious. The translation of the second term surely does not render fully the complexity of the Greek word.

23. According to Plu. *Mor* 907c, Plato stated that the embryo was a 'living being' because it moves and feeds in the uterus.

24. Plu. *Mor.* 1052f-1053d; see also Chapter 2 §iii. *psuchê*, the Greek word for soul, is derived from *psuchein* 'chill'. The relation of the soul to cold air goes back to Diogenes of Apollonia; cf. also Plato *Cra.* 399d-e; Arist. *De an.* 405b28-9.

25. Philo *De special. legibus* 3,108-9 (V pp. 180-1 Cohn).

26. Philo *De special. legibus* 3, 08-9 (V pp. 152-4 Cohn).

27. I would rather speak about 'conception' than 'fertilisation' (rendering the Greek word *sullêpsis*) because the latter, even though more precise, is a modern term and may convey the wrong impression about the degree of understanding of the genetic process by the ancient world.

28. See e.g. Clement *Ecl.* 50,11-3, Lactantius *De opificio dei* 17,7: *anima ... insinuatur in corpus ... post conceptus protinus*.

29. See Chapter 2 §iv, where the views of Christian gradualists are explored.

30. Edelstein *Oath* passim, Carrick *Medical ethics* 110-12. There are several important studies of Pythagorean beliefs concerning the body-soul relationship; see W. Burkert *Lore and science in ancient Pythagoreanism* (Cambridge, Mass. 1972); G.E.R. Lloyd *Magic, reason and experience*.

31. DL 8,24 = b1a 29-36 D-K

32. Galen 6,701-2. The relevant passage is quoted in §iv. See also R.J. Hankinson in *Phronesis* 36 (1991) 197-233; H. von Staden 'Hellenistic theories of body and soul' in J.P. Wright & P. Potter (ed.) *Psyche and soma* 87-105;

33. Virgil *Aen.* 6,427 *infantumque animae flentes*.

34. Juv. *Sat.* 6,596 *homines in ventre*.

35. Dem. 43,75 (*verbatim* quotation of the law); D.S. 1,77,9-10.

36. Galen 19,330; on Empedocles in the Hippocratic Corpus see J. Jouanna

'Présence d' Empédocle dans la collection hippocratique' *Bulletin de l'Association Guillaume Budé* 452-63.

37. Diog. Apoll. fr. 4 D-K = Simp. *In Phys.* 151,28.

38. Diog. Apoll. fr. 5 D-K.

39. Plu. *Mor.* 907d. E. Nardi *Aborto* 129 and n. 257 identifies the person mentioned here with Diogenes the Cynic, but the evidence cited above unambiguously suggests that he should be identified with Diogenes of Apollonia.

40. On Anaximenes' theory of the soul as air see: Simp. *Phys.* 6r 24, 26; *Dox.* 476; Hippo *Philos.* 7; *Dox.* 560.

41. H. von Staden *Herophilos* 298; see also 257-8.

42. Plu. *Mor.* 907c-d = Herophilus fr. 202b von Staden, cf. also. fr. 202a and 202c. Translation by H. von Staden.

43. The views of Herophilus on the soul are explored in greater detail by H. von Staden in his contribution 'Hellenistic theories of body and soul' in J.P. Wright & P. Potter *Psyche and soma* 87-91.

44. Ps.-Gal. *To Gauros* 14,4.

45. In the words of Lactantius who summarises such views in *De opificio* 17,5; cf. Tertullian *De anima* 25,2-6.

46. The views of the Stoics are presented in considerable detail by E. Nardi *Aborto* 206-18; see also H. von Stadten in J.P. Wright & P. Potter *Psyche and soma* 96-105.

47. Galen 19,330, Philo 5,251.

48. Philo 5,154 Cohn.

49. The assimilation of nature with an artist can also be found in Dem. 59,113 and Arist. *Pol.* 1454b10.

50. According to Ps.-Gal. 19,451 ff.

51. See e.g. the views and methods of Aristotle on the matter presented by J.M. Oppenheimer, *Arethusa* 8 (1975) 331-43.

52. As in Hip. *Nat. puer.* 7,490-2 (13).

53. Galen 4,631 (*CMG* 2,5,226).

54. See e.g. *Nat. puer.* 7,468 (12), 7,496-8 (17), *Vict.* 6,428-84 and 6,500 (1,9 and 27); see also Appendix 1, especially 19,170-1; I.M. Lonie *Hippocratic Treatises* (Berlin 1981) 147-55; B. Gundert 'Soma and psyche in Hippocratic medicine' in P.J. Wright & P. Potter (ed.) *Psyche and soma*, 13-35.

55. Galen 19,337. Various theories about the stages of foetal development are built around the numbers 7, 9, 40 and their multiples, but these are based on philosophical theories about numbers rather than accurate scientific observation. Cf. the studies of W.H. Roscher 'Die enneadischen und hebdomadischen Fristen und Wochen der ältesten Griechen' in *Abhandlungen der phil.-hist. Klasse der königl. Sächs. Ges. Wiss.* 21.4 (1903); 'Die hippokratische Schrift von der Siebenzahl in ihrer vierfachen Überlieferung' in *Studien zur Geschichte und Kultur des Altertums* vol. 6, Hefte 3 & 4 (Paderborn 1913); 'Die Tessarakontaden und Tessarakontadenlehren der Griechen und anderer Völker. Ein Beitrag zur vergleichenden Religionswissenschaft, Volkskunde und Zahlenmystik, sowie zur Geschichte der Medizin und Biologie' in *Berichte über die Verhandl. der königl. Sächs. Ges. Wiss., Leipzig* 61, 17-204 (1909). In saying that, one must admit that these numbers are approximately true in most cases.

56. *kata tous tês harmonias logous*. The passage is quoted in Chapter 2 §ii.

57. Hip. *Alim.* 9,112-16 (42), cf. Gal. 15,407-8.

58. Ps.-Gal. *Philosoph. hist.* 125; cf. also 111. Diogenes of Apollonia fr. 9 D-K (= Galen 17,106). Galen, however, states that he found no trace of this view in Diogenes' book. Censorinus *De die natali* 9,2 reports that, according to Diogenes, a boy is formed by the fourth month and a girl by the fifth. For the opposite view see Hip. *Epid.* 5,116 (2,3,17), *Nat. puer.* 7,498-500 (18), Arist. *GA* 775a10 ff., Galen 4,631 (*CMG* 2,5,26); further references to ancient authors can be found in the commentary of P. de Lacy *Galen: On semen* (*CMG* vol. 5,3,1) (Berlin 1992) p. 244.

59. The quote is from R. Flemming *Medicine* p. 86.

60. For example, the author of the Pseudo-Galenic study *Whether what is carried in the womb is a living being* (see Appendix 1) does not differentiate between a male and a female foetus, I believe simply because such a distinction would serve no purpose for his argument.

61. Hip. *Nat. puer.* 7,498-500 (18). The same views are attributed to Polybus 'the pupil' of Hippocrates by Galen 17,445.

62. Hip. *Nat. puer.* 7,504 (18,7)

63. Hip. *Nat. puer.* 7,504 (18,8).

64. Hip. *Nat. puer.* 7,500 ff. (18,1 ff.).

65. Galen 4,631 (*CMG* 2,5,26). Cf. 17,444.

66. Greek *sullêpsis*: the term needs to be understood literally as 'capture' in this passage

67. Sor. I 43.

68. Hip. *Nat. puer.* 7,500 ff. (18,1). Galen 4,238-9. E. Nardi (*Aborto* pp. 100-1) notes that the books mentioned here can be found in 19,19-20, and 5,181-805 respectively.

69. Hip. *Septim.* 7,448-50 (9).

70. Arist. *HA* 583b11-23. Cf. 583a24-6; *GA* 758b2-6. The same definition is repeated by Galen 17,445.

71. Sor. I 64.

72. Exodus 21:22-4. On this passage see also J. Riddle *Eve's herbs* 70 ff.

73. See J.T. Noonan 'An almost absolute value in history' in *The morality of abortion: legal and historical perspectives* ed. J.T. Noonan (Cambridge 1970); J.T. Noonan *Contraception*.

74. Y. Courtone *St Basile: Lettres* vol. 2 (Paris: Les belles lettres, 1961), Letter to Amphilochios 188,2: *akribologia exeikonismenou kai anexeikonistou*.

75. Ibid. *hê phtheirasa kath' epitêdeusin phonou dikên hupechei.*

76. E. Nardi *Aborto* 160-81, J.T. Noonan *Contraception*.

77. Theodoret Bishop of Cyrrhus *Opera omnia* ed. J.L. Schulze, vol. 1, 48 = Migne *PG* 80, col. 272.

78. *Théodoret de Cyr: Thérapeutique des maladies helleniques* ed. P.Canivet, 1, p. 243.

79. Augustine *Quaestionum in heptateuchum libri VII, vol. II, quaestiones Exodi* LXXX.

80. See e.g. Cyril of Alexandra *De adoratione in spiritu et veritate* 8 (= Migne *PG* 68,545), Maximus the Confessor *Contra eos qui corpora ante animas ...* Migne *PG* 91,1340.

81. Galen 17,1006.

82. Hip. *Nat. puer.* 7,510 ff. (21,1 ff.); cf. Hip. *Mul.* 7,150; *Steril.* 7,446.

83. Hip. *Alim.* 9,114 (42).

84. Galen 17,447.

85. Sor. I 45.

86. See the passage of Clement of Alexandria (*Strom.* 8,4) quoted in Chapter 2 §i. The causal connection of self-motion and life in Plato would be a notion shared by most of his contemporaries, as T.M. Robinson points out in J.P. Wright & P. Potter *Psyche and soma* 52.

87. Galen 4,542-3 (*CMG* 1,9): *gonê, kuêma, embruon, paidion*. The same distinction is made in other studies of his, such as 15,402 and in 17,345. The attribution

of the distinction into these four stages to Hippocratic medicine is disputable: see
P. de Lacy *Galen: On semen (CMG* vol. 5,3,1) (Berlin 1992) 218.

88. Galen 4,543.

89. See Church of England, Board for Social Responsibility *Abortion: an ethical
discussion* (Church Information Office for the Board, 1973) 24-32.

90. On Aristotle's medical and biological knowledge see C. Oser-Grote *Aristoteles und das Corpus Hippocraticum* (Stuttgart 1999), and also the valuable
collection of essays edited by W. Kullmann & S. Föllinger *Aristotelische Biologie,
Intentionen, Methoden, Ergebnisse* (Stuttgart 1997); W. Jaeger in *JHS* 77 (1957)
54-61.

91. See E. Nardi *Aborto* 123-32; J.M. Oppenheimer in *Arethusa* 8 (1975) 331-43;
M.C. Horowitz in *Journal of the History of Biology* 9 (1976) 183-213; G.E.R. Lloyd
& G.E.L Owen (ed.) *Aristotle on mind and the senses* (Cambridge 1978); A. Preus
'Science and philosophy in Aristotle's *Generation of Animals*' *J. Hist. Biol.* 3 (1970)
1-52; M.C. Nussbaum & A. Oksenberg Rorty (ed.) *Essays on Aristotle's De anima*
(Oxford 1992).

92. See for example the arguments of A.V. Campbell in *Abortion: medical
progress and social implications* (Ciba Foundation Symposium, London 1985)
228-45, and the heated arguments in J. Jarvis Thomson 'A defense of abortion' in
Philosophy and public affairs vol. 1, no. 1 (1971) 47-66; M. Tooley *Abortion and
infanticide* (Oxford 1983); Church of England, Board for Social Responsibility
Abortion: an ethical discussion (London: Church Information Office for the Board,
1973); J.T. Noonan *Contraception.*

93. P. van der Eijk, 'Aristotle's psycho-physiological account of the soul-body
relationship' in J.P. Wright & P. Potter (ed.) *Psyche and soma* 57-77. The study
contains rich bibliography on the subject; see esp. p. 61 n. 13.

94. Arist. *Pol.* 1335b24-6.

95. See above, n. 70.

96. See the passage quoted in n. 16.

3. The Doctor's Dilemma

1. For modern literature exploring some of the doctor's dilemmas in our times
see *The Abortion Act 1967* (London 1969) esp. pp. 1-8, 21-30, 41-9, 64-72; I.
MacGillivray & K.J. Dennis in G. Horobin (ed.) *Experience with abortion* 47-67; C.
McCance, P.C. Olley & V. Edward in *Experience* 245-300; C. Farmer in *Experience*
333-57; 'Abortion and the law in Britain' in M. Potts, P. Diggory & J. Peel (ed.)
Abortion (Cambridge 1977) 277-97; G.I. Zatuchni, J.J. Sciarra & J.J. Speidel
Pregnancy termination (Northwestern University, Evanston 1978) passim; P.
Frank in *Abortion: medical progress and social implications* (Ciba Foundation
Symposium 115, London 1985) 67-82; Z. Matéjcek, Z. Dytruch & V. Schüller in
Abortion: medical progress 136-49; H.P. David in *Abortion: medical progress*
150-64; J. Mattinson in *Abortion: medical progress* 165-77; S.A.M. McLean (ed.)
Legal issues in human reproduction (Dartmouth 1989) passim; J.C. Callahan (ed.)
Reproduction, ethics and the law (Bloomington 1995) passim.

2. See R.F.R. Gardner *Abortion: the personal dilemma; a Christian gynaecologist examines the medical, social, and spiritual issues* (Grand Rapids 1972).

3. See I. MacGillivray & K.J. Dennis in G. Horobin (ed.) *Experience with
abortion* 47-67.

4. Aleck Bourne: see Church of England, Board for Social Responsibility *Abortion: an ethical discussion* (London: Church Information Office for the Board, 1973)
15-16.

5. C. Browder *The wickedest woman in New York* provides interesting perspectives on the phenomenon of illicit abortions.

6. See Church of England, Board for Social Responsibility *Abortion: an ethical discussion* (London: Church Information Office for the Board, 1973), 7. A thorough account of the developments concerning abortion in England is provided by B. Brookes *Abortion in England, 1900-1967*.

7. J.A. Stallworthy in *The Abortion Act 1967* (London 1969), 41-9; K. Simpson in *The Abortion Act 1967* 61-4; S. Wangala, N.M. Murugu & J.G.K Mati in *Abortion: medical progress* 41-53; P. Frank in *Abortion: medical progress* 67-82.

8. More detailed accounts of medical education in the ancient world can be found in I.E. Drabkin in *BHM* 15 (1944) 333-51; F. Kudlien 'Medical education in Classical antiquity' in C.D. O'Malley (ed.) *The history of medical education*.

9. J. Longrigg *Medicine* 2. For a more detailed exploration of the bond between Greek medicine and philosophy see also L. Edelstein in *BHM* 26 (1952) 299-316; R.J. Hankinson (ed.) *Method, medicine and metaphysics: studies in the philosophy of ancient science* (Edmonton 1988).

10. Longrigg (*Medicine* 49-51) argues against this connection of Alcmaeon with the Pythagoreans, probably correctly.

11. Hip. *NH* 6,32 (1).

12. See Longrigg *Medicine* 104-48; W. Kullmann & S. Föllinger (ed.) *Aristotelische Biologie: Intentionen, Methoden, Ergebnisse* (Stuttgart 1997) passim, with rich bibliography; C. Oser-Grote *Aristoteles und das Corpus Hippocraticum* (Stuttgart 1999); W. Jaeger in *JHS* 77 (1957) 54-61.

13. W. Detel 'Why all animals have a stomach' in *Aristotelische Biologie* 63-84, esp. p. 65.

14. See Longrigg *Medicine* 149-76; J. Kollesch 'Die anatomischen Untersuchungen des Aristoteles und ihr Stellenwert als Forschungsmethode in der Aristotelischen Biologie' in *Aristotelische Biologie* 367-74.

15. The exact date of Diocles and his precise relationship with Aristotle are controversial. Some argue that he was a pupil of Aristotle (thus Phillips *Greek medicine* 128-35), others that he was his contemporary and co-operator (thus Longrigg *Medicine* 162-76). The fragments of Diocles can now be found in the new edition by P.J. van der Eijk *Diocles of Carystus: a collection of the fragments with translation and commentary* (Boston 2000). A second volume with commentary is to follow.

16. See Longrigg *Medicine* 177-226; H. von Staden *Herophilus* passim; and 'Teleology and mechanism: Aristotelian biology and early hellenistic medicine' in *Aristotelische Biologie* 183-208; R.T. Hankinson in *CQ* 39 (1989) 206-27.

17. For further information on the Methodist school see M. Frede 'The method of the so-called Methodical School of Medicine' in J. Barnes et al. (ed.) *Science and speculation* 1-23; J. Pigeaud 'Les fondements théoriques du méthodisme' in P. Murdy & J. Pigeaud (ed.) *Les Écoles médicales à Rome* 8-50; G. Rubinstein *The riddle of the Methodist Method*.

18. See also P. Carrick *Medical ethics* 30-1; E.D. Phillips *Greek medicine* 128 ff.; K. Dreichgräber *Die griechische Empirikerschule: Sammlung der Fragmente und Darstellung der Lehre* (Berlin & Zurich 1965); M. Frede 'The empiricist attitude towards reason and theory' in R.J. Hankinson (ed.) *Method, medicine and metaphysics* 79-97.

19. Hom. *Od.* 19,456-7; Pi. *Pyth.* 3,52-3.

20. The Greeks also owed to Egyptian and Babylonian medicine some of their pharmacopoeia, gynaecological knowledge and possibly surgical techniques: see Longrigg *Medicine* 9-11; G. Ebers *Papyros Ebers: Das hermetische Buch über die Arzneimittel der alten Ägypter in hieratischer Schriften* (Leipzig 1875); J.H.

Breasted *The Edwin Smith surgical papyrus* (Chicago 1930); J.B. de C.M. Saunders *The transition from ancient Egyptian to Greek medicine* (Kansas 1963); P. Ghalioungui 'The relation of Pharaonic to Greek and later medicine' *Bulletin of the Cleveland Medical Library* 15.3 (1968) 96-107; P. Carrick *Medical ethics* 3-6. On Babylonian medicine see R. Campbell Thomson *The devils and evil spirits in Babylonia* (London 1903-4).
    21. On the incantations as part of the healing process see Hom. *Od.* 19,457-8; Pi. *Pyth.* 3,51.About the gods as creators of disease and healers see Hom. *Il.* 5,99 ff. 305 ff. 447 ff.; *Od.* 5,394 ff., 9,411 ff.; Hes. *Op.* 100-4; 238-45.
    22. Hip. *VM* 1,572 (2).
    23. The distinction between Cnidian and Coan medicine is a controversial issue, a proper discussion of which is outside the purposes of this study (see H. von Staden *Herophilos* 487 n. 15 for a brief presentation of the main opinions and bibliography). However, these terms, accurate or not, have been established as the embodiment of two different types of medicine, one with emphasis upon theoretical principles (Coan), and one closer to traditional popular medicine and more practical in nature (Cnidian). I use the terms here within this context, and not necessarily because I am convinced that they represent two actual schools.
    24. R.D. Steuer & J.B. de C.M. Saunders *Ancient Egyptian and Cnidian medicine* (Berkeley Ca. 1959) passim; *La Collection Hippocratique et son rôle dans l' histoire de la médecine* (Leiden 1975) (Acts of the Conference held in Strasbourg, 23-27 October 1972) 95-170.
    25. O. Temkin 'Greek medicine as science and craft' *Isis* 44 (1953) 213-25.
    26. See also P. Carrick *Medical ethics* 3-14; H.F.J. Horstmanshoff in *Journal of the History of Medicine and Allied Sciences* 45 (1990) 176-97; V. Nutton 'Murders and miracles: lay attitudes towards medicine in classical antiquity' in R. Porter (ed.) *Patients and practitioners* (Cambridge 1985); R. Flemming *Medicine* 33-124.
    27. Hip. *Acut.* 2,240-2 (3).
    28. See also O. Temkin *Hippocrates* 18 ff.; R. Flemming *Medicine* 253-87.
    29. On Hippocrates as an almost mythical figurehead and moral guide for doctors in subsequent centuries see O. Temkin *Hippocrates* passim.
    30. For a number of issues related to ancient medical ethics P. Carrick *Medical ethics* and F. Kudlien in *Clio Medica* 5 (1970), 91-121 remain useful. See also the old but insightful article by L. Edelstein in *BHM* 30 (1956) 391-419.
    31. Just to mention a couple of well-known examples, in Athens all the members of the incoming Council were obliged to take an oath (*horkos bouleutikos*) outlining their basic duties as councillors, and the same applied to all citizens who served as jurors in the popular law-courts. See J. Plescia *The oath and perjury in ancient Greece* (Tallahassee 1970) 25-6 and P.J. Rhodes *The Athenian boule* (Oxford 1972) 191-8.
    32. Hip. *Praec.* 9,258 (6)
    33. Galen 5,750-1 (*De placitis* 9,5); cf. Pl. *R.* 336b-394c.
    34. Galen 5,750-1 (*De placitis* 9,5).
    35. Hip. *De arte* 6,46 (3).
    36. Hip. *Praec.* 9,258 (6).
    37. Hip. *Praec.* 9,254-6 (4).
    38. Hip. *Decent.* 9,232-4 (5).
    39. E.J. and L. Edelstein *Asclepius: a collection and interpretation of the Testimonies* (2 vols; Baltimore 1945); F. Graf in O. Reverdin & B.G Grange (ed.) *Le Sanctuaire grec* (Geneva 1992); H. King *Hippocrates' woman* 99-113; S.B. Aleshire *The Athenian Asklepieion.*
    40. On public doctors see L. Cohn-Haft *The public physicians of ancient Greece.* On Democedes see A. Griffiths 'Demokedes of Croton: a Greek doctor at the court

of Darius' in H. Sancisi-Weerdenburg & A. Kuhrt (ed.) *Achaemenid history II: the Greek sources* (Leiden 1987) 37-51.

41. Hip. *Med.* 9,204 (1); cf. also Gal. 13B, 144-52 (Hip. *Epid.* 6,4,19).

42. Hip. *Med.* 9.204-6 (1), 9,236 (*Decent.* 7).

43. Hip. *Decent.* 9,238 (11) and 9,242 (16).

44. Namely: 'yes, unless you are an immortal god'.

45. See Hip. *Vict.* 6,512-22 (1,35); Iamb. *VP* 196 ff., O. Temkin *Hippocrates* 13-14, G. Wöhrle *Studien zur Theorie der antiken Gesundheitslehre* (Stuttgart 1990) passim.

46. R. Flemming *Medicine* 64 ff.

47. Galen 6,18 (*San.* 1,5)

48. Galen 6,40 (*San.* 1,8). Regarding this psychosomatic perception of health in Galen see L. Garcìa Ballester, 'Soul and body, disease of the soul and disease of the body in Galen's medical thought' in P. Manuli & M. Vegetti (ed.) *Le opere psichologiche di Galeno* 117-52; R.T. Hankinson in *Phronesis* 36 (1991), 197-233.

49. See R. Flemming *Medicine* 256-72.

50. Galen 13B,146 (Hip. *Epid.* 6,4,9); on Callianax see above.

51. Hip. *Med.* 9,206 (1).

52. Hip. *Decent.* 9,232-4 (5).

53. See I. Shapiro (ed.) *Abortion: the Supreme Court decisions, 1965-2000* 2nd ed. (Indianapolis 2001).

54. Scribonius Largus *Compositiones,* Praef. 5,20-3; Sor. I 60; Priscianus *Euporiston* 3,6,23. See also P. Mudry 'Éthique et médecine à Rome: la Préface de Scribonius Largus ou l'affirmation d'une singularité', in H. Flashar & J. Jouanna (ed.) *Médecine et morale dans l'antiquité*; V. Nutton in *Pharmaceutical Historian* 25 (1995) 5-9.

55. On the long debate concerning the authorship of the Hippocratic Corpus see Chapter 1 n. 9.

56. S. Nittis 'The authorship and probable date of the Hippocratic Oath' *Bull. Hist. Med.* 8 (1940) 1012-21. Nittis' views are criticised in considerable detail by P. Carrick (*Medical ethics* 69-96), who largely agrees with Edelstein.

57. L. Edelstein *Hippocratic oath*.

58. C. Lichtenthaeler *Der Eid des Hippokrates: Ursprung und Bedeutung* (Cologne 1984) 286.

59. D.W. Amundsen *Medicine* 39.

60. Hip. *Epid.* 1,11.

61. See for example L. Edelstein *Hippocratic oath* 8, C. Lichtenthaeler *Eid* 137.

62. In Sophocles' play Antigone is found hanging in the grave where she was buried alive after disobeying Creon's orders and burying her dead brother. In Sophocles' *Oedipus Rex* Jocasta hangs herself after it is revealed that she has been living with her own son and had children by him. Deianeira in Sophocles' *Women of Trachis* commits suicide after she realises that she has given her husband Heracles poison instead of a love philtre. On suicide in Greek thought see R. Hirzel 'Die Selbstmord' *ARW* 11 (1908) 75-104, 243-84, 417-76. The Stoics defend suicide as an honourable alternative with particular vigour: see Seneca *Lucil.* 77, D.L. 4,3; 6,18.

63. See also D. Gourevitch 'Suicide among the sick in classical antiquity' *BHM* 43 (1969); P. Carrick *Medical ethics* 39-56 and 127-50.

64. Hip. 9,258-62 (*Praec.* 7), 1,588-90 (*AM* 9), *Art.* 69, *De arte* 8, Aesop. 189, Oribasius 8,8.

65. See Pl. *R.* 406c; 407d; 408b, E. *S.* 1109 ff., Arist. *Rh.* 1361b, Plu. *Mor.* 231a.

66. Arist. *NE* 1138; cf. D.W. Amundsen *Medicine* 46-7 n. 35.

67. See J.C.C. Strachan 'Who did forbid suicide in *Phaedo* 62B?' *CQ* 20 (1970) 216-20.

68. L. Edelstein *Hippocratic oath* 7-18.

69. Iamblichus *De vita Pythagorica* 196 ff., 205-6.

70. See Chapter 6 and D.M. MacDowell *Athenian homicide law* 3-5, 141-50.

71. If ancient views on the sanctity of human life appear to be inconsistent and contradictory, I must point out that our views on it may appear equally confused to future historians. To give one striking example, the present legal systems of many countries advocate the sanctity of human life, but at the same time allow the execution of people. Evidently the majority view in our times does not recognise the sanctity of human life unconditionally and without qualifications, and neither did the Greeks and the Romans.

72. P. Carrick *Medical ethics* 39.

73. See also J.M. Rist *Human value: a study in ancient philosophical ethics*; O. Temkin 'The idea of respect for life in the history of medicine' in O. Temkin, W.K. Krankena & S.H. Kaddish *Respect for life in medicine, philosophy and the law* 1-23.

74. See Lichtenthaeler op. cit. in n. 58, esp. ch. 16, pp. 279-86.

75. K. Dreichgräber 'Die ärtzliche Standesethik des hippokratischen Eides' in H. Flashar (ed.) *Antike Medizin* 94-120, esp. 118.

76. When, for example, Galen (14,114 ff.) speaks about the antidote of Caesar, he mentions various therapeutic purposes, but also states that it could easily be used as an undetectable lethal poison, if administered in low dosages over a long period of time.

77. Scribonius Largus *Compositiones, Praef.* 5,20-3.

78. A brief account of Scribonius Largus can be found in Flemming *Medicine* 140-3; see also 'Professio Medici: Zum Vorwort des Scribonius Largus' *Abhandlungen der Akademie der Wissenschaften und der Literatur, geistes- und sozialwissenschaftliche Klasse*, 9 (Wiesbaden 1950).

79. Sor. I 60; see also John of Alexandria *Commentary on Hippocrates 'On the Nature of the Child'* 18 (=2,216); Priscianus *Gyn.* 6,23 (=241,4-15 Rose).

80. See K. Dreichgräber op. cit. in n. 75, 108-9, L. Edelstein *Hippocratic oath* passim; E. Nardi *Aborto* 59-66; O. Temkin op. cit. in n. 73; C. Lichtenthaeler op. cit in n. 58, 145-6, P. Carrick *Medical ethics* 84.

81. J. Riddle *Contraception* 7-10; id. 'Ever since Eve' *Archaeology* (April/May 1994) 33; H. King (*Hippocrates' woman* 139) shares this view that the Oath did not impose a general ban on abortion.

82. E. Nardi *Aborto* 61.

83. Galen 12,252 (*De simplicibus medicamentorum* 9,1).

84. Prisc. *Eup.* 3,6,23.

85. K. Hopkins in *Comparative Studies in Society and History* 8 (1965-6) 132.

86. R. Flemming *Medicine* 168-9.

87. Hip. *Superf.* 8,490 (27), Galen 2,183 (*De naturalibus facultatibus* 3,12), Sor. I 60, Prisc. *Eup.* 3,6,23.

88. Hip. *Nat. mul.* 7,380 (37), *Mul.* 8,176 (78); *Mul.* 218-20 (91). See also Chapter 1 §v.

89. Sor. I 60, Galen 16,180 (Hip. *Hum.* 1,19), 19,456 (Hip. *Def.* 458).

90. John of Alexandria *Commentary on Hippocrates 'On the nature of the child'*, 18 (=2,216); cf. also Priscianus *Gyn.* 6,23 (=241,4-15 Rose).

91. See O. Temkin *Hippocrates* 14-15.

92. Galen 17,438 (Hip. *Epid.* 2,27).

93. E. Eyben in *AncSoc* 11/12 (1980-81) 12.

94. Juv. *Sat.* 6,594-7

95. J. Riddle *Eve's herbs.*

96. R. Flemming (*Medicine,* Appendix 2, pp. 383-91) has collected the inscriptions referring to Greek and Roman medical women. See also the references to medical women in Hip. *Mul.* 8,144 (68), Hyginus *Fabulae* 274 (the case of Hagnodice). Unfortunately this important evidence attesting the presence of a respectable number of female medical practitioners in the Roman empire does not help to solve any of our problems, as it does not tell us much about these women. Other important studies include H. King's *Hippocrates' woman* 172-87 and 'Agnodike and the profession of medicine' *Proceedings of the Cambridge Philological Society* 32 (1986) 53-77.

97. R. Flemming *Medicine* 36-7.

98. See Gal. 14,641 ff.; R. Flemming *Medicine* 256-72.

99. A thorough account of midwifery in the ancient world is provided by H. King *Hippocrates' woman* 157-87; see also V. French in *Helios* 13 (1986) 69-84; J. Achterberg *Woman as healer*; R. Flemming *Medicine* 129 ff.

100. Pl. *Tht.* 149c-d.

101. Socrates was the son of the midwife Phainarete in real life.

4. The Woman's Point of View

1. Stratis Myrivilis *Life in the Tomb*, ch. 17, translated by Peter Bien.

2. There is a number of recent studies relating the actual experience of women with abortion; see e.g. P.E. McCormick, *Attitudes toward abortion;* H. J. & J.D. Osofsky *The abortion experience*; M. Denes *In necessity and sorrow*; M.K. Zimmerman *Passage through abortion*; N.L. Stotland *Abortion: facts and feelings*; J. Wilt *Abortion, choice, and contemporary fiction.*

3. In R.E. Hall (ed.) *Abortion in a changing world* (New York 1970) 183-7; see also G. Devereux *A study of abortions in primitive societies.*

4. V.G. Valaoras & D. Trichopoulos in R.E. Hall (ed.) *Abortion* 284-90.

5. See Church of England, Board for Social Responsibility *Abortion: an ethical discussion* (London: Church Information Office for the Board, 1973) 45-9.

6. L. Thomson, in R.E. Hall *Abortion* 188-211.

7. P.C. Olley in G. Horobin (ed.) *Experience with abortion* 99 ff.; G. Howard in *The Abortion Act* 64-72.

8. Since the employment of scans and tests during pregnancy that can determine whether the foetus has some form of serious disability, parents have been confronted with the dilemma of knowingly bringing a disabled child into the world or destroying the disabled foetus. This is a very serious question in modern medical ethics, but since such technology was unknown to the ancient world, the issue will not be discussed here. The ancient Greeks had to face a similar dilemma after the birth of a disabled child, and this issue I explore further in Chapter 5.

9. On the importance of the concept of legitimacy see D. Ogden *Greek bastardy in the classical and hellenistic period* (Oxford 1996); K. Kapparis *Against Neaira* 8-13, 198-206; R. Sealey 'On lawful concubinage in Athens' *ClAnt* 3 (1984) 111-33; C. Patterson 'Those Athenian bastards' *ClAnt* 9 (1990) 40-73; P. Rhodes 'Bastards as Athenian citizens' *CQ* 28 (1978) 89-92; D.M. MacDowell 'Bastards as Athenian citizens' *CQ* 26 (1976) 88-91.

10. A brief yet comprehensive account of the *oikos* can be found in V.J. Hunter *Policing Athens: social control in Attic lawsuits* (Princeton 1994) 9-42.

11. See C. Patterson 'Marriage and the married woman in Athenian law' in S. Pomeroy (ed.) *Women's history and ancient history* (Chapel Hill & London 1991) 48-72.

12. See H. Licht *Sexual life in ancient Greece* (Eng. tr.; London 1932).

13. See E. Cantarella *Bisexuality in the ancient world* (Eng. tr.; New Haven & London 1992); K.J. Dover *Greek homosexuality* 2nd ed. (London & Cambridge Mass. 1989).

14. S.B. Pomeroy *Xenophon Oeconomicus* (Oxford 1994) 297-300, commenting on X. *Oec.* 9,5-6 argues that slaves were not allowed to have sexual relationships without the permission of their masters, who as owners of the slaves' bodies were also owners of their sexual desires. But this point of view takes into account only the desire of masters to control their slaves, not the actual realities of the lives of slaves. See also Pomeroy 'Slavery in the light of Xenophon's *Oeconomicus*' *Index* 17 (1989) 11-18.

15. Cf. Aesch. 1,124: 'If a doctor occupies one of the workshops in the street it is called a clinic, ... if a mason occupies it, then it is called a masonry, if a pimp and prostitutes occupy it, then it is immediately called a brothel by the type of work performed in it.'

16. The standard work on the lives of alien residents in Athens is D. Whitehead *The ideology of the Athenian metic* (Cambridge 1977). See also a useful collection of articles in R. Lonis (ed.) *L'etranger dans le monde* grec (Nancy 1988).

17. Pl. *R.* 460e-461b

18. On Persian and Roman perceptions see Chapter 5.

19. Dem. 23,53; see also Lys. 1,30, 13,66; X. *Hier.* 3,3; Men. fr. 306 Körte. On adultery see K. Kapparis *Against Neaira* 295-307, and 'When were the Athenian adultery laws introduced? *RIDA* 42 (1995) 97-122; C. Carey 'Rape and adultery in Athenian law' *CQ* 45 (1995) 407-18; E.M. Harris 'Did the Athenians regard seduction as a worse crime than rape?' *CQ* 40 (1990) 370-7; D. Cohen 'The Athenian law of adultery' *RIDA* 31 (1984) 147-65; U.E. Paoli *SDHI* 16 (1950) 123-82.

20. See Lys. 1,49; X. *Mem.* 2,2,5; Ar. *Nub.* 1083 and Scholia, Iuven. 10,37; K. Kapparis in *RIDA* 42 (1995) 101-2, 112-13, and also 'Humiliating the adulterer: the law and the practice in classical Athens' *RIDA* 43 (1996) 63-77.

21. Arist. *Ath.* 26,4; see K. Kapparis *Against Neaira* 198-206 for further sources and bibliography.

22. Dem. 59,87; see also the commentary on this passage in K. Kapparis *Against Neaira* 354-60.

23. Aesch. 1,183.

24. Ael. *HA* 11,15.

25. Ael. *HA* 8,20.

26. Ael. *VH* 13,24.

27. K. Kapparis 'Has Chariton read Lysias 1 "On the murder of Eratosthenes"?', *Hermes* 128 (2000) 380-3.

28. *Anth. Pal.* 4,3; 5,41.

29. C. Edwards *Politics of immorality* 34.

30. For a more detailed presentation of the provisions of this law and further discussion on its objectives see S. Treggiari *Roman marriage;* T.A.J. McGinn *Prostitution* 70-247; C. Edwards *Politics of immorality* 1-62; E. Grubbs *Law and family* 103-12; J. Gardner *Being a Roman citizen* 123 ff.; S. des Bouvrie 'Augustus' legislation on morals – what morals and what aims' *Symbolae Osloenses* 59 (1984) 93-113; K. Galinsky, 'Augustus' legislation on morals and marriage' *Philologus* 125 (1981) 126-44; F. Cairns 'Propertius on Augustus' marriage law (II.7)' *GB* 8 (1979) 185-205; D. Nörr 'Planung in der Antike: über die Ehegesetze des Augustus' in H. Baier (ed.) *Freiheit und Sachzwang: Beiträge zu Ehren Helmut Schleskys* (Opladen 1977) 309-34; P. Csillag, *The Augustan laws on family relations* (Budapest 1976); P.A. Brunt *Italian manpower 225 BC – AD 14* (Oxford 1971) 558-66.

31. E. Grubbs *Law and family* 101-39.

32. These measures are expounded by S. Dixon *Roman mother* (London & Sydney 1988) ch. 4.

33. Plu. *Mor.* 242c.

34. Plu. *Lyc.* 18,1.

35. See X. *Lac.* 2,6-8; Isoc. 12,211-12; MacDowell *Spartan law* 59-61.

36. Aesch. 1,182.

37. Plu. *Sol.* 23,2.

38. This is the expression used in the law of adultery quoted in Dem. 59,87 to define a woman caught committing adultery, whether married or unmarried: see my commentary on this document in K. Kapparis *Against Neaira* 354-60.

39. G.A. Ralles & M. Potles *Syntagma tôn Theiôn kai Hierôn Kanonôn* (Athens 1852-1859) vol. 4, p. 96. On Zonaras as a commentator on canons see P. Pieler 'Johannes Zonaras als Kanonist' in N. Oikonomides (ed.) *To Byzantio kata ton 12o aiôna* (Athens 1991) 601-20. On the development of Byzantine canon law and its relationship to imperial law see R. Morris (ed.) *Church and people in Byzantium*, (Birmingham 1990), especially the brief and informative account of R. Macrides '*Nomos* and *kanon* on paper and in court' 61-85. I am grateful to Ruth Macrides and Margaret Mullett for their help with Byzantine canon law.

40. Canon 91 reads as following: 'Concerning penalties for those who give or take drugs to cause abortion: Those women who give drugs that cause abortion, as well as those who take poisons to kill the foetus, shall be subject to the penalty for a murderer.' I am quoting the translation of G. Nedungatt & M. Featherstone (ed.) *The council in Trullo revisited* (Rome 1995). For the relevant literature and further references to abortion in canon law see E. Nardi *Aborto* 605-82.

41. Tertullian *De virginibus velandis* 19,4 ff.

42. For a brief presentation of the debate see Gamel in *Helios* 16 (1989) 184-5.

43. Juv. *Sat.* 2,36-40; Pliny *Ep.* 4,11,6; Suet. *Dom.* 22.

44. Juv. *Sat.* 2,34-40 (Penguin translation by P. Green).

45. Juvenal's remark that she had a series of abortions need not be taken seriously; it could just be an exaggeration. Meanwhile the fact that he does not mention Julia's death probably suggests that he has distorted the incident to suit his own purposes. Pliny and Suetonius make clear that she died as a result of this one attempt; cf. E. Nardi *Aborto* 284, n. 218.

46. Ogden op. cit in n. 8, 161-2.

47. Juv. *Sat.* 6,594-600.

48. Ael. *NA* 8,20.

49. Aristaenet. 2,15.

50. Juv. *Sat.* 6,594-600.

51. See the lucid account of the social context of adultery by D. Cohen in P. Cartledge, P. Millett & S.C. Todd (ed.) *Nomos: essays in Athenian law, politics and society* (Cambridge 1990) 147-65, and the response by C. Carey 'Rape and adultery in Athenian law' *CQ* 45 (1995) 407-18.

52. On the significance of slave names see M. Lambertz *Die griechischen Sklavennamen* (Vienna 1907-8); S. Copalle *De servorum Graecorum nominibus capita duo* (Diss. Marburg 1908).

53. See Dem. 57,42.

54. Galen 17,438 (Hip. *Epid.* 2,27). The excessive consumption of wine might itself be considered suspicious, as several passages from medical authors suggest that it was perceived as detrimental to the pregnancy (Sor. I 64, and Chapter 1 on the famous wine of Keryneia).

55. Sor. I 60; a more detailed discussion of the passage is provided in Chapter 3. See also Clement *Paed.* 2,10,96,1; Quintilian *Declamationes* CXLV.

56. Tac. *An.* 14,63.

57. For further information on prostitution and its forms in ancient Greece see K. Kapparis *Against Neaira*, esp. 4-8; N.J. Davidson *Courtesans and fishcakes* (London 1997); A. Rousselle *Porneia*.

58. In the festival of the Haloa their presence was so prominent that some scholars have argued that decent women did not attend the festival, I think erroneously: see K. Kapparis *Against Neaira* 413-17. The Adoneia was another festival where courtesans made their presence felt: see M. Detienne *The gardens of Adonis* (Sussex 1977).

59. See Dem. 59,67; Lys. 10,19, and K. Kapparis *Against Neaira* 311-13.

60. Aesch. 1,119, Hyp. 3,4, Arist. *Ath.* 50,2, and Rhodes *AP* 574.

61. See Aeschines 1, *Against Timarchos*, passim.

62. Theophylact is probably drawing from Ovid's two abortion poems (*Amores* 13 and 14: see Chapter 4 §iii) the example of Medea and her justification for killing her children (*Amores* 14), the idea that the woman had the abortion in order to retain her figure, and the concept that the entire operation was done furtively with the assistance of potent drugs. Apart from that, the letter is modelled on Alciphron's *Letters of courtesans*, and it is possible that Theophylact echoes the view of Soranus (I 61) when he states that childbirth is safer than abortion.

63. The character of the 'good courtesan' (*chrêstê hetaira*) was a standard literary theme in New Comedy and in later literature influenced by it: see M.M. Henry *Menander's courtesans and the Greek comic tradition* (Frankfurt a.M. 1985) passim.

64. Theophylact *Ep.* 30, p. 772 Hercher.

65. Philemon *PCG* fr. 3, Eubulus *PCG* frr. 67 and 82.

66. Sor. I 61.

67. Some scholars have been rather surprised by the fact that the *coitus interruptus*, perhaps the most effective of the contraceptive methods known to the ancient world, is hardly mentioned. But this, along with non-vaginal forms of sexual activity, prolonged breast feeding (which inhibits ovulation), homosexual relationships and so on, do not consist contraceptive methods *per se*; they are basically low-risk or no-risk activities that one would hardly expect to be included in a list of *contraceptive* methods. See also McLaren *Contraception* 25 ff.

68. L. Dean-Jones *Women's bodies* 148-224.

69. Hip. *Carn.* 8,610 (19).

70. See K. Kapparis *Against Neaira* 217-21; N.J. Davidson op. cit. in n. 57 passim; G.W. Arnott 'Aulêtrida pezên' *Glotta* 68 (1990) 91-2.

71. Hip. *Nat. puer.* 7,488-90 (13).

72. Aristaenet. 1,19: 'Melissarion was costly and associated with very rich men. She should avoid conceiving a child, so as not to become cheaper, prematurely losing her looks during childbirth. This musician had heard the things that women tell each other, that once a woman is about to conceive, the semen does not come out, but is withheld by nature. Listening to this, wisely she put it into her mind and remembered what she was told. When she became aware of the fact that the semen was not coming out of her, she told her mother and word came to me, as I was more experienced. And as soon as I heard and advised her to do what I knew, I set her free from the expected hope.' In Aristaenetus the woman has a name (Melissarion), she is free, not a slave, and tells her mother, not a mistress or procuress, about the early signs of the pregnancy. The woman in Aristaenetus has more of a personality and surely this was partly the purpose of the epistolographer when he introduced these modifications to the Hippocratic passage.

73. A phrase that clearly implies a pregnancy, but in a euphemistic manner words such as 'pregnancy' or 'childbirth' are avoided. On the pregnancy as a 'hope' see E. Nardi *Aborto* 354-60.

74. See L. Dean-Jones *Women's bodies* 173-6 and esp. n. 95; I.M. Lonie *The Hippocratic Treatises 'On generation'; 'On the nature of the child'; 'Diseases'* (Berlin 1981) 161.

75. In *Ant.* 1,14-15 a woman accidentally causes the death of her lover and master when she hears that he intended to establish her in a brothel. See also Dem. 59,30 and my commentary in *Against Neaira* 228-9.

76. L. Dean-Jones (*Women's bodies* 28) understands the Greek word *gonê* literally as 'seed', but I think here it is used for 'period'. Menstrual blood is identified as crude semen in Arist. *GA* 728a26-31; see also Dean-Jones 200-9. Every woman would know that a missed period is a fairly sure sign of a pregnancy. If I am right, then the pregnancy terminated here was not six days old, as the author claims, but more than a month old.

77. On women's awareness of their bodies see L. Dean-Jones *Women's bodies* 26-1.

78. Sor. I 60; cf. John of Alexandria *Commentary on Hippocrates 'On the nature of the child'*, 18 (=2,216); Priscianus *Gyn.* 6,23 (=241,4-15 Rose). See also the discussion of the Oath in Chapter 3.

79. Clem. *Ped.* 2,10,96,1, Plu. *Mor.* 134 f.

80. Ar. *Lys.* 29-48.

81. See Athen. 13, passim (with numerous references to classical poetry and prose); S.B. Pomeroy *Xenophon Oeconomicus* (Oxford 1994) 304-6; B. Grillet *Les Femmes et les fards dans l'antiquité grecque* (Lyon 1975); M. Dayagi-Mendeles *Perfumes and cosmetics in the ancient world* (Jerusalem 1989); R. Garland *The eye of the beholder* (London & Ithaca NY 1995) 105-22; M. Alden 'The beguilement of Zeus – in all the better shops' *Costume* 33 (1999) 68-73.

82. See M. Kilmer 'Genital phobia and depilation' *JHS* 102 (1982) 104-12.

83. Eubulus *PCG* fr. 97. In my translation I adopt masculine gender for the participle in line 1 (*peripeplasmenoi*). The reasons are explained in a forthcoming independent article.

84. Alexis *PCG* fr. 98.

85. I owe this remark partly to Dr Maureen Alden's observation that women would often dress up and try to look beautiful not in order to impress their husbands, but their peers, that is other women in their community. See also Dem. 48,55, Luc. *D. meret.* 5,4, 6,2; Alciphr. 4,17,5; D.M. Schaps *Economic rights of women in ancient Greece* (Edinburgh 1979) 7-11 and 101-5.

86. Dem. 59,87, Aesch. 1,183, K. Kapparis *Against Neaira* 354-60.

87. *Poetae Melici Graeci*, fr. 1 (843) Page; cf. also Arist. fr. 96 Rose.

88. *TrGF* 71 fr. 3. For my purposes I have translated the text as it is reconstructed in the Loeb edition of Athenaeus. The text of the *TrGF* does not attempt to reconstruct this desperately damaged passage.

89. See for example Lys. 1,7: Euphiletos says of his wife: 'at the beginning she was the best among women, a good housekeeper, thrifty, and looking after everything carefully'. Ischomachos in Xenophon *Oeconomicus* 7,11 summarises to his wife the purpose of their union as following: 'Tell me, wife, have you ever thought about why I married you and why your parents gave you to me? It must be quite obvious to you, I'm sure, that there was no shortage of partners with whom we might sleep. I, on my part, and your parents, on your behalf, considered who was the best partner we could choose for managing the estate and for children' (tr. S.B. Pomeroy). See also Dem. 59,122; V.J. Hunter *Policing Athens* 38; S. Blundell *Women in ancient Greece* (Cambridge, Mass. 1995) 119-24.

90. See Eub. *PCG* fr. 97, Alexis *PCG* fr. 98, S.B. Pomeroy *Xenophon Oeconomicus* 304-5.

91. Dem. 59,122; see also my commentary ad loc.

92. See D.M. MacDowell *Andocides: On the mysteries* (Oxford 1962) 12-13, 147. It is beyond doubt that male pride and ego also played its part in this dispute, not least because Callias was not claiming the woman for himself, but for his son.

93. Dem. 59,113.

94. See C. Patterson 'Marriage and the married woman in Athenian law' in S.B. Pomeroy (ed.) *Women's history and ancient history* (Chapel Hill & London 1991) 40-73.

95. X. *Oec.* 7,6 seems to me to be a reference to the good cooking skills of Ischomachos' young wife. I think Pomeroy misunderstands the phrase *ta ge amphi gastera ... pepaideumenê* when she translates 'she had been very well trained to control her appetites'. She understands it as a reference to 'a common misogynistic complaint that women were insatiable' (p. 271). I think the passage refers to the training of the young wife of Ischomachos as a cook in her parental home; her husband commends her skills, and thinks that it is a very useful thing for a woman, as well as for a man, to know how to cook well. On cooking as a traditional woman's task see Ar. *Ec.* 221-3.

96. Hyp. *Aparasema* fr. 10 Blass.

97. X. *Oec.* 10. S.B. Pomeroy (*Xenophon Oeconomicus* 305) suggests that Xenophon reflects at this point Spartan ideals, where natural beauty was considered to be superior to make up and ornaments (X. *Lac.* 5,8; Plu. *Lyc.* 1,4,4). This is possibly correct, but not necessarily the case for the reasons mentioned above: this form of disapproval could be equally Athenian.

98. Quintilian *Declamationes* 145.

99. See L. Dean-Jones *Women's bodies* 95-6 and 148 ff. Jokes about how much women love sex can be found in Arist. *Lys.* 124 ff.; *Th.* 383-573.

100. For an insight into the activities and lifestyles of upper-class women see Juv. *Sat.* 6, Sen. *Ad Helv.* passim, Cic. *Cael.* 13-16.

101. Juv. *Sat.* 6,594-600.

102. S. Dixon *Roman mother* (London & Sydney 1988) 21-30.

103. See.M. Cobrier 'Ideologique et pratique de l'héritage' *Index* 13 (1985) 501-28.

104. See *RG* 6,8,5; Hor. *Carm.* 4,5,21-4; Ovid *Fasti* 2,139; Dio 54,16; Suet. *Aug.* 34; Ulpian 21,20; *Dig.* 23,2, 44-6; McLaren, *Contraception*, 43-7; S. Treggiari *Roman marriage*; T.A.J. McGinn *Prostitution* 70-247; C. Edwards *Politics of immorality* 1-62; J. Gardner *Being a Roman citizen* 123 ff.; S. des Bouvrie 'Augustus' legislation on morals – what morals and what aims' *Symbolae Osloenses* 59 (1984) 93-113; K. Galinsky, 'Augustus' legislation on morals and marriage,' *Philologus* 125 (1981) 126-44; F. Cairns 'Propertius on Augustus' marriage law (II.7)' *GB* 8 (1979) 185-205; D. Nörr 'Planung in der Antike: über die Ehegesetze des Augustus' in H. Baier (ed.) *Freiheit und Sachzwang: Beiträge zu Ehren Helmut Schleskys* (Opladen 1977) 309-34; P. Csillag, *The Augustan laws on family relations* (Budapest 1976); P.A. Brunt *Italian manpower 225 BC – AD 14* (Oxford 1971) 558-66.

105. On the measures of the Roman state to encourage maternity see Dixon *Roman mother* 71-104.

106. Whether this condemnation is genuine or not is another matter, and I do not wish to engage into this long and controversial discussion here.

107. Gellius *NA* 12,1,8.

108. On motherhood in the Roman empire see S. Dixon *Roman mother* passim.

109. Ovid *Nux* 23-4.

110. See especially W.J. Watts in *AC* 16 (1973) 89-101.

111. See E. Nardi *Aborto* 233 n. 72 on this interpretation of the poems.

112. Sen. *Helv.* 16,3.

240   *Notes to pages 119-129*

113. Ovid *Fasti* 1,619-28; Plu. *Mor.* 278b; see also the discussion in Chapter 4 §v.

114. Dixon *Roman mother* 92-4.

115. Rouselle *Porneia* 43.

116. Sor. I 60.

117. Chariton *Chaireas and Callirhoe* 2.8.6-2.9.6.

118. R. Johne in G. Schmeling (ed.) *The novel in the ancient world* (Leiden 1996) 180. On Chariton's novel *Chaireas and Callirhoe* see the recent article by B.P. Reardon in the same volume, pp. 309-35, and for older bibliography see T. Hägg *Narrative technique in ancient Greek romances* (Stockholm 1971).

119. Callirhoe was obviously already pregnant by Chaireas when she was thought dead and was buried alive.

120. Her father: the glorious Syracusan general who defeated the Athenians in the Sicilian expedition (Thucydides 6-7) is the father of the heroine in the novel.

121. As we have already noted, Medea killed her children to have revenge on her unfaithful partner Jason (E. *Med.* 792-1414). In this respect she is the archetype of the cruel mother, but ancient authors (Ovid. *Am.* 2,14, Theophylact *Ep.* 30 Hercher) are prepared to excuse her because she was blinded by her love for Jason and incensed by a deep feeling of betrayal.

122. Amphion and Zethus, sons of Zeus and Antiope, were re-united with their lost mother, freed her from long-term captivity, and took her under their protection: see Eur. fr. 179-227 Nauck. Cyrus the Great was exposed to die but later reunited with his true parents, Cambyses and Mandane, daughter of Astyages, king of the Medes: see Hdt. 1.107-22.

123. Galen 17.1, 635; 17.2, 653.

124. Ovid *Her.* 11,39-46.

125. The laws governing the main issues related to inheritance are quoted in Dem. 46,14.8.20.22.24, and Dem. 43,51.

126. See for example the case of Phile in Isaeus 3, *On the estate of Pyrrhus*. Phile was accepted as a legitimate daughter of Pyrrhus for many years, but at some point lateral relatives brought a lawsuit claiming that she was not legitimate, because allegedly she was the daughter of a courtesan. If the prosecution succeeded in persuading the jury that she was illegitimate, then she would be removed from the inheritance line, and in the absence of any other direct descendant the property of Pyrrhus would be inherited by lateral relatives.

127. See K. Kapparis *Against Neaira* 16-19. Important studies of women's property and inheritance rights in classical Athens include D.M. MacDowell *Law in classical Athens* 92-108; V.J. Hunter *Policing Athens: social control in Attic lawsuits* (Princeton 1994) 20-9; L. Rubinstein *Adoption in IV Century Athens*; E.M. Harris 'Women and lending in Athenian society: a horos re-examined' *Phoenix* 46 (1992) 309-21; L. Foxhall 'Household, gender and property in Classical Athens' *CQ* 39 (1989) 22-44; D.M. Schaps *Economic rights of women in Ancient Greece* (Edinburgh 1979); J.E. Karnezis *Hê Epiklêros* (Athens 1972); D. Asheri in *Historia* 12 (1963) 1-21; L.J. Kuenen-Janssens 'Some notes on the competence of the Athenian woman to conduct a transaction' *Mnemosyne* 9 (1941) 199-214.

128. The law is quoted *verbatim* in Dem. 43,75.

129. See D.M. MacDowell, *Spartan law*, 89-110.

130. Cic. *Clu.* 32; see also E. Nardi *Aborto* 214-28.

131. Cic. *Clu.* 34: *spem illam, quam in alvo commendatam a viro continebat, ... vendidit*.

132. See E. Nardi *Aborto* 623-6, 638-47.

133. L. Thomson *Fijian frontier* (San Francisco & Honolulu 1940).

134. Ovid *Fasti* 1,619-28; Plu. *Mor.* 278b.

135. Plutarch uses rather neutral vocabulary that only implicitly indicates that the matrons resorted to abortions in order to avoid giving birth: he says *sunethento oun allêllais mê kuiskesthai mêdê tiktein*. Ovid shows no such restraint; he says *visceribus crescens excutiebat onus*.

136. Sen. *Contr.* 2,5,2.

5. The Man's Point of View

1. See for example some of the articles in A. Smyth *The abortion papers, Ireland* (Dublin 1992), and especially the intriguing paper by the editor herself entitled 'The politics of abortion in a police state', pp. 138-48. A insightful perspective into the gender politics of abortion is provided by M. Boyle *Re-thinking abortion*.

2. See e.g. S. Faludi *Backlash: the undeclared war against American women* (New York 1991).

3. A good introduction to modern male concerns and perspectives on abortion is provided in A.B. Shostak, G. McLouth & L. Seng *Men and abortion*.

4. Cic. *Clu.* 32.

5. G. Raepsaet 'Les motivations de la natalité à Athènes aux Ve et IVe siècles avant notre ère' *AC* 40 (1971) 80-100.

6. See also Isaeus 2,1.7.10.23.46; Lacey *Family* 97-8; L. Rubinstein *Adoption* 64-77; K. Kapparis *Against Neaira* 286-7.

7. Lys. 13,91; Aesch. 1,28; Dem. 24,103-17; Arist. *Ath.* 55,3; 56,6; D.M. MacDowell *Law in classical Athens* 92; Rhodes *AP* 618 and 629; S.B. Pomeroy *Families* 194 and 222; C. Patterson *The family in Greek history* (Cambridge Mass. 1998); see M. Golden *Children and childhood in classical Athens* (Baltimore 1990) 23-50, 80-114; B.S. Strauss *Fathers and sons in Athens* (London 1993).

8. B.S. Strauss *Fathers and sons* 82-97.

9. Aesch. 1,13 *tên onesin tês paidopoiias*; S.B. Pomeroy *Families* 38, 141, 143. For a more detailed study of the relationship of parents and children in Athenian society, and the rights and duties resulting from this relationship for each side, see M. Golden *Children and childhood* and B.S. Strauss *Fathers and sons*.

10. Aesch. 1,13-14.

11. See Dem. 43,62.57-8; Plu. *Sol.* 21; Donna C. Kurtz & J. Boardman *Greek burial customs* (Ithaca, NY 1971); M. Alexiou *The ritual lament in Greek tradition* (Cambridge 1974); S.C. Humphreys *The family, women and death* (London 1983); R. Rehm *Marriage to death: the conflation of wedding and funeral rituals in Greek tragedy* (Princeton 1994); S.B. Pomeroy *Families* 100-40.

12. For the sources and bibliography see my note in K. Kapparis *Against Neaira* 286-7; B.S. Strauss *Fathers and sons* 33-72; L. Rubinstein *Adoption* passim; S.B. Pomeroy *Families* 25 and 121-2.

13. M. Golden *Children and childhood* 93.

14. M. Golden *Children and childhood* 82-114, B.S. Strauss *Fathers and sons* 72-6.

15. See e.g. E. *Med.* 914-21 (Jason speaks), and 1021-80 (Medea speaks); *Supp.* 1101-3; *Heracl.* 408-14; Aesch. 2,152, 3,77-8; Ar. *Nub.* 1380-5; *Ach.* 326-9; *Th.* 289-91; X. *Smp.* 3,12; M. Golden *Children and childhood* 82-114; B.S. Strauss *Fathers and sons* 72-6.

16. Lysias frr. 19-24 Carey; see the discussion in Chapter 6.

17. E. *Andr.* 355-60.

18. M. Lloyd *Andromache* (Warminster 1994) ad loc.

19. For a discussion of the role of the Roman father within the family see J.A. Crook 'Patria potestas' *CQ* 17 (1967) 113-22; K.R. Bradley 'Child care at Rome: the role of men' *Historical reflections/Réflections historiques* 12 (1985) 485-523; B.

Rawson (ed.) *The family in ancient Rome: new perspectives* (London & Sydney 1988); R.P. Saller *'Patria potestas* and the stereotype of the Roman family' *Continuity and Change* 1 (1986) 7-22; id. *'Pietas*, obligation and authority in the Roman family' in P. Kneissl & V. Losemann (ed.) *Alte Geschichte und Wissenschaftsgeschichte: Festschrift für Karl Christ zum 65. Geburtstag* (Darmstadt 1988) 393-410; J.F. Gardner *Family and familia in Roman law and life* (Oxford 1998).
20. Cic. *Clu.* 31-5.
21. Tertullian *De anima* 25,5; *Ad nationes* 1,15,8; *De virginibus velandis* 14,4; *De exhortatione castitatis* 12,5; Methodius *Symposion* 2,6.
22. For the foetus as 'a hope' see E. Nardi *Aborto* 354-60.
23. D.M. MacDowell in his important article 'The oikos in Athenian law' (*CQ* 39 [1989] 10-21) has rightly argued that Athenian law did not address groups, but individuals. However, the *oikos* was a key concept in public life, especially in relation to traditional institutions such as genos and phratry, and played an important role when it came to legal matters such as inheritance and adoption. See also K. Kapparis 'Was atimia for debts to the state inherited through women?' *RIDA* 41 (1994) 113-21.
24. See Dem. 57,54.67; Din. 2,17; Arist. *Ath.* 55,2 and Rhodes *AP* 617-18; H.J. Rose 'The religion of a Greek household' *Euphrosyne* 1 (1957) 95-116.
25. The most comprehensive account of conflict among men in the household is provided by B.S. Strauss *Fathers and sons* 130-78.
26. See also K. Kapparis *Against Neaira* 14-16; L. Foxhall 'Household, gender and property in classical Athens' *CQ* 39 (1989) 22-44; V.J. Hunter *Policing Athens* 9-42; P.G. McC Brown 'Love and marriage in Greek comedy' *CQ* 43 (1993) 189-205; Lacey *Family* passim, M. Golden *Children and childhood* 23-50; B.S. Strauss *Fathers and sons* 33-53; S.B. Pomeroy *Xenophon Oeconomicus* passim, *Families* 17-66; C. Patterson *Family* passim.
27. Arist. *EE* 1241b24-32.
28. See e.g. Dem. 43,19 and B.S. Strauss *Fathers and sons* 68-9; the law is quoted by Apollodorus (Dem. 46,14) word for word. See also Chapter 4 §i.
29. On adoption and the continuation of the *oikos* see L. Rubinstein *Adoption* passim.
30. See esp. 19,178-81.
31. Philo 5,154 Cohn.
32. See Musonius *Diss.* 15, and Chapter 5 §iii.
33. Hip. *Epid.* 5,238 (5,53); see also Demand *Birth* 57-8.
34. Pl. *Lg.* 5,737c-d
35. Enlightened *turannoi* such as Peisistratus in Athens or Dionysius I in Syracuse would do their best to give an appearance of legitimacy to their rule by respecting constitutional formalities such as inviting assemblies. However, they were not bound to respect the wishes of the people unless they chose to do so, and sometimes they did.
36. Arist. *Ath.* 26,4; see also *Pol.* 1275b31, 1278a34; Plu. *Per.* 37; C. Hignett *A history of the Athenian Constitution to the end of the fifth century* BC (Oxford 1952) 343-7; Rhodes *AP* 331-5; C. Patterson *Pericles' citizenship law of 451-50 BC* (Salem N.H. 1981) esp. 140-50; R. Sealey 'On lawful concubinage in Athens' *ClAnt* 3 (1984) 111-33; K.R. Walters 'Pericles' citizenship law' *ClAnt* 2 (1983) 314-36; A.L. Boegehold in *Athenian identity and civic ideology* ed. A.L. Boegehold & A. Scafuro (Baltimore 1994) 57-67; D. Ogden *Greek bastardy in the classical and hellenistic period* (Oxford 1996) 59-69.
37. Th. 8,67-9; Arist. *Ath.* 29,2-5, 32,1 and Rhodes *AP* 362-415; Lys. 12,65.
38. D.S. 18,18.
39. Arist. *Pol.* 1271a6-37.

40. Arist. *Pol.* 1270a29-32.

41. See X. *Lac.* 1,6; Plu. *Lys.* 30,7; *Lyc.* 15,1-3; D.M. MacDowell *Spartan law* 71-88; D. Daube 'The duty of procreation' *Proceedings of the Classical Association* 74 (1977) 10-25.

42. On Sparta's population problems see Hdt. 7,234,2 in combination with Th. 5,68, X. *HG* 4,2,16; 4,15,17; 6,1,1; P. Cartledge *Sparta and Laconia* (London 1979) 307-18.

43. Pl. *R.* 460a-461c.

44. See E. Nardi *Aborto* 116-22; M. Moissides *Janus* 18 (1913) 413-22, 643-9; 19 (1914) 289-311; G. van N. Viljoen in *Acta Classica* 2 (1959) 60-3; H.D. Rankin in *Hermes* 93 (1965) 407-20; W.W. Fortenbaugh in *Arethusa* 8 (1975) 283-305; M. Golding & M. Naomi in *Arethusa* 8 (1975) 345-58; J.J. Mulhern in *Arethusa* 8 (1975) 265-81.

45. See. Ps-Plu. *Placit. Philosoph.* 5,15,1; cf. Chapter 2.

46. Tertullian *De anima* 25,2.

47. Arist. *Pol.* 1335b19-26.

48. Aristotle agrees with Plato (*R.* 460c, *Th.* 160e) that disabled children should not be reared: see the discussion in Chapter 5 §v.

49. Cic. *Clu.* 32.

50. On the measures of the Roman state to encourage maternity see S. Dixon *Roman mother* (London & Sydney 1988) 71-104.

51. On the laws of Augustus see Chapter 4 §iv.

52. See the interesting article by M.K. Gamel in *Helios* 16 (1989) 183-206; L. Cahoon in *TAPhA* 118 (1988) 293-307; O. Steen Due in *C&M* 32 (1980) 133-50; W.J. Watts in *AC* 16 (1973) 89-101.

53. That is, the lover of a woman who had the abortion. Literary scholars use the term *amator* (lover) in order to avoid getting involved in the eternally controversial issue whether the views expressed are really those of the poet himself. I am much less concerned with such issues. Although stylisation and literary purposes cannot be ignored, the historian primarily needs to search for a reflection of the ideology of the Augustan era in Ovid's work.

54. According to the poet here, even the child-killing Medea could be excused because her actions were dictated by love for her husband, while women like Corinna in the poem, having abortions secretly and for no good reason, have no such excuse. As we have seen, Procne killed her son Itys to take vengeance on her husband Tereus (S. fr. 580-95 Radt [*Tereus*], Ovid *Met.* 6,424 ff.).

55. The two abortion poems in the *Amores* (13, 14) have been considered distasteful by some, while others feel that 'these poems do Ovid credit' (E. Eyben in *AncSoc* 11 [1980] 51-3); see also J. Booth *Ovid Amores II* (Warminster 1991) com. ad. loc. Booth characterises this account of the topic of abortion as 'startlingly new to personal love poetry'.

56. Musonius Rufus *Diss.* 15.

57. For further discussion of Musonius' views see E. Nardi *Aborto* 12-16 and 283.

58. Important studies on Achaemenid Persia are I. Gershevitch (ed.) *The Cambridge history of Iran* vol. 2 (Cambridge 1985); A.T. Olmstead *History of the Persian empire* (Oxford 1948); J. Wiesehöfer *Ancient Persia from 550 BC to 650 AD* (New York 1996); P. Briant *Histoire de l' Empire Perse: de Cyrus à Alexandre* (Paris 1996); M. Brosius *Women in Ancient Persia 559-331 BC* (Oxford 1998).

59. Hdt. 1,136-7.

60. See A.T. Olmstead *History* 133; on the *Videvdad* see *Cambridge history* 664-97.

61. The reader will probably find interesting the modern perspectives on the issue as presented by J. Woods in *Engineered death*.

62. The standard study on adoption is L. Rubinstein *Adoption in IV century Athens*.

63. For example, the speaker in Isaeus 2,25 says that Menecles, when he adopted a son, was hoping that the adoptee would take care of him while he was alive, and perform the appropriate burial rites when he was dead.

64. S. *OT* 774-93.

65. The primary source suggesting that the adoptee had to be a citizen, and perhaps legitimate, is Isaeus 7,16. The interpretation of this source creates several problems, briefly presented by A.R. Harrison (*Law of Athens* 1,84-9). See also L. Rubinstein *Adoption* 18-19.

66. Adoption of girls was perfectly possible (e.g. Isaeus 7,9, 11,8. 41), but as D.M. MacDowell (*Law in classical Athens* 101) puts it ' it was obviously more efficient to adopt a male at once than to adopt a female and hope that she would produce a son eventually'.

67. See for example the tale of Herodotus (1,108-21) on how baby Cyrus was a replacement for the dead baby of the couple who adopted him, and the joke in the *Thesmophoriazousai* (502-16) that the baby boy of the slave would be presented to the husband by the conspiring women as his own son.

68. See e.g. Hdt. 1,116; E. *Ion* 956; Pl. *Tht.* 149a-151c and 160e-161a; Arist. *Pol.* 1335a19; Isoc. 5,66; Ar. *Nub.* 531; *Th.* 502 ff.; Sch. Ar. *V.* 286 ff.

69. See e.g. Terence *Hauton Tim.* 626-7, Ovid *Met.* 9,678, Apul. *Met.* 10,23.

70. *P.Oxy.* 11,744.

71. Law of Gortyn *IC* 4,72.

72. S.J. Milligan's PhD thesis *Treatment of infants*. The list of all known cases of exposed children, which contains mythological as well as allegedly actual cases, can be found in her Table 2, p. 229 ff. Unfortunately the excellent thesis of Dr Milligan has not yet been published. I am grateful to Professor D.M. MacDowell for allowing me to borrow the copy that belongs to the Department of Classics in Glasgow.

73. H. Bolkestein in *CPh* 17 (1922) 222-39.

74. A. Cameron in *CR* 46 (1932) 105-14.

75. A.W. Gomme *The population of Athens*; D. Engels in *CPh* 75 (1980) 112-20.

76. W.V. Harris in *CQ* 32 (1982) 114-16; M. Golden in *Phoenix* 35 (1981) 316-31.

77. E. Eyben in *AncSoc* 11 (1980) 5-82. See also R. Odenziel 'The history of infanticide in antiquity' in J. Block & P. Mason (ed.) *Sexual asymmetry* 87-107; R.H. Feen 'Abortion and exposure in ancient Greece' in Bondeson et al. (ed.) *Abortion* 283-300; L.P. Wilkinson 'Population and family planning' in *Classical attitudes to modern issues*; A. Cameron in *CR* 46 (1932) 105-14; H. Bolkestein in *CPh* 17 (1922) 222-39; La Rue Van Hook in *TAPhA* 51 (1920) 134-43.

78. C. Patterson in *TAPhA* 115 (1983) 103-23.

79. Milligan's table of all attested cases would confirm Patterson's conclusion that girls probably did not fare worse than boys; however, one should bear in mind that this table could not really accommodate anonymous true incidents.

80. Plu. *Lyc.* 16,1-2. The translation is that of D.M. MacDowell *Spartan law* 52-4. See also M. Huys in *AncSoc* 27 (1996) 47-74; P. Roussel in *REA* 45 (1943) 5-17.

81. P. Cartledge (*Agesilaos and the crisis of Sparta* [London & Baltimore 1987] 22-3) provides various explanations as to why a boy with congenital disabilities was allowed not only to live, but also go through full training (*agôgê*), and finally become king. None of these explanations is convincing: things would be much simpler if we assumed that the exposure of disabled babies in Sparta was nothing more than an exaggeration which became a legend.

82. See e.g. A. Powell *Athens and Sparta* (London & New York 1988) 219.

83. E. *Ion* 10-56 (Loeb translation with minor modifications).

84. S. *OT* 711-22.

85. Hdt. 1,107-13.

86. In one of these dreams Mandane urinates so much that the whole of Asia sinks in a sea of urine, and in another a vine tree springs out of the genitalia of Mandane and overwhelms the whole of Asia.

87. Seneca *Moral Essays I,* Loeb p. 144

88. Juv. *Sat.* 2,36-40; see also Pliny *Ep.* 4,11,6; Suet. *Dom.* 22.

89. On adultery in ancient societies see Chapter 4 §i.

90. See the discussion of the law-code of Darius in Chapter 5 §iv.

6. Abortion and the Law

1. And. 1,83.

2. See e.g. Dem. 24,139-43.

3. Particularly informative on the legal and social struggle regarding abortion in Ireland and other European countries are the following: B. Rolston & A. Eggert (ed.) *Abortion in the new Europe*; T. Hesketh *The second partitioning of Ireland?*; B. Brookes *Abortion in England, 1900-1967*; B. Girvin 'Ireland and the European Union' in M. Githens & D.M. Stetson (ed.) *Abortion politics* (New York & London 1996) 165-86.

4. A substantial number of studies explores the relationship of attitudes towards abortion and the law in modern times. See M. Boyle *Re-thinking abortion*; P. Cozic & J. Petrikin *The abortion controversy*; R. Dworkin *Life's dominion*; C.N. Flanders *Abortion*; L.T. Lee *Brief survey of abortion laws*; A.F. Guttmacher (ed.) *The case for legalized abortion now*; J.E. Bates & E.S. Zawadzki *Criminal abortion*; P. Ramsey *Ethics at the edges of life*; R. Solinger *Abortion wars*; J. Woods *Engineered death*; D.T. Smith (ed.) *Abortion and the law*; A. Kulczycki *The abortion debate*; J. Van der Tak *Abortion, fertility, and changing legislation*; D. Callahan *Abortion*; K. Hindell & M. Simms *Abortion law reformed*.

5. Among numerous studies discussing abortion and Christian views on human life the reader may find the following particularly useful: S.J. Heaney (ed.) *Abortion: a new generation of Catholic responses*; R.F.R. Gardner *Abortion: the personal dilemma*; W.O. Spitzer & C.L. Saylor (ed.) *Birth control and the Christian*; J.T. Noonan *Contraception: a history of its treatment by Catholic theologians and canonists*; P. Cozic & J. Petrikin *The abortion controversy*; M.J. Gorman *Abortion and the early church*.

6. The authorship of the tetralogies is contested, but Antiphon could have written them, and this is sufficient for my point.

7. Ant. 4,a,2-4.

8. The main studies on Athenian homicide law are D.M. MacDowell *Athenian homicide law in the age of the orators*; M. Gagarin *Drakon and early Athenian homicide law* (New Haven 1981); A. Tulin *Dike Phonou: the right of prosecution and Attic homicide procedure* (Stuttgart 1996); E. Carawan *Rhetoric and the law of Draco*.

9. E. Nardi *Aborto* 132-4, 191-3, 213-4, 394-5; id. 'Antiche prescrizioni greche di purità culturale in thema d'aborto' in *Eranion in honorem G.S. Maridakis* (Athens 1963) vol. 1, 43-85; id. 'Altre antiche prescrizioni greche di purità culturale in thema d'aborto' in *Studi in onore di Edoardo Volterra* (Milan 1969) vol. 1, 141-8.

10. The referee for Duckworth suggested that I use the word 'miscarriage' in the translation of the documents, not 'abortion', since most of the documents probably have in mind a spontaneous abortion. This is a good point; however, the Greek original does not make such distinctions. The verb is usually *ektitrôskein* (or sometimes *ambliskein* or *ambloun*) and the nouns are *ektrôsis, trôsmos, trôma, amblôsis*. All these can be used indiscriminately for a spontaneous or an induced abortion. *apoballein/ apobolê* on the other hand, exclusively used for a miscarriage, are never employed in any of these documents. I wonder whether this is significant, but probably we should not read too much in this vocabulary.

11. *SEG* 9,72, vv. 106-9.

12. R. Herzog 'Heilige Gesetze von Kos' in *Abhandlungen der preussischen Akademie der Wissenschaften, Jahrgang 1928, philosophisch-historische Klasse* p. 15.

13. Herzog 14.20; and also R. Herzog 'Aus dem Asklepeion von Kos, II *Hagneiai* und *Katharmoi* im koischen Demeterdienst' in *ARW* 10 (1907) 401.

14. *SEG* 14,529.

15. P. Roussel 'Règlements rituels' in *Mélanges Holleaux: Recueil de mémoires concernant l'antiquité grecque offert a Maurice Holleaux* (Paris 1913) 268.

16. The actual point in the text where words such as 'birth' or 'abortion' would be included is not preserved, but I agree with previous scholars that these words must have been part of the missing text. See E. Nardi 'Antiche prescrizioni greche' in *Eranion* 1, 60-2.

17. See F. Preisigke, F. Bilabel & E. Kiessling *Sammelbuch griechischer Urkunden aus Ägypten* (Strassburg 1915) 1-2.

18. An alternative name for Dionysus.

19. Sokolowski, *LSA* 84.

20. Ziehen in *SIG* 3, 148.

21. Sokolowski, *LSG* 159.

22. *IGA* 74.

23. R. Parker *Miasma: pollution and purification in early Greek religion* (Oxford 1983) passim.

24. Athenagoras Apol. *Legatio sive supplicatio pro Christianis* 35,6.

25. Y. Courtone *St Basile: Lettres* vol. 2 (Paris: Les belles lettres, 1961) Letter to Amphilochios 2.

26. See e.g. E. Caillemer 'Amblôseôs graphê' in *Dictionnaire des antiquités grecques et romaines* 224-5; A.R. Harrison *Law* 1, 72-3 (the views of Harrison are discussed in greater detail in Chapter 6 §iii.). N. Demand (*Birth, death and motherhood* esp. 55-7, 103-7) argues that it was the father's right, not the life of the infant which was violated.

27. Dem. 43,75

28. D.S. 1,77,9. See also E. Nardi *Aborto* 225 n. 53; G. Glotz *Solidarité* 352.

29. I quote here the results of lexicographic research using the *Latin Texts* (PHI 5) CD-Rom.

30. C.H. Brecht in *RE* 18,4 2046-8; G. Glotz *Solidarité* 351-5.

31. E. Eyben *AncSoc* 11 (1980) 21-2; E. Nardi *Aborto* 33-41.

32. See Aesch. 2,93; 3,51.212; Dem. 40,32; 54,18; Lys. 3,38-48; 4,18; 6,15; D.M. MacDowell *Law in classical Athens* 123-4.

33. Ps.-Gal. 19,179.

34. R. Crahay *AC* 10 (1941) 12; E. Nardi *Aborto* 33-41.

35. There is a striking example of this practice in Aesch. 1,26, where the orator attributes to Solon the procedure of the fourth-century Assembly. See also D.M. MacDowell *Spartan law* 1-22; E. Ruschenbusch *Solonos Nomoi* (Wiesbaden 1966).

36. Ps.-Gal. 19,179-180.

37. Plu. *Alex.* 77.

38. Curt. 10,6-10; D.S. 17,117,3; 18,2-4. Neither Philip III nor Alexander IV was in a position to govern. The first had a serious mental disability, while the second never lived to reach adulthood. Both fell victim to the power struggle among the Diadochoi.

39. Musonius Rufus *Diss.* 15.

40. See Chapter 5 §ii.

41. See e.g. J.S. Murray 'The alleged prohibition of abortion in the Hippocratic Oath' *EMC* 35 (1991) 293-311; J. Gardner *Women in Roman law and society* 158-9; R. Flemming, *Medicine* 169; cf. also N. Demand *Birth, death and motherhood* esp. 55-7, 103-7.

42. Caracalla enfranchised the entire population of the Roman empire through the *Constitutio Antoniana* in AD 212, that is, perhaps only a year or two after the law of Severus-Caracalla banned abortion. See Chapter 5 §iv.

43. Sauppe considered this speech to be a rhetorical exercise with the above-mentioned Hippocratic and Galenic passages (8a and b) providing the basic materials. E. Nardi (*Aborto* 86 n. 135) disagrees, and so do I. Some of the rhetoricians thought that it might not be authentic Lysias, but all ancient sources understand that it was a true law-court speech from the classical period.

44. The evidence of this passage on the penalties for failure to pursue a public prosecution seems to be contradicted by Dem. 59,53 and 68. Twice Stephanus is able to reach a private reconciliation with men against whom he had submitted a *graphê* (Phrastor and Epainetus) without any penalty. Probably the state did not penalise someone who decided well in advance of the trial to drop the public prosecution in favour of a private compromise, either through direct conciliation or through private arbitration. I cannot see why the state would force a trial if a resolution like this could be effected, which ultimately would save jury time and money. If so, then it is clear that Antigenes II and the woman's adult sons from a previous marriage who were speaking in her defence, could not reach a compromise. Perhaps the words from the defence speech quoted here refer to an unsuccessful attempt to find an alternative solution before going to court. If Antigenes II, as the prosecutor, unilaterally abandoned proceedings and did not turn up for the trial on the set date, either because he did not want to, or because he was afraid that he might lose very badly (less than a fifth of the votes with the resulting penalty of 1000 drachmas), understandably he should be liable to a fine for wasting the court's time and resources. On this issue see also D.M. MacDowell *Demosthenes: Against Meidias* edited with introduction, translation and commentary (Oxford 1989) 327-8.

45. A.R. Harrison *Law* 1, 72-3. Harrison seems to imply that Antigenes was claiming the woman as an *epiklêros*. But since she had adult male brothers, those who are defending their mother, she could not be an *epiklêros*.

46. G. Glotz *Solidarité* 351.

47. Lipsius *Recht* 608 ff.; E. Nardi *Aborto* 82-93.

48. *paradoxos* is the word he uses in no. 3.

49. With regard to the debate on the title of the speech see E. Nardi *Aborto* 85 n. 134. I consider this debate to be irrelevant, since, according to my interpretation, we have two different speeches.

50. All Athenian magistrates underwent an auditing of their conduct in office when their term expired. During this auditing, called *euthuna*, any citizen could come forward and accuse them of not performing their duties properly. In that case the magistrate under scrutiny would face trial for misconduct. The Athenian *demos* was a strict supervisor of its officials.

51. On the reputation of the Areopagus see R. Wallace *The Areopagos Council* *to 307 BC* (Baltimore 1988) 126-7; O. de Bruyn *La compétence de l'Areopage en matière de procès publics* (Stuttgart 1995) 155-64.

52. The aforementioned studies of Wallace and O. de Bruyn provide excellent accounts of the difficult evidence on the functions of the Areopagus.

53. Especially sections 178-80 (see Appendix 1).

54. Cic. *Brutus* 313.

Appendix 1

1. Gal. 6,701-2. On the issue of the authorship of this study see further Hermann Wagner *Galeni qui fertur libellus 'Ei zoon to kata gastros'* (Diss. Madburg 1914) xiv-xix.

2. On rhetoric in ancient medical literature see A.M. Battegazzore (ed.) *Dimostrazione, argomentazione dialettica e argomentazione retorica nel pensiero antico* (Genoa 1993).

3. On the sources see also Wagner op. cit. in n. 1, pp. xix-xxiii. A systematic account of these (and more) sources is outside my purposes at this point; a forthcoming independent article explores this issue and other aspects of this fascinating treatise in greater detail. Here I simply present an overview and some basic explanatory notes intended to serve as an orientation to the difficult issues that this study explores.

4. This translation is mainly based upon the text of Kühn, which broadly represents the tradition of L (Laurentianus 74,3), the most complete, and arguably the most authoritative, among the manuscripts of Galen. H. Wagner (op. cit. in n. 1) considers P (Parisinus 3035) a very important manuscript and consequently adopts in his edition many of the readings of P. (See the detailed discussion in his introduction, and the stemma on p. xii.) However, it seems to me that the readings of L are closer to the ancient tradition of the text, even though this manuscript has many shortcomings and often cries out for scholarly intervention. That is why I have used the text of Kühn, aware of its shortcomings and prepared to follow Wagner where his text appears to be more satisfactory, or even introduce my own emendations. However, this appendix is not the place for textual criticism or detailed philological arguments. Some of my observations on this text and its history are presented in a forthcoming independent article, while a proper critical edition with detailed commentary is among my long-term plans. Here it will suffice to say that I have tried to present as accurate, correct and fluent an English version of a very difficult Greek text as I can.

Appendix 2

1. For the text see F. Sokolowski *Lois sacrées de l'Asie Mineure* (Paris 1955) pp. 53-8, no. 20 (*LSA* 20). For rich bibliography on this document see E. Nardi in *Eranion* vol. 1, pp. 65-71, and more recently Parker *Miasma* 355-6.

2. E. Nardi *Aborto* 194-4.

3. Scribonius Largus *Compositiones,* Praef. 5,20-3

4. Especially sections 64-87, where Apollodorus expounds the alleged impieties of Phano against the god Dionysus. After she was caught committing adultery, and in spite of this she acted as priestess on behalf of the city at the festival of the Anthesteria. Not only she entered the temple of the god, from which she ought to have refrained, but also saw and performed sacred and secret rituals. The orator states that a punishment from the god is imminent, and unless the jury imposes it, the anger of the god will be directed against the entire city.

5. For a detailed presentation of the relevant documents see Chapter 6 §i.

Select Bibliography

Achterberg, J. *Woman as healer* (London 1991).

Aleshire, S.B. *The Athenian Asklepieion: the people, their dedications, and the inventories* (Amsterdam 1991).

Amundsen, D.W. *Medicine, society and faith in the ancient and medieval worlds* (Baltimore 1996).

Asheri, D. 'Laws of inheritance, distribution of land and political constitutions in ancient Greece' *Historia* 12 (1963) 1-21.

Balss, H. 'Die Zeugungslehre und Embryologie in der Antike' *Quellen und Studien zur Geschichte der Naturwissenschaften und der Medizin* 5 (1934) 1-82.

Bates, J.E. & Zawadzki, E.S. *Criminal abortion: a study in medical sociology* (Springfield, Il. 1964).

Beagon, M. *Roman nature: the thought of Pliny the Elder* (Oxford 1992).

Bequaert Holmes, H. *Issues in reproductive technology: an anthology* (New York & London 1992) esp. 113-92.

Bérard, J. 'Problèmes démographiques dans l'histoire de la Grèce antique' *Population* 1 (1947) 303-12.

Bolkestein, H. 'The exposure of children at Athens and the *enchytristriai*' *CPh* 17 (1922) 222-39.

Bondeson, W.B, Engelhardt, H.T., Spicker, S.F. & Winship, D.H. (ed.) *Abortion and the status of the foetus* (Dordrecht 1983).

Boyle, M. *Re-thinking abortion: psychology, gender, power, and the law* (London & New York 1997).

Brecht, C.H. 'Partus abactio' *RE* 18,4, 2046-8.

Brody, B.A. *Abortion and the sanctity of human life: a philosophical view* (Cambridge, Mass. 1975).

Brookes, B. *Abortion in England, 1900-1967* (London & New York 1988).

Browder, C. *The wickedest woman in New York: Madame Restell, the abortionist* (Hamden 1988).

Burguière, P., Gourevitch, D. & Malinas, Y. *Maladies des femmes*, tome 1, livre 1: *Soranos d'Éphèse: texte établi, traduit et commenté* (Paris: Les belles lettres, 1988).

Byl, S. 'Les grands traités biologiques d'Aristote et la collection Hippocratique' in *Corpus Hippocraticum: actes du Colloque Hippocratique de Mons*, ed. R. Joly (Mons 1977) 313-32.

Cahoon, L. 'The bed as battlefield: erotic conquest and military metaphor in Ovid's *Amores*' *TAPhA* 118 (1988) 293-307.

Caillemer, E. '*Amblôseôs graphê*' in *Dictionnaire des antiquités grecques et romaines*, ed. C. Daremberg & E. Saglio, vol. 1 (1877) 224-5.

Callahan, D. *Abortion: law, choice, and morality* (New York 1970).

Cameron, A. 'The exposure of children and Greek ethics' *CR* 46 (1932) 105-14.

Carawan, E. *Rhetoric and the law of Draco* (Oxford 1998).

Carrick, P. *Medical ethics in antiquity: philosophical perspectives on abortion and euthanasia* (Dordrecht 1985).

Cohn-Haft, L. *The public physicians of ancient Greece*, Smith College Studies in History 42 (1956).

Cooke, C.W. & Dworkin, S., *The Ms Guide to a woman's health* (New York 1979) esp. pp. 187-206.

Cornell, D. *The imaginary domain: abortion, pornography & sexual harassment* (New York 1995).

Cozic, P. & Petrikin, J. *The abortion controversy* (San Diego 1995).

Crahay, R. 'Les moralistes anciens et l'avortement' *AC* 10 (1941) 11.

Craik, E.M. *Hippocrates: Places in man*, Greek text and translation with introduction and commentary (London 1988).

Daly A., *Women under the knife: a history of surgery* (New York 1991).

Dean-Jones, L. *Women's bodies in classical Greek science* (Oxford 1994).

—— 'The cultural construct of the female body' in S.B. Pomeroy (ed.) *Women's history and ancient history* (Chapel Hill & London 1991) 111-37.

De Lacy, P. 'Galen's Platonism' *AJP* 93 (1973) 27-39.

Delcourt, M. *Stérilités mystérieuses et naissances maléfiques dans l'antiquité classique* (Liege 1938).

Demand, N. *Birth, death and motherhood in classical Greece* (Baltimore 1994).

DeMause, L. (ed.) *The history of childhood* (New York 1974).

Den Boer, W. 'Private morality in Greece and Rome' in *Abortion and family planning* (Leiden 1979) 272-88.

Denes, M. *In necessity and sorrow: life and death in an abortion hospital* (New York 1976).

Devereux, G. *A study of abortion in primitive societies* (New York 1955).

Dickison, S.K. 'Abortion in antiquity' *Arethusa* 6 (1973) 159-66.

Drabkin, I.E. 'On medical education in Greece and Rome' *BHM* 15 (1944) 333-51.

Dreichgräber, K. *Der Hippokratische Eid* (Stuttgart 1955).

—— 'Die ärtzliche Standesethik des hippokratischen Eides' *Quellen und Studien zur Geschichte der Naturwissenschaften und der Medizin* 3 (1933) 79-99, reprinted in H. Flashar (ed.) *Antike Medizin* (Darmstadt 1971) 94-120.

—— *Die griechische Empirikerschule: Sammlung der Fragmente und Darstellung der Lehre* (Berlin & Zurich 1965).

—— 'Professio Medici: Zum Vorwort des Scribonius Largus' *Abhandlungen der Akademie der Wissenschaften und der Literatur, geistes- und sozialwissenschaftliche Klasse*, 9 (Wiesbaden 1950).

Dölger, M.F.J. 'Das Lebensrecht des ungeborenes Kindes und die Fruchtabtreibung in der Bewertung der heidnischen und christlichen Antike' *Antike und Christentum* 4 (1933) 1-61.

Due, O.S. 'Amores und Abtreibung' *C&M* 32 (1980) 133-50.

Duke, J.A. *Handbook of medicinal herbs* (Boca Raton 1985).

Dworkin, R. *Life's dominion: an argument about abortion, euthanasia and individual freedom* (New York 1993).

Edelstein, L. *The Hippocratic oath* (Baltimore 1943).

—— 'The relation of ancient philosophy to medicine' *BHM* 26 (1952) 299-316.

—— 'The professional ethics of the Greek physician' *BHM* 30 (1956) 391-419.

Edwards, C. *The politics of immorality in ancient Rome* (Cambridge 1993).

Engels, D. 'The problem of female infanticide in the Graeco-Roman world' *CPh* 75 (1980) 112-20.

Eyben, E. 'Family planning in Graeco-Roman antiquity' *AncSoc* 11 (1980) 5-82.

Feen, R.H. 'Abortion and exposure in Ancient Greece: assessing the status of the fetus and the "newborn" from classical sources' in Bondeson et al. (ed.) *Abortion* 283-300.

Flanders, C.N. *Abortion* (New York 1991).

Flashar, H. (ed.) *Antike Medizin* (Darmstadt 1971).

—— & Jouanna, J. (ed.) *Médecine et morale dans l'antiquité* (Geneva 1997) 297-322.

Flemming, R. *Medicine and the making of Roman women: gender, nature and authority from Celsus to Galen* (Oxford 2000).

Fortenbaugh, W.W. 'Plato: temperament and eugenic policy' *Arethusa* 8 (1975) 283-305.

Fournier, P. 'A propos des "expositi" ' *Revue historique de droit français et étranger* 5 (1926) 302-8.

Frede, M. 'The method of the so-called Methodical School of Medicine' in J. Barnes et al. (ed.) *Science and speculation: studies in hellenistic theory and practice* (Cambridge 1982) 1-23.

—— 'The empiricist attitude towards reason and theory' in R.J. Hankinson (ed.) *Method, mdicine and mtaphysics: sudies in the philosophy of ancient science* (Edmonton 1988) 79-97.

French, R. & Greenaway, F. (ed.) *Science in the early Roman empire: Pliny the Elder, his sources and influence* (London 1986).

French, V. 'Midwives and maternity care in the Roman world' *Helios* 13 (1986) 69-84.

Gamel, M.K. '*Non sine caede*: abortion politics and poetics in Ovid's *Amores*' *Helios* 16 (1989) 183-206.

Garcìa Ballester, L. 'Soul and body, disease of the soul and disease of the body in Galen's medical thought' in P. Manuli & M. Vegetti (ed.) *Le opere psichologiche di Galeno: Atti del terzo colloquio Galenico Internazionale, Pavia, 10-12 settembre 1986* (Pavia 1988) 117-52.

Gardner, J.F. *Women in Roman law and society* (London 1986).

—— *Being a Roman citizen* (London & New York 1993).

Gardner, R.F.R. *Abortion: the personal dilemma* (Grand Rapids 1972).

Garnsey, P. *Famine and food supply in the Graeco-Roman world: responses to risk and crisis* (Cambridge 1988).

Germain, L.R.F. 'Aspects du droit d'exposition en Grèce' *Revue historique de droit français et étranger* 47 (1969) 177-97.

—— 'L'exposition des enfants nouveau-nés dans la Grèce ancienne. Aspects sociologiques' *Recueils de la Société Jean Bodin pour l'histoire comparative des institutions. L'Enfant.* 1er partie: *Antiquité – Afrique – Asie* (Brussels 1975).

—— 'Le mythe et le droit: l'exposition des enfants nouveau-nés dans la mythologique grecque' *Revue historique de droit français et étranger* 56 (1978) 699-700.

Gernet. L. *Droit et société dans la Grèce ancienne* (Paris 1955).

Githens, M. & Stetson, D.M. (ed.) *Abortion politics* (New York & London 1996).

Glotz, G. *La solidarité de la famille dans le droit criminel en Grèce* (Paris 1904).

Golden, M. 'Demography and the exposure of girls at Athens' *Phoenix* 35 (1981) 316-31.

Golding, M. & Naomi, H. 'Population policy in Plato and Aristotle: some value issues' *Arethusa* 8 (1975) 345-58.

Gomme, A.W. *The population of Athens in the fifth and fourth centuries BC* (Oxford 1933).

Gorman, M.J. *Abortion and the early Church: Christian, Jewish and pagan attitudes in the Graeco-Roman world* (Downers Grove 1982).

Green, P.M. *Prolegomena to the study of magic and superstition in the Natural History of Pliny the Elder* (PhD thesis, University of Cambridge 1954).

Grensemann, H. *Hippokrates über Achtmonatskinder, über das Siebenmonatskind (unecht). Corpus Medicorum Graecorum* 1,2,1.

—— *Hippokratische Gynäkologie: die gynäkologischen Texte des Autors nach den pseudoHippokratischen Schriften de Mulieribus I, II und de Sterilibus* (Wiesbaden 1982).

Grubbs, E. *Law and family in late antiquity* (Oxford 1995).

Guttmacher, A.F. (ed.) *The case for legalized abortion now* (Berkeley 1967).

Hahn, J. 'Plinius und die griechischen Ärze im Rom: Naturkonzepten und Medizinkritik in der Naturalis Historia' *Sudhoffs Archiv* 75 (1991) 209-39.

Hands, A.R. *Charities and social aid in Greece and Rome* (London 1968).

Hankinson, R.T. 'Galen and the best of all possible worlds', *CQ* 39 (1989) 206-27.

—— 'Galen's anatomy of the soul' *Phronesis* 36 (1991) 197-233.

Hanson, A.E. 'Graeco-Roman gynecology' *SAMPh Newsletter* 17 (1989) 83-92.

—— 'The logic of the gynaecological prescriptions' in Juan Antonio López Férez (ed.) *Tratados Hipocráticos* (Madrid 1992) 235-50.

—— 'The medical writers' woman', in D. Halperin, J. Winkler & F. Zeitlin (ed.) *Before sexuality: the construction of erotic experience in the ancient Greek world* (Princeton 1990) 309-38.

Harris, W.V. 'The theoretical possibility of extensive infanticide in the Graeco-Roman world' *CQ* 32 (1982) 114-16.

Harrison, A.R. *The law of Athens* (Oxford 1968).

Hartmann, H. 'Abortio' *RE* 11 (1877) 7-8.

Hatcher, R.A. et al. *Contraceptive technology 1990-1992* (15th edition; New York 1990).

Heaney, S.J. (ed.) *Abortion: a new generation of Catholic responses* (Braintree, Mass. 1992).

Hesketh, T. *The second partitioning of Ireland?: the abortion referendum of 1983* (Dun Laoghaire 1990).

Himes, N. *Medical history of contraception* (Baltimore 1936).

Hindell, K. & Simms, M. *Abortion law reformed* (London 1971).

Hodkinson, S. 'Land tenure and inheritance in classical Sparta' *CQ* 36 (1986) 378-406.

Hopkins, K. 'Contraception in the Roman empire' *Comparative Studies in Society and History* 8 (1965-6) 124-51.

Horobin, G. (ed.) *Experience with abortion: a case study of north-east Scotland* (Cambridge 1973).

Horowitz, M. C. 'Aristotle and woman' *Journal of the History of Biology* 9 (1976) 183-213.

Horstmanshoff, H.F.J. 'The ancient physician: craftsman or scientist?' *Journal of the History of Medicine and Allied Sciences* 45 (1990) 176-97.

Humbert, G. 'Abigere partum' *Dictionnaire des antiquités grecques et romaines* ed. C. Daremberg & G. Saglio, vol. 1 (1877) 7-10.

Huys, M. 'The Spartan practice of selective infanticide and its parallels in ancient Utopian tradition' *AncSoc* 27 (1996) 47-74.

Ilberg, J. 'Zur gynäkologischen Ethik der Griechen' *ARW* 13 (1910) 1-18.

Illingworth, R.S. *The normal child: some problems of the early years and their treatment* (7th edition; Edinburgh, London & New York 1979).

Jaeger, W. 'Aristotle's use of medicine as a model of method in his *Ethics*' *JHS* 77 (1957) 54-61.

Jöchle, Wolfgang 'Menses-inducing drugs: their role in antique medieval and renaissance gynaecology and birth control' *Contraception* 10 (1974) 425-39.

Joly, R. 'La structure du Foetus de huit mois' *AC* 45 (1976) 173-80.

Jones, W.H.S. *The doctor's oath: an essay in the history of medicine* (Cambridge 1924).

Jouanna, J. 'Tradition manuscrite et structure du traité hippocratique Sur le foetus de huit mois' *REG* 86 (1973)1-16.

────── 'Présence d' Empédocle dans la collection hippocratique' *Bulletin de l'Association Guillaume Budé* (1961) 452-63.

Just, R. *Women in Athenian law and life* (London 1989).

Kalmar, R. (ed.) *Abortion: the emotional implications* (Dubuque, Iowa 1977).

Kapparis, K. *Apollodoros 'Against Neaira' [D.59], edited with introduction, translation and commentary* (Berlin & New York 1999).

────── 'Humiliating the adulterer: the law and the practice in classical Athens' *Revue internationale des droits de l'antiquité* 43 (1996) 63-77.

────── 'When were the Athenian adultery laws introduced?', *Revue internationale des droits de l'antiquité* 42 (1995) 97-122.

Keller, A. *Die Abortiva in der römischen Kaiserzeit* (Stuttgart 1988).

King, H. *Hippocrates' woman: reading the female body in ancient Greece* (London & New York 1998).

────── 'Medical texts as a source for women's history' in A. Powell (ed.) *The Greek world* (London 1995) 199-218.

────── 'Food and blood in Hippocratic gynaecology' in J. Wilkins et al. (ed.) *Food in antiquity* (Exeter 1995) 351-8.

────── 'Agnodike and the profession of medicine' *Proceedings of the Cambridge Philological Society* 32 (1986) 53-77.

Krenkel, W.A. 'Erotica I. Der Abortus in der Antike' *Wissenschaftliche Zeitschrift der Universität Rostock: Reihe Gesellschaft und Sprachwissenschaften* 20 (1971) 443-52.

Kudlien, F. 'Medical ethics and popular ethics in Greece and Rome' *Clio Medica* 5 (1970), 91-121.

────── 'Medical education in classical antiquity' in C.D. O'Malley (ed.) *History of medical education* (Berkeley & Los Angeles 1970).

────── 'Galen's religious belief', in V. Nutton (ed.) *Galen: problems and prospects: a collection of papers submitted at the 1979 Cambridge conference* (London 1981) 117-30.

Kulczycki, A. *The abortion debate in the world arena* (New York 1999).

Lacey, W.K. *The family in classical Greece* (Ithaca, NY 1968).

Langslow, D.R. *Medical Latin in the Roman empire* (Oxford 2000).

Lapidge, M. 'Stoic cosmology' in J. Rist (ed.) *The Stoics* (Berkeley & Los Angeles 1978) 161-85.

Lecrivain, C. 'Notes de droit penal grec. II. L'avortement' *Mélanges Gustave Glotz* II (Paris 1932).

Lee, L.T. *Brief survey of abortion laws of five largest countries* (Medford, Mass. 1973).

Lineau, C. 'Die Behandlung und Erwähnung von Superfetation in der Antike' *Clio Medica* 6 (1971) 275-85.

Lipsius, J.H. *Das Attische Recht und Rechtsverfahren* (Leipzig 1915).

Lloyd, G.E.R. *Science, folklore and ideology: studies in the life sciences in ancient Greece* (Cambridge 1983).

────── *Magic, reason and experience: studies in the origin and development of Greek science* (Cambridge 1979).

Long, A.A., 'Soul and body in Stoicism' *Phronesis* 27 (1982) 34-57.

Longrigg, J. *Greek Rational Medicine* (London 1993).

MacDowell, D.M. *The law in classical Athens* (London 1978).

────── *Spartan law* (Edinburgh 1986).

—— *Athenian homicide law in the age of the orators* (Manchester 1963).

McCormick, P.E. *Attitudes toward abortion: experiences of selected black and white women* (Lexington, Mass. 1975).

McGinn, T.A.G., *Prostitution, sexuality and the law in ancient Rome* (Oxford 1998).

McLaren, A. *A history of contraception from antiquity to the present day* (Oxford 1990).

Mayer-Maly, T. 'Abortio' *Kleine Pauly* 1 (1964) col. 16-17.

Milligan, S.J. *The treatment of infants in classical and hellenistic Greece* (PhD thesis; University of Glasgow 1989).

Minuli, P., 'Elogio della castità: la Ginecologia di Sorano' *Memoria* 3 (1982) 39-49.

—— 'Donne mascoline, femmine, sterile, vergini perpetua: ginecologia greca tra Ippocrate e Sorano' in S. Campese, P. Manuli & G. Sissa, *Madre materia: sociologia e biologia de la donna greca* (Turin 1983) 147-92.

—— 'Galen and Stoicism' in J. Kollesch & D. Nickel (ed.) *Galen und das hellenistische Erbe: Verhandlungen des IV. internationalen Galens-Symposium, veranstaltet vom Institut für Geschichte der Medizin am Bereich Medizin (Charite) der Humboldt Universität zu Berlin, 18-20 September 1989*, Sudhoffs Archiv Beihefte 32 (Stuttgart 1993) 53-61.

Moissides, M. 'La puérculture et l'eugenique dans l'antiquité grecque' *Janus* 18 (1913) 413-22, 643-9; 19 (1914) 289-311.

—— 'Contribution à l'étude de l'avortement dans l'antiquité grecque' *Janus* 25 (1921) 59-85.

Morowitz, H.J. & Trefil, J.S. *The facts of life: science and the abortion controversy* (New York 1992).

Muldoon, M. *Abortion: an annotated indexed bibliography* (New York 1980).

Mulhern, J.J. 'Population and Plato's *Republic*' *Arethusa* 8 (1975) 265-81.

Murdy, P. (ed.), *La Preface du De medicina de Celse* (Lausanne 1982).

—— 'Éthique et médecine à Rome: la Préface de Scribonius Largus ou l'affirmation d'une singularité' in H. Flashar & J. Jouanna (ed.) *Médecine et morale dans l'antiquité* (Geneva 1997) 297-322.

Nardi, E. *Procurato aborto nel mondo greco-romano* (Milan 1971).

—— 'Antiche prescrizioni greche di purità culturale in tema d'aborto' *Eranion in honorem G.S. Maridakis* I (Athens 1963) 43-85.

Nickel, D. 'Stoa und Stoiker in Galens Schrift De foetuum formatione' in J. Kollesch & D. Nickel (ed.) *Galen und das hellenistische Erbe: Verhandlungen des IV. internationalen Galens-Symposium, veranstaltet vom Institut für Geschichte der Medizin am Bereich Medizin (Charite) der Humboldt Universität zu Berlin, 18-20 September 1989*, Sudhoffs Archiv Beihefte 32 (Stuttgart 1993) 79-86.

Noonan, J.T. *Contraception: a history of its treatment by Catholic theologians and canonists* (Cambridge 1966) 1-139.

Nutton, V. 'Scribonius Largus, the unknown pharmacologist' *Pharmaceutical Historian* 25 (1995) 5-9.

—— 'The drug trade in antiquity' *Journal of the Royal Society of Medicine* 78 (1985) 138-45.

—— 'Murders and miracles: lay attitudes towards medicine in classical antiquity' in R. Porter (ed.) *Patients and practitioners* (Cambridge 1985).

—— 'The perils of patriotism: Pliny and Roman medicine' in R. French & F. Greenaway (ed.) *Science in the early Roman empire: Pliny the Elder, his sources and influence* (London 1986).

Odenziel, R. 'The history of infanticide in antiquity; a literature stillborn' in *Sexual asymmetry: studies in ancient society* ed. J. Blok & P. Mason (Amsterdam 1987) 87-107.

Oppenheimer, J. 'When sense and life begin: background to a remark in Aristotle's *Politics* (133b24)' *Arethusa* 8 (1975) 331-43.

Osofsky, H.J. & J.D. *The abortion experience: psychological and medical impact* (Hagerstown, Md. 1973).

Patterson, C. 'Not worth the rearing: the causes of infant exposure in ancient Greece' *TAPhA* 115 (1983) 103-23.

Peck, A.L. 'The connate pneuma: an essential factor in Aristotle's solution to the problem of reproduction and sensation' in E.A. Underwood (ed.) *Science, medicine and history: essays in honour of Charles Singer* (London 1953) 111-21.

Phillips, E.D. *Greek medicine* (London 1973).

Pigeaud, J. 'Les fondements théoriques du méthodisme' in P. Murdy & J. Pigeaud (ed.) *Les écoles médicales à Rome: actes du 2ème colloque international sur les textes medicaux latins antiques, Lausanne, septembre 1986* (Geneva 1991) 8-50.

Pomeroy, S. 'Infanticide in hellenistic Greece' in A. Cameron & A. Kuhrt (ed.) *Images of women in antiquity* (London 1983) 207-22.

⸻ *Families in classical and hellenistic Greece* (Oxford 1997).

Porter, I.H. & Hook, E.B. (ed.) *Human embryonic and fetal death* (New York 1980).

Post, L.A. 'Dramatic infants in Greek' *CPh* 34 (1939) 193-208.

Preus, A. 'Biomedical techniques for influencing human reproduction in the fourth century BC' *Arethusa* 8 (1975) 237-63.

Prioreeschi, P. 'Quandoque bonus dormitat Hippokrates: induced abortion and embryo's age in the Hippocratic Corpus' *Acta belgicae historiae medicinae* 5 no. 4 (1992) 181-4.

Raepsaet, G. 'Les motivations de la natalité à Athènes aux Ve et IVe siècles avant notre ère' *AC* 40 (1971) 80-100.

Ramsey, P. *Ethics at the edges of life: medical and legal intersections* (New Haven 1978).

Rankin, H.D. 'Platon's eugenic Euphemia and apothesis in *Republic* book V' *Hermes* 93 (1965) 407-20.

Redford, D.B. 'The literary motif of the exposed child' *Numen* 14 (1967) 209-28.

Reiman, J. *Abortion and the ways we value human life* (Lanham, Md. 1999).

Reinach, S. 'Aôroi biaiothanatoi' *Archiv für Religionswissenschaft* 10 (1906) 320.

Rhodes, P.J. *A commentary on the Aristotelian Athenaion politeia* (Oxford 1981).

Riddle, J.M. *Contraception and abortion from the ancient world to the Renaissance* (Cambridge 1992).

⸻ *Eve's herbs: a history of contraception and abortion in the west* (Cambridge, Mass. 1997).

⸻ *Dioscorides on pharmacy and medicine* (Austin, Tx 1985).

⸻, Worth Estes, J. & Russel, J.C. 'Ever since Eve ... birth control in the ancient world' *Archaeology* (April/May 1994) 29-35.

Rolston, B. & Eggert, A. (ed.) *Abortion in the new Europe: a comparative handbook* (Westport, Conn. 1994).

Roscher, W.H. 'Die enneadischen und hebdomadischen Fristen und Wochen der ältesten Griechen' *Abhandlungen der phil.-hist. Klasse der köningl. Sächsischen Gesellschaft der Wissenschaften* 21.4 (1903).

⸻ 'Die hippokratische Schrift von der Siebenzahl in ihrer vierfachen Überlieferung' *Studien zur Geschichte und Kultur des Altertums* vol. 6, Hefte 3 and 4 (Paderborn 1913).

⸻ 'Die Tessarakontaden und Tessarakontatenlehren der Griechen und anderen Völker' *Berichte über die Verhandl. der köningl. Sächsischen Gesellschaft der Wissenschaften, Leipzig* 61 (1909) 17-204.

Rose, J.H. 'The religion of the Greek household' *Euphrosyne* 1 (1957) 95-116.

Rostofjeff, M. *The social and economic history of the hellenistic world* (Oxford 1941).

Roussel, P. 'L'exposition des enfants à Sparte' *REA* 45 (1943) 5-17.

Rousselle, A. *Porneia: on desire and the body in antiquity* (Oxford 1988).

Rubinstein, G. *The riddle of the Methodist Method: understanding a Roman medical sect* (PhD thesis, University of Cambridge 1985).

Rubinstein, L. *Adoption in IV century Athens* (Copenhagen 1993).

Rudhaardt, J. 'La reconnaisance de la paternité, sa nature et sa portée dans la société athénienne. Sur un discours de Démostene' *MH* 19 (1962) 39-64.

Sabbah, G. & Mudry, P. (ed.) *La Médecine de Celse: aspects historiques, scientifiques et littéraires* (Saint-Étienne 1994).

Samter, E. *Familienfeste der Griechen und Römer* (Berlin 1901).

Scarborough, J. 'Contraception in antiquity: the case of Pennyroyal' *Wisconsin Academy Review* 35 (1989) 19-25.

────── 'Pharmacy in Pliny's *Natural History*: some observations on substances and sources' in R. French & F. Greenaway (ed.), *Science in the early Roman empire: Pliny the Elder, his sources and influence* (London 1986) 59-85.

Schmidt, A. *Drogen und Drogenhandel im Altertum* (Leipzig 1924).

Schmidt, M. 'Hephaistos lebt – Untersuchungen zur Frage der Behandlung behinderter Kinder in der Antike' *Hephaistos* 5-6 (1983-4) 133-61.

Shostak, A.B., McLouth, G. & Seng, L. *Men and abortion: lessons, losses and love* (New York 1984).

Skowronksi, M *Abortion and alternatives* (Millbrae, Ca. 1977).

Sifakis, G.M. 'Children in Greek tragedy' *BICS* 26 (1979) 67-80.

Singer, P. et al. (ed.) *Embryo experimentation* (Cambridge 1990).

Smith, D.T. (ed.) *Abortion and the law* (Cleveland 1967).

Smith, W.D. *The Hippocratic Tradition* (Ithaca 1979).

Sokolowski, F. *Lois sacrées de l'Asie mineure* (Paris 1955) 187-8: epigraphic evidence on impurity of exposure.

────── *Lois sacrées des cités grecques* (Supplement, Paris 1962) p. 57, text 54,6, p. 202, text 119,4: references to abortion.

Solinger, R. *Abortion wars: a half century of struggle, 1950-2000* (Berkeley, Ca. 1998).

Speckhard, A.C. *The psycho-social aspects of stress following abortion* (PhD thesis, University of Minnesota 1985).

Spitzer, W.O. & Saylor, C.L. (ed.) *Birth control and the Christian: a Protestant symposium on the control of human reproduction* (Wheaton, Il. 1969).

Steen Due, O. 'Amores und Abtreibung' *C&M* 32 (1980) 133-50.

Still, G.F. *The history of paediatrics* (London 1931).

Stotland, N.L. *Abortion: facts and feelings: a handbook for women and the people who care about them* (Washington, DC 1998).

Temkin, O. *Soranus's Gynaecology* (Baltimore 1956) esp. 62 ff.

────── *Hippocrates in a world of Pagans and Christians* (Baltimore 1991).

──────, Krankena, W.K. & Kaddish, S.H. (ed.) *Respect for life in medicine, philosophy and the law* (Baltimore 1997).

Thalheim, T. 'Amblosis' *RE* I,2 (1894) 1804-5.

Treggiari, S. *Roman marriage: iusti conjuges from the time of Cicero to the time of Ulpian* (Oxford 1991).

Van der Eijk, P.J. (ed.) *Ancient histories of medicine: essays in medical doxography and historiography in classical antiquity* (Leiden, Boston & Cologne 1999).

────── (ed. with H.F.J. Horstmanshoff and P.J. Shrijvers) *Ancient medicine in its sociocultural context* (Amsterdam 1995).

────── 'Antiquarianism and criticism: forms and functions of medical doxography in Methodism (Soranus, Caelius Aurelianus)' in P.J. van der Eijk (ed.) *Ancient histories* 388-452

Van der Tak, J. *Abortion, fertility, and changing legislation: an international review* (Lexington 1974).

Van Geytenbeek, A.C. *Musonius Rufus and Greek diatribe* (Assen 1963).

Van Hook, La Rue, 'The exposure of infants at Athens' *TAPhA* 51 (1920) 134-43.

Von Staden, H. *Herophilus: the art of medicine in early Alexandria* (Cambridge 1989).

———— 'Celsus as historian?' in P.J. van der Eijk (ed.) *Ancient histories of medicine* 251-94.

Vaughan, A.C. *The genesis of human offspring: a study in early Greek culture* (Northampton, Mass. 1945).

Viljoen, G. van N. 'Plato and Aristotle on the exposure of infants at Athens' *Acta Classica* 2 (1959) 60-3.

Wagner, H. *Galeni qui fertur libellus 'Ei zoon to kata gastros'* (Diss., Madburg 1914).

Watt, H. *Life and death in healthcare ethics: a short introduction* (London 2000).

Watts, W.J. 'Ovid, the law and Roman society on abortion' *AC* 16 (1973) 89-101.

Wright, J.P. & Potter, P. (ed.) *Psyche and soma: physicians and metaphysicians on the mind-body problem from antiquity to enlightenment* (Oxford 2000).

Wilkinson, L.P. 'Population and family planning' in *Classical attitudes to modern issues* (London 1979).

Wilt, J. *Abortion, choice, and contemporary fiction: the armageddon of the maternal instinct* (Chicago 1990).

Winter, E.B. *Psychological and medical aspects of induced abortion: a selective, annotated bibliography 1970-1986* (New York 1988).

Woods, J. *Engineered death: abortion, suicide, euthanasia and senecide* (Ottawa 1978).

Zancarol, J.D. *L'évolution des idées sur l'avortement provoqué* (Diss., Paris 1934) esp. 45-54.

Ziehen, L. 'Das Spartanische Bevölkerungsproblem' *Hermes* 68 (1933) 218-37.

Zimmerman, M.K. *Passage through abortion: the personal and social reality of women's experiences* (New York 1977).

Index of Ancient Authors

Index of Topics